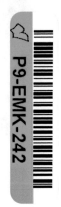

The Natural Diet Solution
for
PCOS and Infertility

FIRST EDITION

The Natural Diet Solution

for

PCOS and Infertility

How to Manage Polycystic Ovary Syndrome Naturally

Nancy Dunne, N.D.
&
Bill Slater

HEALTH SOLUTIONS PRESS
P.O. BOX 30034
SEATTLE, WA 98113

First edition printing, March 2006

Published by:
Health Solutions Press
P.O. Box 30034
Seattle, WA 98113
Contact: www.ovarian-cysts-pcos.com/db/contact
Web: www.ovarian-cysts-pcos.com

Disclaimer: The information in this book is not intended to treat, diagnose, cure or prevent any disease, including PCOS or infertility, and is provided for educational purposes only. Always seek the advice of your physician with any questions you have regarding a medical condition and before undertaking any diet, exercise or other health program. The authors have made their best effort to produce a high quality, informative and helpful book. But they make no representation or warranties of any kind with regard to the completeness or accuracy of the contents of the book. They accept no liability of any kind for any losses or damages caused or alleged to be caused, directly or indirectly, from using the information contained in this book.

ISBN: 097722290X

ISBN: 978-0-9772229-0-2

Cover design by Anne Mustappa
Layout/production by Bob Paltrow Design (www.bobpaltrow.com)
Book production coordination by E.G. Harris (www.bcwriting.com)

Acknowledgments

Nancy Dunne would like to acknowledge all of the women who have trusted themselves to take their health into their own hands, supported by the principles and practices of naturopathic medicine. Dr. Dunne also especially thanks her daughter, Tassia Tkatschenko, for her example of courageous compassion and her (usually) cheerful tackling of the hard work of self responsibility. And finally, a profound thanks to Bill Slater, whose scholarship and deep, tenacious caring is the heart of the work that puts this book into your hands.

Bill Slater wishes to give special thanks to Elizabeth Harris and Marilyn Lewis for their invaluable contributions to this book.

TABLE OF CONTENTS

Why a PCOS Diet? 9

What's In This Book 12

PART 1: The Fundamentals

1. A Word About PCOS

1.1 What Is PCOS? 22

1.2 What Causes PCOS? 26

2. How We Developed the Healthy Diet for PCOS

2.1 The 'Food Pyramid' 37

2.2 Low-Carb Diets 40

2.3 The Other Diets 46

2.4 What Did Your Ancestors Eat? 52

2.5 The Basis of the PCOS Diet 55

2.6 Healthy PCOS Diet vs. Low-Carb Diet 57

3. A Word About Your Weight

3.1 Diet and Long-Term Weight Management 60

3.2 Thrifty Genes and Your 'Set Point' 64

3.3 Hormones, Inflammation and Your Weight 67

3.4 How Calorie Density Makes You Fat 68

3.5 Portion Control 71

3.6 Is Calorie Restriction a Good Idea? 73

3.7 Weight vs. Body Composition 76

3.8 What if You're NOT Overweight? 80

4. Carbohydrates

4.1 What's a Carbohydrate? 82

4.2 Glycemic Index 87

4.3 Anti-Nutrients in Grains and Legumes 95

4.4 To Soy or Not to Soy 100

4.5 What Is Fiber? 105

4.6 Plant Foods 109

4.7 Guidelines for Eating Carbohydrates 112

5. Protein

5.1 What's a Protein? 115

5.2 The Problem with Milk 121

5.3 Guidelines for Eating Animal Protein 128

6. Fats and Oils

6.1 What's a Fat? 131
6.2 Essential Fats and Eicosanoids 141
6.3 Other Fatty Information 151
6.4 Guidelines for Eating Fats 158

PART 2: The Healthy PCOS Diet

7. Introduction to the Diet

7.1 PCOS Diet Levels 164
7.2 What to Eat 168
7.3 What Not to Eat 170

8. Main Components of the Diet

8.1 Meats 174
8.2 Seafood 177
8.3 Poultry 180
8.4 Eggs 182
8.5 Dairy Products 186
8.6 Legumes 189
8.7 Grains 192
8.8 Vegetables 194
8.9 Sprouts 198
8.10 Fruits 201
8.11 Nuts and Seeds 204
8.12 Fats & Oils 207

9. Water and Beverages

9.1 Water 210
9.2 Purified Water 216
9.3 Coffee 218
9.4 Tea 220
9.5 Soft Drinks 222
9.6 Alcoholic and Other Beverages 224

10. Other Elements of Your Diet

10.1 Herbs, Spices, Seasonings and Condiments 228
10.2 Sweeteners 234
10.3 Snacks 238
10.4 Meal Replacement Shakes 240

11. More Dietary Tips

11.1 Eat Organic 245
11.2 Eating in Restaurants 247
11.3 Eating Away from Home 254
11.4 Healthy Eating Habits 257
11.5 When Should You Eat? 258
11.6 Tips for Increasing Your Fertility 260
11.7 Advice for Vegetarians 264
11.8 If You're Pregnant 267

12. Getting Started

12.1 Prepare for Success 271
12.2 Shopping List for Recommended Diet Level 276
12.3 Handy Cooking Tips 281

13. Meal Plans and Recipes

13.1 Daily Meal Plans for 30 Days 287
13.2 Recipes 321
    13.2.1 Basic Meals 325
    13.2.2 Meat 329
    13.2.3 Seafood 343
    13.2.4 Poultry 351
    13.2.5 Eggs 360
    13.2.6 Salads 363
    13.2.7 Vegetables 380
    13.2.8 Soups 396
    13.2.9 Juices and Smoothies 405
    13.2.10 Snacks and Handhelds 409
    13.2.11 Sauces and Dressings 414

PART 3: Additional Steps To Take

14. Other Things You Can Do

14.1 Exercise 431
14.2 Stress Management 440
14.3 Emotional Factors 450
14.4 Liver Health 455
14.5 Your Health Care Team 458
14.6 Check for Food Allergies 460
14.7 Measure Your Progress 462

15. Nutritional Supplements

15.1 Why You Need Nutritional Supplements 467
15.2 Nutritional Supplement Quality 472
15.3 Supplements for PCOS, Infertility and Insulin Problems 474

16. More about Hormones, Weight and Inflammation

16.1 What Makes You Hungry? 487
16.2 'Evil Twins': Insulin Resistance and Leptin Resistance 493
16.3 Inflammation and Your Weight 502

17. Resources and Feedback

17.1 Resources 510
17.2 Feedback from You 514

About the Authors 515
References 517

Introduction
Why a PCOS Diet?

Polycystic ovary syndrome is a chronic hormonal and metabolic disorder that presents a bewildering array of health problems such as infertility, overweight, hirsutism, hair loss, depression, dark skin patches and lack of energy.

As serious as these symptoms are, the consequences of not dealing effectively with PCOS are even more serious, including heart disease, diabetes, reduced quality of life and shortened lifespan.

Our review of published research on PCOS and our clinical experience strongly indicates that a healthy diet can favorably influence the outcome of this disorder. In other words, what you eat and drink will either improve or worsen the symptoms and consequences of PCOS.

Yet the hundreds of emails we receive from visitors to our website (www.ovarian-cysts-pcos.com) indicate that many women are unsure or confused about their diet. The primary goal of this book is to provide clear guidelines for those who aren't sure what to eat or not to eat.

Which Diet Is Best?

Not all women with PCOS are overweight, although being overweight is a major diagnostic clue for PCOS. Research shows that a loss of 7%-10% of body weight will often restore normal menstrual cycles in women with PCOS, making successful pregnancy more likely.

The serious chronic diseases associated with PCOS include diabetes, high blood pressure and heart disease. These conditions are related to abdominal obesity, blood sugar, cholesterol levels and systemic inflammation. We have therefore designed our recommendations to include long-term weight loss that will reliably correct some of the metabolic causes of PCOS.

Women report to us that they have had success losing weight by following any number of different diet programs. Indeed, we will always lose weight whenever we sufficiently decrease our calories. However, losing weight is only the beginning step. Achieving and maintaining a lifelong healthy lean-to-fat tissue ratio is the ultimate goal. In recent years we have learned a great deal of new information about what elements are necessary for losing fat, gaining muscle and permanently maintaining optimal body composition.

We have reviewed all of the popular diets as well as much medical research on diet and PCOS. We have distilled the healthiest elements from the various diets and research articles and have developed a diet that we believe will benefit most women with PCOS.

Our conclusion, based on an extensive review of medical research and Dr. Dunne's clinical experience treating women with PCOS, has convinced us the key to success is to start with a ketogenic weight loss diet (if you are overweight). When a suitable amount of weight has been lost, you can make a transition to greater variety of foods and latitude in portion sizes. Your diet should be accompanied by regular exercise and increased self awareness and self care to ensure that you maintain your healthy habits and live a long and fully functional life free of chronic disease.

We advocate a restriction of refined carbohydrate-rich foods and improvement in the quality of all carbohydrates. It's insufficient to focus solely on grams of fat or calories. We are aware of many women who have achieved good results by limiting their carbohydrate intake. There is also a growing body of scientific evidence supporting low or controlled carbohydrate diets. The medical community is starting to realize that a lower carbohydrate, ketogenic diet may be a viable option to add to other well-known approaches, such as the traditional low calorie, high carbohydrate and low-fat diet.

The controlled carbohydrate approach is particularly valuable for women with high serum triglycerides, low HDL ("good" cholesterol) levels, abdominal obesity, or insulin resistance (metabolic syndrome or hyperinsulinemia). Reducing carbohydrate intake has been shown to improve these health indicators without adverse clinical effects.

One diet approach will never fit all women with PCOS. However, you will likely do best by restricting carbohydrates initially and then adding back healthy unrefined carbohydrates until a metabolic balance is achieved and you can maintain your health with the diet and regular exercise.

The recommendations in this book provide a basic foundation for success. Some will need ongoing emotional support and practical "how to" advice from health professionals for improving food and exercise habits. Others have unique needs and health conditions that should be evaluated by a qualified health professional. Please see our resource section for information on how to find a naturopathic physician who can guide and support your personal, lifelong healthcare strategy.

The purpose of our healthy PCOS diet is to help you rebuild your health and maintain a high level of vibrant health for the rest of your life. Nothing is more precious than your health. A healthy body allows you to enjoy your life and be the woman you want to be.

Expanding Universe of Knowledge

An enormous amount of research is going on in the areas of PCOS, fertility, hormones and diet. Hundreds of new, relevant research articles are published every month.

Please understand that we are not aware of the entire universe of medical and health knowledge. We have tried our best to review as much research data as possible so that we could provide relevant and useful information to you. However, this book may contain errors or omissions. For example, in the area of diet, what is "right" today may be "wrong" tomorrow as new research comes to light. What we think is the best and most correct information today may be incorrect in the future. So, essentially we are sharing with you what we know today. Next year, we will know more than we know today. Gradually, parts of this book may become dated or obsolete. We hope to revise this book from time to time to keep it current with the latest research.

The Modern American ('Western') Diet

A huge body of evidence shows that most people living in North America eat foods and drink beverages that do not provide the nutrition they need for good health. By "nutrition," we're referring to essential food elements required to sustain life and good health: the macronutrients fat, protein and carbohydrates, as well as micronutrients such as vitamins, minerals, amino acids, essential fatty acids and fiber.

The typical American diet is becoming much less nutritious. Everything from agricultural practices, transport and storage, to our families' busy daily schedules have contributed to changes that are making it harder to eat a truly healthy diet. We eat in restaurants or buy takeout more often than we cook from scratch. We rely on processed foods that contain all kinds of artificial ingredients, such as monosodium glutamate (MSG), preservatives, artificial colorings, artificial flavors, artificial sweeteners and more. Processed foods also contain large quantities of adulterated or damaged food substances, such as partially hydrogenated vegetable oils or rancid (oxidized) oils. All of these elements are a burden to your digestion and elimination functions. Many of our foods contain pesticides and other petrochemicals that disrupt hormone function and may seriously damage your health.

Please understand that good nutrition is just as important as breathing clean air and drinking pure water. As far as your body is concerned, eating French fries is the same thing as smoking a cigarette or drinking water out of a well contaminated with dioxin. Either way, you damage your body, endanger your health and adversely impact your quality of life.

If you intend to manage your PCOS symptoms, have a successful pregnancy and enjoy a healthy and long life, you'll want to master the art of nutritious, healthy eating.

What's In This Book?

This book in divided into three basic parts. The first part includes Sections 1 through 6 and provides you with some fundamental knowledge about PCOS, weight issues, carbohydrates, protein and fats.

The second part includes Sections 7 through 13 and describes our recommended diet.

The third part of this book includes Sections 14 through 17 and describes other things you can do to deal with PCOS and better your health. It also gives you a listing of possibly helpful nutritional supplements, some in-depth information about hormones and inflammation and some helpful resources.

Section 1: A Word about PCOS

Chapter 1.1: What is PCOS? This chapter tells you what polycystic ovary syndrome (PCOS) is and what its symptoms are. It also describes the long-term health consequence of PCOS.

Chapter 1.2: What Causes PCOS? PCOS is a disorder that is not well understood nor are its causes fully known. To most individuals and doctors, PCOS is a "medical mystery." It appears to be partly a genetically inherited disorder. However, genetic inheritance does not fully explain the causes of PCOS. This chapter describes possible environmental and other causes of this syndrome.

Section 2: How We Developed the Healthy Diet for PCOS

Chapter 2.1: The 'Food Pyramid'. The Food Pyramid has done much to make America fatter. However, the revised Pyramid, issued in early 2005, is a big improvement, although it didn't go far enough.

Chapter 2.2: Low-Carb Diets. Low-carb diets have both benefits and risks. Although they clearly can lead to short-term weight loss, their long-term health effects are unclear. A high-carb, high-fiber diet has some benefits. The type of carbohydrate and the total calories consumed are important factors in weight control.

Chapter 2.3: The Other Diets. This chapter is a review of eight of the most well known diets other than the popular low-carb diets such as Atkins or South Beach. The success of any weight loss diet is due to three factors: (1) long-term adherence, (2) portion size control and (3) restricted number of calories.

Chapter 2.4: What Did Your Ancestors Eat? The genes of your ancestors are virtually the same as yours. But our food today is nothing at all like what your ancestors ate. The few remaining hunter-gatherers are mostly free of cardiovascular disease, diabetes or obesity, in contrast to people who consume a "modern" diet.

Chapter 2.5: The Basis of the PCOS Diet. We propose a diet that is more suited to your genes. This chapter describes the basic elements of a healthy diet for PCOS and improved fertility.

Chapter 2.6: Healthy PCOS Diet vs. Low-Carb Diet. This chapter compares our healthy PCOS diet to a typical low-carb diet. A primary distinction between the PCOS and a low-carb diet is that we place much greater emphasis on *the type* of carbohydrate.

Section 3: A Word about Your Weight

Chapter 3.1: Diet and Long-Term Weight Management. The right diet will greatly help you to lose weight and keep it off. This chapter describes a ketogenic diet that will aid your weight loss efforts.

Chapter 3.2: Thrifty Genes and Your 'Set Point.' There's evidence to indicate that PCOS women tend to gain more weight with the same amount of calories when compared to "normal" women. This chapter reviews two mechanisms that may cause this to happen.

Chapter 3.3: Hormones, Inflammation and Your Weight. There are dozens of hormones and other signaling molecules in your body that influence your weight by regulating your appetite and metabolism. In addition, chronic inflammation is a common characteristic of PCOS and is closely associated with excessive weight and hormone dysregulation.

Chapter 3.4: How Calorie Density Makes You Fat. Consumption of processed foods tricks us into eating more calories than we realize. The calorie density in foods — not the fat by itself — may be responsible for the excessive total calories we consume in a meal.

Chapter 3.5: Portion Control. Americans are eating larger meal portions than ever before. The result is a big increase in total caloric intake. A large portion of high calorie density foods is especially troublesome. Portion control is an important component of any healthy diet.

Chapter 3.6: Is Calorie Restriction a Good Idea? Reduction of total caloric intake has been shown to cause weight loss and to restore menstrual cycling. However, "crash diets" are unwise.

Chapter 3.7: Weight vs. Body Composition. Many women seem obsessed about "losing weight." However, we think that "body composition" is a better indicator of your health. The weight you want to lose is fat, while retaining lean muscle mass.

Chapter 3.8: What if You're NOT Overweight? The diet in the book will benefit you, regardless of your body dimensions.

Section 4: Carbohydrates

Chapter 4.1: What's a Carbohydrate? Some aren't clear on just what a "carbohydrate" is. This chapter reviews various aspects of carbohydrates.

Chapter 4.2: Glycemic Index. Foods with a low "glycemic index" appear to be beneficial for PCOS complications such as diabetes, insulin resistance, cardiovascular disease and chronic inflammation. This chapter explains terms such as "glycemic index," "glycemic load" and "available carbohydrate."

Chapter 4.3: Anti-Nutrients in Grains and Legumes. Anti-nutrients are substances in foods that may not be beneficial to us and may possibly be harmful. We consume these substances every day and should be more aware of them.

Chapter 4.4: To Soy or Not to Soy. The food industry strongly promotes the consumption of soy. But it's questionable whether consumption of genetically modified soy products is healthy.

Chapter 4.5: What Is Fiber? Fiber is the part of a plant that is not digested. Most Americans don't consume nearly enough fiber even though it will help balance estrogen, reduce insulin resistance, reduce glucose levels, curb appetite and provide a host of additional health benefits.

Chapter 4.6: Plant Foods. The substances in plant foods are absolutely essential for good health. They also contribute to better hormonal balance and may improve ovarian function.

Chapter 4.7: Guidelines for Eating Carbohydrates. This chapter is a brief summary of what type of carbohydrates you should consume.

Section 5: Protein

Chapter 5.1: What Is a Protein? This chapter describes the value and uses of protein in your body.

Chapter 5.2: The Problem with Milk. Consumption of high levels of dairy products from cows is a fairly recent phenomenon. This chapter discusses the health implications of consuming milk and dairy products.

Chapter 5.3: Guidelines for Eating Protein. This chapter provides guidelines for eating proteins.

Section 6: Fats

Chapter 6.1: What's a Fat? Dietary fats are a complex and confusing topic. This chapter provides a basic introduction to the topic of fats.

Chapter 6.2: Essential Fats and Eicosanoids. Essential fatty acids and eicosanoids are poorly understood…yet they are absolutely crucial for good health and controlling health problems associated with PCOS. This chapter explains what essential fats and eicosanoids are and how they work in your body.

Chapter 6.3: Other Fatty Information. This chapter discusses saturated fats, medium chain triglycerides, unsaturated fats and monounsaturated fats.

Chapter 6.4: Guidelines for Eating Fats. This chapter outlines the types of fats and oils to consume and describes the problems with bottled oils.

Section 7: Introduction to the Diet

Chapter 7.1: PCOS Diet Levels. This chapter describes the mechanism of the diet in this book. You'll want to read this chapter in order to make sense of the rest of the book.

Chapter 7.2: What to Eat. Here we tell you what to eat in very basic terms. There is no "one size fits all" diet that works for PCOS. To some extent, you will want to customize our diet to your specific needs.

Chapter 7.3: What Not to Eat. In this chapter, we describe (in general terms) all the foods you should always avoid regardless of your PCOS symptoms.

Section 8: Main Components of the Diet

Chapter 8.1: Meats. List of acceptable and unacceptable meats, plus additional comments.

Chapter 8.2: Seafood. List of acceptable and unacceptable seafood, plus additional comments.

Chapter 8.3: Poultry. List of acceptable and unacceptable poultry, plus additional comments.

Chapter 8.4: Eggs. List of acceptable and unacceptable eggs, plus additional comments.

Chapter 8.5: Dairy Products. List of acceptable and unacceptable dairy products, plus additional comments.

Chapter 8.6: Legumes. List of acceptable and unacceptable legumes, plus additional comments.

Chapter 8.7: Grains. List of acceptable and unacceptable grains, plus additional comments.

Chapter 8.8: Vegetables. List of acceptable and unacceptable vegetables, plus additional comments.

Chapter 8.9: Sprouts. List of sprouts, plus suggestions on how to grow sprouts.

Chapter 8.10: Fruits. List of acceptable and unacceptable fruits, plus additional comments.

Chapter 8.11: Nuts and Seeds. List of acceptable and unacceptable nuts and seeds, plus additional comments.

Chapter 8.12: Fats and Oils. List of acceptable and unacceptable fats and oils, plus additional comments.

Section 9: Water and Beverages

Chapter 9.1: Water. This chapter reviews the numerous health benefits that water offers. Water is what your body wants, not a manufactured beverage. Drinking pure water is an important part of our diet.

Chapter 9.2: Purified Water. Chlorinated tap water may impair ovarian function and the menstrual cycle. Always drink purified water.

Chapter 9.3: Coffee. The evidence on coffee is conflicting. In general, however, you may wish to avoid coffee because it may unfavorably influence fertility and pregnancy.

Chapter 9.4: Tea. Green tea may reduce estrogen, inhibit the action of testosterone and reduce appetite. It is also well known as a cancer preventative.

Chapter 9.5: Soft Drinks. Under no circumstances should you ever consume soft drinks. This chapter tells you why.

Chapter 9.6: Alcoholic & Other Beverages. In this chapter, we briefly review alcoholic and other beverages not discussed in previous chapters. Moderate consumption of wine or beer appears to be mildly beneficial.

Section 10: Other Elements of Your Diet

Chapter 10.1: Herbs, Spices, Seasonings and Condiments. This is a listing of numerous spices and seasonings that you can use to make you food more flavorful in a healthy way. Also included is a discussion of salt.

Chapter 10.2: Sweeteners. The best source of something sweet is fresh fruit. If you need an added sweetener, use stevia. This chapter has a list of acceptable and not acceptable sweeteners, along with some descriptions of various sweeteners.

Chapter 10.3: Snacks. This chapter contains a list of acceptable snack foods.

Chapter 10.4: Meal Replacement Shakes. Meal replacement shakes are not a substitute for a healthy diet. A high-quality product may be used on those occasions when you do not have access to a healthy meal.

Section 11: More Dietary Tips

Chapter 11.1: Eat Organic. Although more expensive, organic foods are well worth the cost in terms of better nutrition and reduction of exposure to pesticides and other chemicals.

Chapter 11.2: Eating in Restaurants. People who eat frequently in restaurants are fatter than people who don't. This chapter gives you some guidelines if you're going to eat in a restaurant.

Chapter 11.3: Eating Away from Home. Because of your job or for social reasons, you may find yourself eating away from home. This chapter gives you some helpful dietary tips for any away-from-home situation.

Chapter 11.4: Healthy Eating Habits. *What* you eat is important. But *how* you eat can also be very beneficial for your health.

Chapter 11.5: When Should You Eat? Eating breakfast and having regular meals appears to reduce caloric intake, improve weight control and help normalize insulin.

Chapter 11.6: Tips for Increasing Your Fertility. This chapter is a summary of sixteen dietary and other tips that will help to improve your fertility.

Chapter 11.7: Advice for Vegetarians. Although a totally vegetarian diet has its benefits, it is not recommended for women who have PCOS, for reasons that we outline in this chapter.

Chapter 11.8: If You're Pregnant. Pregnancy requires a diet that is somewhat different from a diet when you are not pregnant. You are not trying to lose weight while you are pregnant.

Section 12: Getting Started

Chapter 12.1: Prepare for Success. This chapter helps you to actually get started with your new diet. Included are descriptions of our menu plans and recipes, shopping tips, suggestions for on-the-go meals, kitchen tools you'll need and timesaving tips for the cook.

Chapter 12.2: Shopping List for Recommended Diet Level. There are two diet levels in this book. The most restricted is the Recommended Level. The master shopping list in this chapter is limited to Recommended Level foods. If you are at the Maintenance Level of our diet, you can add Maintenance Level foods to this shopping list.

Chapter 12.3: Handy Cooking Tips. This chapter contains a variety of suggestions for easy and healthy cooking or food preparation.

Section 13: Meal Plans and Recipes

Chapter 13.1: Daily Meal Plans for 30 Days. The purpose of this chapter is to show you how you might eat for one month if you are at the Recommended Level, which is the most restricted level of the diet.

Chapter 13.2: Recipes. This chapter contains dozens of recipes that you can use (or modify) as you implement your new diet.

Section 14: Other Things You Can Do

Chapter 14.1: Exercise. Other than diet, regular exercise is the most important thing you can do to control PCOS symptoms. Exercise is helpful for weight loss, including loss of abdominal fat. Exercise can also reduce insulin resistance, which is a primary cause of PCOS.

Chapter 14.2: Stress Management. Chronic stress is an important but under-recognized contributor to PCOS. Stress may have an adverse effect on reproductive hormones, cause an increase in abdominal fat and create a host of other health problems.

Chapter 14.3: Emotional Factors. Dealing effectively with PCOS is not restricted to "physical" things like diet and exercise. There is also a huge emotional component that is ignored by most doctors. It's important to recognize the emotional issues and deal with them.

Chapter 14.4: Liver Health. PCOS is not simply a problem with your ovaries. All of your glands and organs are involved in some way. An essential organ that is almost always overlooked is the liver. Impaired liver function or fatty liver degeneration will make it harder for you to manage PCOS.

Chapter 14.5: Your Health Care Team. PCOS is a complex, poorly understood disorder. You may need more than one health care professional to help you.

Chapter 14.6: Check for Food Allergies. Food allergies cause inflammation and a variety of unpleasant symptoms. Most food allergies are "hidden," so it's wise to get a test. You'll want to avoid allergenic foods, even if they are included in the healthy PCOS diet.

Chapter 14.7: Measure Your Progress. Keeping track of your progress increases the probability of ultimate success. This chapter gives you some guidelines.

Section 15: Nutritional Supplements

Chapter 15.1: Why You Need Nutritional Supplements. You may have heard that you can get 100% of your nutrition from your food. This chapter gives twenty-two reasons why this may not be true.

Chapter 15.2: Nutritional Supplement Quality. This chapter gives you tips and guidelines for choosing the best nutritional supplement.

Chapter 15.3: Supplements for PCOS, Infertility and Insulin Problems. This chapter is a descriptive list of forty supplements you could possibly take for PCOS. Of course, we are not recommending you take all of them. Always consult with a physician about which supplements are appropriate for you.

Section 16. More Information about Hormones, Weight and Inflammation

Chapter 16.1: What Makes You Hungry? Women with PCOS tend to have a bigger appetite than non-PCOS women and they feel hungrier. Numerous hormones are involved in this appetite problem. In this chapter, we describe how the hunger process works and three hormones that are involved in it.

Chapter 16.2: 'Evil Twins': Insulin Resistance and Leptin Resistance. Resistance to the actions of these two hormones is a big reason why you have PCOS, infertility problems and weight/appetite problems.

Chapter 16.3: Inflammation and Your Weight. Chronic inflammation plays an important but under-recognized role in PCOS. It is involved in obesity, insulin resistance and leptin resistance, which are common problems in PCOS.

Section 17: Resources and Feedback

Chapter 17.1: Resources. Here you will find sources of professional help as well as sources for obtaining more information about PCOS and infertility.

Chapter 17.2: Feedback. What you think and feel is just as important as what we think and feel. Go to this chapter to communicate with us and let us know what's on your mind.

Part 1
The Fundamentals

Section 1

A Word About PCOS

1.1 What Is PCOS?

In each menstrual cycle, follicles grow on the ovaries. Eggs develop within those follicles, one of which will reach maturity sooner than the others and be released into the fallopian tubes. This is "ovulation." The remaining follicles will dissolve back into the ovary.

In the case of polycystic ovaries, however, the ovaries are larger than normal and there are a series of undeveloped follicles that appear in clumps, rather like a bunch of grapes. Polycystic ovaries are not necessarily troublesome and may not even affect your fertility.

However, when the cysts cause a hormonal imbalance, a pattern of symptoms may develop. This pattern of symptoms is called a syndrome. These symptoms are the difference between suffering from PCOS and from simply having polycystic ovaries.

So you can have polycystic ovaries without having PCOS. However, all women with PCOS will have polycystic ovaries. Polycystic Ovary Syndrome is the name given to a metabolic condition in which a woman will have polycystic ovaries, along with a certain pattern of other symptoms that reflect imbalances in reproductive and other hormones.

We referred to PCOS as a "metabolic" disorder. By this we mean that there are numerous factors in basic body processes that have gone off track. Because your body is a unified whole, a problem or dysfunction in one area causes dysfunction in other areas. PCOS is a dysfunction that is related to your whole body, not just your ovaries.

What are the Symptoms of PCOS or Polycystic Ovaries?

PCOS presents a complex and baffling array of symptoms. Each woman with PCOS will have some combination of the following symptoms:
- Multiple ovarian cysts
- Polycystic ovaries 2-5 times larger than healthy ovaries
- Irregular or absent menses
- Infertility
- Acne
- Obesity or inability to lose weight
- Excessive body or facial hair (hirsutism)
- Insulin resistance and possibly diabetes
- Thinning of scalp hair
- Velvety, hyperpigmented skin folds (acanthosis nigrans)
- High blood pressure
- Multiple hormone imbalances, commonly including:
  - Androgens (testosterone)
  - Cortisol
  - Estrogens

- FSH (follicle stimulating hormone)
- Insulin
- LH (luteinizing hormone)
- Progesterone
- Prolactin
- Thyroid hormones

How Common Is PCOS?

PCOS is the most common hormonal disorder occurring in women during their reproductive years. It is thought that 4% to 10% of all women have PCOS. However, since many women don't know they have PCOS or some aspect of it, the actual number probably exceeds 10%. PCOS is a leading cause of infertility. Symptoms of PCOS frequently start to show up soon after puberty.

PCOS Is a Threat to Your Health if Left Untreated

The long-term health consequences of PCOS may include but are not be limited to:
- Cardiovascular disease
- Diabetes
- Pregnancy-associated disorders
- Cancers
- Seizure disorders

A Sampling of What Medical Studies Have to Say

- Evidence of pancreatic exhaustion is seen frequently in women with PCOS. Insulin resistance normally forces the pancreas to overwork to secrete lots of insulin. This leads to cellular dysfunction, an inability to produce enough insulin to control blood sugar and diabetes.

- 40% of women with PCOS have abnormal blood sugar levels and 10% already have Type 2 diabetes.

- The incidence of diabetes in adolescents with PCOS is comparable to that seen in adults.

- Women with PCOS have blood sugar imbalances at rates as high as those in the highest risk ethnic groups in the world, such as the Pima Indians.

- PCOS is associated with elevated LDL "bad" cholesterol, regardless of weight.

- PCOS and obesity together lead to chronically elevated triglycerides, which contribute to heart disease.

- High blood pressure is commonly seen in women with PCOS.

- PCOS is associated with indicators of cardiovascular disease, including increased blood clot formation, increased inflammation and thickening of blood vessel walls and abnormal cholesterol and triglycerides.

- 77% of women with abnormally infrequent or scanty menstrual flow have evidence of PCOS and 33% have abnormal blood sugar levels.

- Using menstrual cycle length of 40 days or more as an indicator, the Nurses' Health Study showed a 2.2-fold increase in the risk of Type 2 diabetes development. The study also showed that irregular menses was associated with a 53% increase in cardiovascular disease events.

- Women with PCOS have reproductive abnormalities, including increased gestational diabetes in both obese and non-obese women, pregnancy-induced hypertension and preeclampsia. Preeclampsia is a condition that can develop in late pregnancy. It is characterized by a sudden rise in blood pressure, excessive gain in weight, generalized swelling, protein in the urine, severe headache and visual disturbances.

- PCOS women also have an increased endometrial cancer risk. The risk of ovarian cancer is increased 2.5-fold, particularly among women who had never used oral contraceptives. Breast cancer risk is not clearly increased with PCOS.

- Women with seizure disorders have increased risk of PCOS.

As you can see, PCOS is not something you want to ignore. "Watchful waiting" is not your best option.

Can PCOS Be Treated by Diet?

Improvements in diet, exercise and lifestyle are essential methods of dealing with PCOS.

A mere 7%-10% weight loss may lead to regular ovulatory cycles in many women. A healthy diet is a vital component of a successful weight loss program.

Several recent studies have shown that a calorie-restricted diet tends to normalize hormones, induce ovulation, improve fertility and reduce other PCOS problems.[1] [2] [3] [4] [5] Whether the "best" diet for PCOS is low-fat or low-carb is not so clear; the studies suggest that either diet works, provided the calories are kept low.

The problem with a calorie-restricted diet is that it is hard to maintain over the long term. After all, who wants to have to "count calories" for the rest of her life?

Another problem with using these restricted diets is that, according to one recent study, women with PCOS have an impaired satiety mechanism.[6] In other words, it may be harder for PCOS women to feel that they have eaten enough. Impaired satiety makes it doubly difficult to stay on an artificially restricted calorie diet.

This book will outline a diet that you can comfortably live with the rest of your life — and that also reduces your PCOS symptoms and greatly improve your overall health.

1.2 What Causes PCOS?

There is uncertainly and no conclusive agreement as to what causes PCOS.

The most common reasons given for PCOS are:
- Genetic predisposition
- Excess insulin production, insulin resistance and obesity
- Environmental petrochemical pollution

Additional possible contributory causes of PCOS may be:
- Food adulteration
- Autoimmune disorders
- Chronic inflammation
- Some medications

Most of these proposed causes of PCOS can be changed for the better by improving your diet. In other words, if you change your diet, you may be able to lessen or remove some of the factors that are causing your PCOS. Your symptoms will be reduced and you will be much healthier.

PCOS is Partly a Genetic Disorder

Most researchers agree the polycystic ovary syndrome is at least partly caused by the set of genes you were born with. Your genetic pattern is somewhat different compared to women who don't have PCOS. [7] [8]

For example, a study recently conducted at Nanjing Medical University examined the ovarian DNA of women with or without PCOS.[9] Out of 9,216 DNA strands examined, 290 of those in the PCOS ovaries were different from those in normal ovaries. Some of these genes were active when they shouldn't have been and some of those that should have been active were inactive. Improperly operating genes lead to cell dysfunction and abnormal metabolism.

Diet and Your Genetic Predisposition

Many women with PCOS have been told that their condition is a genetically inherited trait and that there's not much that can be done except possibly to take birth control pills to reduce symptoms. Most people believe that genes are set of blueprints that determine your physical characteristics, how you behave, what diseases you get (or don't get) and how long you live. They are like rules set in stone — they can't be altered.

This is a myth.

You are not genetically "doomed" to an outcome over which you have no control. Your health destiny is not preordained. "Genetic determinism" has been completely discredited by recent research.

Genetic research has revealed that your traits or characteristics are not forever cast in stone the instant you were conceived. Rather, how they behave is modified by their environment. The nature of the environment will strongly influence what actually does happen.[10]

For example, suppose your mother had taken DES (a synthetic estrogen) while you were in her womb. Her doctor would have given DES to her to prevent miscarriage, or just to have a healthier pregnancy and healthier baby. You would have been born as an apparently healthy baby. However, you would have had a vastly higher risk of developing reproductive tract deformities and abnormalities, including a rare form of vaginal cancer, because of subtle changes in the cellular environment brought there when the DES chemistry entered the picture.

Think of your genetic blueprint as "written in pencil." In this case, DES was like a big eraser that erased part of your blueprint and replaced it with a different blueprint. The same is true for anything else in your environment, from the moment of conception until you die. You are continually under the influence of your environment, whether it's inside your body or outside.

You can't change what has already happened to you. If your mother took DES, smoked cigarettes, drank alcohol and ate a lot of fried food while you were in her womb, you have turned out to be a different person than you would have if she had not done those things.

However, you still have the rest of your life. You *do* have a lot of control over your environment and therefore you can greatly influence your genetic blueprints.

One of those control mechanisms is your diet.

We think of our height as genetically locked in stone. However, whole populations change when the quality of nutrition changes. The average height of adult Japanese men and women has increased nearly six inches since World War II. Why? Their diet has changed drastically over the years, thus leading to changes in a physical trait that many people previously thought was unchangeable.

An individual woman's genetic blueprint may shape her with rounded hips, backside and thighs and delicate shoulders with small breasts. Depending on diet choices, that basic shape can be lived in at 135 pounds or 195 pounds, with significant differences in her daily experience and lifelong health.

Another important consideration is that you are genetically and biochemically unique from anyone else. So what you eat will affect you differently from someone else. That's why a "one size fits all" diet will not work for many women.

Example: Health authorities have told you to reduce salt intake if you have high blood pressure. However, studies show that only 30%-50% of people can reduce their blood pressure by restricting salt intake. Salt restriction does not reduce blood pressure for the others. Your current genetic blueprint will determine whether salt restriction will reduce your blood pressure or not.

Insulin Resistance

At least 30% of women with PCOS have insulin resistance, although some investigators think the number may be higher than 50%.

The symptoms of insulin resistance are acne, apple-shaped obesity, difficulty losing weight, high blood pressure, hirsutism, carbohydrate cravings and elevated blood glucose and triglycerides.

Insulin resistance means that cells in your body are less responsive to the insulin hormone. It's as if insulin knocks on the door, but no one answers. As a consequence, the many insulin-dependent processes in your body are impaired. For example, you have a reduced ability to receive molecules of blood sugar into your cells, to burn fat and to regulate the liver's production of blood sugar.

To solve this problem, your pancreas gland produces extra insulin to get all these necessary metabolic tasks done. The effect is a condition called "hyperinsulinemia," which means an abnormally high level of insulin in the blood. But too much insulin causes the cells to become even more insulin resistant than they were before.

Meanwhile, your pancreas is working very hard to produce all this insulin. It eventually gets tired out and starts producing less and less insulin. Then there is less insulin to store and regulate blood sugar and your blood sugar goes out of control. This is diabetes. Your pancreas is shot. You must take insulin injections for the rest of your life to keep your blood sugar under control.

Chronically high levels of insulin and insulin resistance lead to hyperandrogenism[11] (excessive levels of certain male hormones such as testosterone) by stimulating ovarian androgen production and by reducing serum sex-hormone binding globulin (SHBG). This process worsens PCOS symptoms.

This condition is called "hyperinsulemic hyperandrogenism" and is estimated to be the cause of lack of menstruation and infertility in at least half of PCOS women, whether they are overweight or lean.[12]

We now have a vicious cycle:
- High levels of insulin help to create insulin resistance and hyperandrogenism.
- Insulin resistance causes insulin levels to be too high, leading to hyperinsulinemia and hyperandrogenism.
- Hyperandrogenism tends to increase insulin levels.

Both hyperandrogenism and insulin resistance will contribute to excessive insulin levels. The high insulin levels in turn increase insulin resistance and hyperandrogenism. It's like a closed loop, with each of the variables making each other worse.

What Causes Insulin Resistance?

Insulin resistance syndrome is thought to be caused by several factors:
- Genetic abnormalities
- Poor nutrition when you were a fetus
- Too much body fat, especially around the middle
- Your diet[13]

Diet and Insulin Resistance

A number of studies have suggested a link between what you eat and insulin resistance.[14] [15] [16] [17] Two factors are at play:

First of all, when a diet made up of a lot of refined or processed foods is consumed, insulin spikes to high levels. Insulin levels increase in order to control the sudden increase in blood sugar resulting from rapid assimilation of refined starches and sugars. Each meal or snack made up of refined or pre-packaged food represents another substantial increase in insulin. Too much insulin triggers the cells to protect themselves from excessive exposure by becoming "insulin resistant."

Secondly, there are micronutrients in a healthy diet that make insulin's action more efficient, thus reducing insulin resistance. They include: biotin, calcium, chromium, magnesium, selenium, B-complex vitamins, vitamin C, vitamin E and zinc. The typical highly refined American diet is deficient in many of these micronutrients. Therefore the cells do not have enough of the substances they need in order to work with insulin in an efficient manner.

Either way, you create a condition of insulin resistance.

Insulin Resistance and Aborigines and Diet

A fascinating study was conducted with Australian aborigines, comparing their traditional hunter-gatherer diet with their modern Westernized diet.[18]

Dr. Kerin O'Dea, an Australian physician, gathered ten middle-aged, hyperinsulinemic, diabetic, mildly overweight aborigines who had been living on a typical urban, Western diet of refined foods. He sent them to an isolated area and had them live as hunter-gatherers for seven weeks.

Dr. O'Dea monitored what they ate as they wandered about in inland and coastal areas. Their diet varied, depending on where they were. Their diet ranged from 54%-80% protein, 13%-40% fat and 5%-33% carbohydrate. Even though 64% of the diet was of animal origin, it was relatively low in fat due to the very low fat content of the wild animals that were eaten. About 1,200 calories were consumed daily, which would qualify this diet as "low calorie."

How did these men fare? Their blood glucose fell from a dangerous 210 to a slightly elevated 118. Insulin dropped from 23 to 12, nearly normal. Triglycerides dropped from a highly elevated 354 down to 106.

And here's the real kicker...they were less active in the wild than in the city. In other words, their level of exercise actually declined, but they were still able to improve their health.

This study suggests to us that a hunter-gather type of diet is effective in reducing chronic health problems, regardless of exercise. By eating a diet that had *no* processed foods, they were able to recover much of their lost health in only seven weeks.

A diet consisting of whole, unrefined foods will reduce your need for insulin because you do not have a large quantity of sugars and simple carbohydrates entering your bloodstream and forcing a rapid increase in insulin. A diet of whole foods will also reduce your inclination to gain weight, which in itself contributes to insulin resistance.

The PCOS diet in this book recommends that you do not consume any processed, fabricated foods. You are overfed and undernourished. The PCOS diet will correct this imbalance.

Diet and Food Adulteration

There are hundreds of chemicals and other substances added to your foods to "improve" the taste, texture or appearance. Although these chemical additives are approved by the FDA, that does not mean they are safe for you to consume.[19]

The most serious example is a family of substances called excitotoxins, which are chemicals that damage nerve cells. They stimulate nerve cells to fire so rapidly that they become exhausted and possibly die.

Unfortunately, the nerve cells in an area of the brain called the hypothalamus are very sensitive to excitotoxins. The hypothalamus is a collection of specialized cells in your brain that provide the primary link between the endocrine (glandular) and nervous systems. Nerve cells in the hypothalamus control the pituitary gland by producing chemicals that either stimulate or suppress hormone secretions from the pituitary.

Therefore, if the nerve cells in your hypothalamus become damaged, your body's ability to keep your hormones balanced is impaired.

Some excitotoxins are natural, such as the amino acids glutamate, aspartate and cysteine. Others are man-made, such as MSG. MSG, a very common flavor additive, is a combination of glutamate and sodium. In mice, high doses of MSG caused a drop in LH (luteinizing hormone) and GH (growth hormone). On the other hand, low doses of MSG were shown to cause abnormally high levels of LH. Elevated LH is one of the primary reproductive problems that PCOS women have.

Administration of MSG to female rats when they were very young significantly reduced ovarian and pituitary gland weights, showed an absence or disruption of ovarian cyclicity after puberty and had significantly higher concentrations of serum prolactin.[20] Luteinizing hormone (LH), follicle stimulating hormone (FSH) and estrogen were also reduced in another study of rats.[21]

Another man-made excitotoxin is "hydrolyzed vegetable protein" or HVP. On food labels, it is sometimes described as "vegetable protein" or "plant protein." HVP is manufactured from plant material treated with acid and caustic soda. It contains glutamate, aspartate and cystoic acid, all of which are excitotoxins.

HVP is found in many foods, including protein drinks, frozen dinners, cereals, diet meals, sauces, soups and salad dressings, to name a few. Be aware that the label may only say "vegetable protein" or "plant protein." "Vegetable protein" may seem like something that is really healthy, when it really isn't.

If your mother was consuming excitotoxins while she was pregnant with you, your developing hypothalamus may have been adversely affected, leading to long-term reproductive problems when you became an adult. You can think of your brain as being "hard-wired" as you develop from an embryo. Your mother may have unintentionally — and permanently — disturbed the "wiring" of your brain by consuming excitotoxins or by being exposed to environmental chemicals that act like hormones.

Excitotoxins and other food additives pose a serious to your health and the future health of your unborn children. Moreover, they appear to contribute to your PCOS symptoms.

Diet and Environmental Pollution

The amount of chemical pollution today is unprecedented in human history. We dump nearly 6,000,000,000 pounds of chemicals into our environment every year. At least 75,000 different chemical have been invented since 1940 and many are scattered throughout our environment — in the air you breathe, the water your drink, the food you eat, the objects you touch. Only a few hundred of these tens of thousands of chemicals have ever been studied for their human health implications.

Should you be concerned?

There is substantial evidence that environmental chemical pollutants are disrupting the reproductive function most living creatures as well as harming our basic health.[22] [23]

Environmental toxins can disrupt your hormones in two basic ways:
- Interfere with the production, transport, acceptance, activity and metabolism of hormones
- Mimic hormones

Of the few hundred chemicals that have been studied, many have been shown to disrupt your hormone and endocrine (glandular) system. Most of them are fat-soluble, meaning that once they enter your body, they will reside for years (or even a lifetime!) in your fat cells. These chemicals confuse your body, since your body's machinery is not designed to metabolize and detoxify these chemicals. Therefore, they are free to do their damage.[24] [25] [26]

Environmental chemical pollution may influence your fertility,[27] your hormonal balance, your general health and even the health of your unborn child.

A substantial number of chemicals have estrogen-like effects, while others suppress estrogen production. [28] [29] Still others may affect testosterone, progesterone, insulin, thyroid and other hormones.[30] [31]

In animal studies and cultures of human ovary cells, many of these chemicals damage or destroy ovarian follicles and thus they can't produce their hormones.[32] These damaged follicles cannot mature in a normal ovulatory cycle and will not produce an egg to be fertilized. Some chemicals can disrupt the maturation of eggs in animals.[33]

Exposure to environmental chemicals may increase the risk of infertility or miscarriage. Concentrations of progesterone, which is necessary to maintain pregnancy, must remain high throughout pregnancy to avoid the loss of the developing embryo. Animal studies show that PCB's cause a reduction in progesterone by accelerating its breakdown in the liver.[34] A study of women who had DDT in their blood showed they had a shortened luteal phase of their menstrual cycle and lower progesterone.[35] It is well known that PCOS women have lower progesterone levels and a higher rate of infertility.

Environmental chemicals have been shown to unfavorably alter the gender development of embryos of many species, including humans, resulting in a whole array of reproductive abnormalities and disorders. One of the primary results is infertility.

Environmental chemical toxins clearly pose an under-recognized but potentially serious threat to your reproductive health, your overall health and longevity and the health of your children, born or not yet born.[36] [37] [38]

The bad news is this: there is no escape from chemical pollution. All of us are exposed daily and already have accumulations of synthetic chemicals in our bodies. Your strategy at this point is to reduce any further exposure.

The PCOS diet will provide you with a diet that is as free as possible from environmental chemicals that will disrupt your hormones and damage your overall health.

Do You Have Chemical Toxins in Your Body?

The problem of environmental toxins is not something that is happening only to somebody else. It is a problem for *you.*

Since 1976 the U.S. Environmental Protection Agency (EPA) has been conducting the National Human Adipose Tissue Survey (NHATS). NHATS is an annual program that collects and chemically analyzes a nationwide sample of human fat tissue specimens for the presence of toxic compounds. The objective of the program is to detect and quantify the prevalence of toxic compounds in the general population.

In 1982 the EPA expanded beyond their normal list to look for the presence of 54 different environmental chemical toxins. Their results were astounding. Five of these chemicals were found in 100% of the samples. Another nine chemicals were found in 91-98% of all samples. In addition, PCBs were found in 83% of all samples and beta-BHC in 87%.

76% of samples had detectable levels of 20 of the 54 chemicals that were measured. In addition, the amounts of these compounds were also alarming.

Bear in mind that only 54 chemicals were assessed out of literally thousand of environmental chemicals and toxins to which you are exposed.

Other studies verify that most of us are carrying some level of environmental toxins in our bodies.

You and your doctor cannot simply ignore the effect of environmental toxins on your hormones and your reproductive and overall health just because you can't see, smell or taste them. You can rest assured that these toxins are everywhere — some are inside your cells and in your blood right now. There is a mountain of evidence to show that environment chemicals and other toxins undoubtedly have a negative impact your health.

If you live in the temperate or colder climates of the northern hemisphere of the planet, you have an especially high risk. Most pollution is created in the northern hemisphere. Much of it goes up into the air. Some of it is carried for thousands of miles by wind and thus is widely dispersed.

The diet we recommend not only is designed to minimize your exposure to toxins, but it also is designed to help you naturally dispose of toxins you already have.

Diet and Autoimmune Disease

Some autoimmune diseases are known to effect fertility. It is not yet clear whether these conditions are a causative factor in PCOS. Autoimmune disease is an inflammatory condition where your immune system mistakenly attacks organs or other tissues in your body, thinking that your cells are "foreign" to your body.

The cause of autoimmune diseases appears to be due to some combination of these factors:
- Gender - Nearly 79% of the 8.5 million autoimmune disease patients in the United States are women;
- Hormone disorders or alterations, including but not limited to: estrogen, progesterone, testosterone, prolactin, growth hormone and insulin-like growth factor-1 (IGF-1);
- Inherited genetic predisposition;
- Environmental factors - substances and microorganisms in your food, water, air and physical environment. The environmental factors could be anything, such as food components, toxic metals, chemicals, viruses, medications, you name it.

All of these factors influence your immune system. There are many autoimmune conditions and they do not have a simple, single cause.

Link Between Hashimoto's Disease and PCOS

A medical study was recently published that showed a relationship between PCOS and Hashimoto's Disease, which is autoimmune thyroiditis.[39] Autoimmune thyroiditis is an inflammatory condition where your immune system attacks and damages your thyroid gland. A healthy thyroid gland is essential to reproductive health and fertility. So if you have Hashimoto's Disease, you are much more likely to have reproductive difficulties such as infertility. The production of adequate thyroid hormones is also necessary for normal fetal and neonatal growth and development.

The study found that 27% of the PCOS women had elevated thyroid-specific antibodies as compared to only 8.3% of the control group. Elevated antibodies suggest an aroused immune system that is causing inflammation. Thyroid ultrasound showed that 42.3% of PCOS women, but only 6.5% of the controls, had thyroid tissue images typical of autoimmune thyroiditis (Hashimoto's Disease). The PCOS women also had higher levels of TSH (thyroid stimulating hormone) than the non-PCOS women, suggesting that the PCOS thyroid is not as successful in making enough thyroid hormone.

Link Between Autoimmunity and PCOS

In another recent study of 108 women with menstrual cycle disturbances, PCOS, endometriosis or chronic lack of ovulation, the researchers found that 40.7% had immune antibodies for autoimmunity vs. only 14.8% for women without any of these conditions.[40]

In other words, the two studies we just mentioned would suggest that as many as 4 of every 10 PCOS women have an autoimmune disorder of some kind.

PCOS - C-Reactive Protein - Autoimmune Connection?

CRP (C-reactive protein) is a protein in the blood that is a general marker of infection and inflammation. It is used to assess how active a body-wide inflammatory condition is.

Women with PCOS have significantly increased CRP concentrations as compared to women with normal menstrual rhythm and normal androgen levels.[41] It appears that low-grade inflammation may be a characteristic of PCOS. We could speculate that the inflammation is, in part, caused by an autoimmune condition.

If the CRP is not caused by an autoimmune condition, it may be due to some other type of chronic infection or inflammation, or from obesity. Or, it may be due to "oxidant stress," which is a condition where your antioxidant defenses are depleted and there is inflammation resulting from free radical damage to your cells.

Inflammatory Cascade in PCOS Ovaries?

A small study conducted at Catholic University Medical School in Rome, Italy showed that ovarian tissue from PCOS women produced a higher level of pro-inflammatory prostaglandins (PGE2) than the ovaries of non-PCOS women.[42] Prostaglandins are hormone-like substances that have very powerful effects on the body. PGE2 is a prostaglandin that creates inflammation.

Role of the PCOS Diet

The PCOS Diet is designed to help you reduce the risk of autoimmune reactions by removing as many inflammatory triggers as possible from your food. We also will suggest foods that support thyroid function.

Section 2

How We Developed the
Healthy Diet for PCOS

2.1 The 'Food Pyramid'

In early 2005, the U.S. Department of Agriculture released official dietary guidelines and key recommendations for healthy eating.[43] The new guidelines are an update to the 1992 Food Guide Pyramid, which has now been discredited by many scientists.

In the past, most of those who followed the Food Guide Pyramid program did not see an improvement in their health. Some of the reasons for this include:

- The Pyramid's failure to draw proper distinctions between "good fats" (i.e., anti-inflammatory omega-3 fats found in fish, flax seed and walnuts) and "bad fats" (i.e., potentially pro-inflammatory omega-6 fats found in most grains). Further, it did it advise against the unhealthy "trans-fats" found in processed foods.
- The USDA 1992 Food Guide Pyramid did not address the effect of various carbohydrates on blood sugar and insulin production, failing to draw critical distinctions between how the body metabolizes diverse carbohydrates such as vegetables, fruits, refined starches and sugars.
- It also promoted over-consumption of dairy products by recommending the equivalent of 2 - 3 glasses of milk a day. The basis for this was presumably its calcium content. Calcium is necessary for bone health. However, the highest rates of bone fractures are found in countries with high dairy consumption.

The New Food Guidelines for 2005

The foundation of the New Food Guidelines consists of weight management and daily exercise recommendations. The Guidelines encourage you to consume a variety of nutrient-dense foods and beverages within and among the basic food groups while choosing foods that limit the intake of saturated and trans-fats, cholesterol, added sugars, salt and alcohol.

In addition, the new guidelines strongly encourage you to maintain body weight in a healthy range by:

- Balancing calories from foods and beverages with calories used in daily activities
- Preventing gradual weight gain over time with small decreases in food and beverage calories and appropriate increases in physical activity

Eating the Right Foods

These are the basic recommendations of the USDA's New Food Guidelines for 2005:

Fruits and Vegetables
- Two cups of fruit and 2 cups of vegetables per day are recommended for a reference 2,000-calorie intake, with higher or lower amounts depending on the calorie level.
- Choose a variety of fruits and vegetables each day. In particular, select from all five vegetable subgroups (dark green, orange, legumes, starchy vegetables and other

vegetables) several times a week.

Grains
Consume 3 or more ounce-equivalents of whole-grain products per day, with the rest of the recommended grains coming from enriched or whole-grain products. In general, at least half the grains should come from whole grains.

Dairy
Consume 3 cups per day of fat-free or low-fat milk or equivalent milk products.

Fats
- Consume less than 10% of calories from saturated fatty acids and less than 300 mg/day of cholesterol and keep trans-fatty acid consumption as low as possible.
- Keep total fat intake between 20%-35% of calories, with most fats coming from sources of polyunsaturated and monounsaturated fatty acids, such as fish, nuts and vegetable oils.
- When selecting and preparing meat, poultry, dry beans and milk or milk products, make choices that are lean, low-fat or fat-free.

Carbohydrates
- Choose fiber-rich fruits, vegetables and whole grains often.
- Choose and prepare foods and beverages with little added sugars.

Sodium and Potassium
- Consume less than 2,300 mg of sodium (approximately 1 teaspoon of salt) per day.
- Choose and prepare foods with little salt. At the same time, consume potassium-rich foods, such as fruits and vegetables.

Alcoholic Beverages
Those who choose to drink alcoholic beverages should do so sensibly and in moderation — defined as the consumption of up to one drink per day for women and up to two drinks per day for men. Alcoholic beverages should not be consumed by some individuals, including those who cannot restrict their alcohol intake, women of childbearing age who may become pregnant, pregnant and lactating women, children and adolescents, individuals taking medications that can interact with alcohol and those with specific medical conditions.

Physical Activity

Engaging in regular physical activity and reducing sedentary activities promotes health, psychological well-being and healthy body weight. Here is some basic information that will help you determine what constitutes a healthy physical activity:
- Engage in at least 30 minutes of moderate-intensity physical activity, above usual activity, at work or home on most days of the week.
- For most people, greater health benefits can be obtained by engaging in physical activity of more vigorous intensity or longer duration.

- To help manage adult body weight and prevent gradual weight gain, engage in approximately 60 minutes of moderate to vigorous activity on most days of the week while consuming less calories than you need.
- To sustain weight loss in adulthood, participate in at least 60 to 90 minutes of daily moderate-intensity physical activity while not consuming more calories than you need. Some people may need to consult with a healthcare provider before participating in this level of activity.

Achieve physical fitness by including cardiovascular conditioning, stretching exercises for flexibility and resistance exercises or calisthenics for muscle strength and endurance.

Customized Food Pyramid

In a huge step towards making the Food Pyramid more useful, the USDA now offers customized pyramids, based on your age, sex and level of physical activity. You can go to the MyPyramid.gov website (www.mypyramid.gov), enter your age, sex and physical activity to get the government's version of the best diet for you.

Summary

The government dietary guidelines are the result of negotiations between scientists and food manufacturers. They resemble a political compromise, not a standard for good health. Under the old guidelines, the food manufacturers and distributors were able to get much of they wanted. The result was that people who followed the Food Guide Pyramid experienced a phenomenal increase in obesity and diabetes.

It is important to keep in mind that the food industry is one of the largest industries in the U.S. It has powerful lobbies and enormous clout with the government. For most food companies, your health is not their primary concern. Their number one priority is to sell you products, not help you get healthy. However, the new government dietary guidelines are a big step forward. This time, the scientists were better able to stand up for themselves against the food lobbies.

Even so, subtle compromises were made. For example, the guidelines say to keep consumption of trans-fats as "low as possible." What is "low as possible" supposed to mean? One gram a day? One ounce a day? One pound a day? Nobody knows. The food lobbies forced this vague language into the new guidelines. The fact is that *no* amount of trans-fat is good for you. There is no such thing as a "good" trans-fat. Had the new guidelines been truly 100% concerned about your health, they would have told you to never to consume any trans-fats at all.

Although the new guidelines are a huge improvement, they are still not sufficient as a dietary plan for women with PCOS.

2.2 Low Carb Diets

Many overweight PCOS women are on a "low-carb" diet, meaning that they carefully restrict the amount of carbohydrates calories they consume.

Low carb diets have also been called, somewhat inaccurately, high-protein diets. Popular "low-carb" diet books advocate what is more accurately described as a moderate or appropriate level of protein. However, some readers and the media have misinterpreted the principles described by the various diet programs.

Careful reading of well-known low-carb diets, including Dr. Atkins New Diet Revolution (3rd edition), Protein Power, South Beach and to a lesser extent, the Zone Diet, reveals these are thoughtful efforts to educate and guide the consumer to a new understanding of how we eat to be well. The recipes in these diets generally have very small portion sizes so that the dieters are restricting their total caloric intake in addition to restricting carbohydrates.

There are two important questions to be answered about these diets:
(1) Do they work?
(2) Are they healthy?

Do Low-Carb Diets Work?

Most of the evidence suggests that low-carb diets cause weight loss, at least in the short term. However, no studies thus far have followed people on this type of diet for longer than nine months. Ongoing comparative research indicates that in general, low-carb diets and calorie restricted, high-carb, low-fat diets are about equally effective for producing short term weight loss.

The important question is: what else happens? Weight loss is only one feature of a successful dietary revision for PCOS. We also want to:
- Maintain and increase lean muscle tissue
- Experience psychological satisfaction and have an improved mood
- Have plenty of energy while we adjust our eating habits
- Make excellent nutrient-dense food choices
- Have our foods taste very good

First, the good news about low carb diets...

Lower carb diets appear to improve body composition in addition to weight loss. In a 10-week study at the University of Illinois, 24 overweight women were divided into two dietary groups.[44] Each group ate the same amount of calories and same amount of fat. However, one group ate twice as much protein as the other group. The two groups lost approximately the same amount of weight, but the high-protein (low-carb) group lost 13.9 lbs of body fat vs.

8.4 pounds for the low protein diet group. This study is significant because it's body fat you want to lose, while retaining muscle mass. We'll discuss this "body fat" issue in detail in the *Weight vs. Body Composition* chapter. The high-protein group also had a lower insulin response to a meal and reported they felt more satisfied after a meal.

A study at the Royal Veterinary and Agricultural University in Denmark compared the effect on a medium or a high protein diet on the body weight of overweight individuals.[45] After one year, each group had lost roughly the same amount of weight, but the high protein group had a 10% greater reduction of abdominal fat. Abdominal fat is the fat that is linked to chronic disease.

A clinical trial at the University of Cincinnati compared overweight women on a very low carbohydrate vs. a calorie-restricted, low-fat diet over 6 months.[46] The low carb diet women lost more weight. Also of interest is that the low carb women, after 2 weeks of dieting, were allowed to consume as many calories as they wished, provided they stayed on a low carb diet. As it turned out, they decreased their intake by an average of 450 calories per day.

Low carb diets appear to cause a spontaneous reduction in calorie intake, probably because protein causes you to feel satisfied sooner than carbohydrates do. Therefore you stop eating sooner.

The Theoretical Basis of Low-Carb Diets

The basic premise of popular "low carb" diet books is three-fold:
- A high-carbohydrate diet makes people fat.
- A low-carb (high-protein) diet leads to weight loss, decreased insulin levels and improved blood sugar control.
- Insulin resistance (the inability to efficiently utilize insulin), a factor that causes carbohydrates to be stored as fat, can be cured with a low-carb, high-protein diet.

However, contrary to these assumptions, critics claim that avoiding carbohydrates is not the reason you lose weight with a low-carb diet.[47] Instead, a low-carb, high-protein diet causes you to lose water, which is heavy.

Another reason for this weight loss is that eating protein diminishes your appetite,[48] so you end up eating fewer calories. Some say that eating too many calories is the primary cause of overweight, not carbohydrates. They say that if you were to eat less fat, you would be eating far fewer calories and thus you would lose weight.

Do Carbs Make You Fat?

Do carbohydrates cause you to become fat? It seems most people think so. Carbs have been blamed for causing excess weight, giving rise to such popular diets as Atkins and Sugar Busters. Let's explore this issue to see what is going on.

There appears to be a preferred sequence for the use of nutrients that is determined by the body's storage capacity and tissues' need for specific fuels.

For example, alcohol has the highest priority for oxidation (burning for energy) because the body has no place to store it, and conversion of alcohol to fat is energetically expensive. The body prefers not to waste energy unless it is absolutely necessary.

Carbohydrates and amino acids (the building blocks of protein) are next in line in the fuel-burning hierarchy.

There are no storage depots for amino acids. Amino acids are used to build proteins that perform critical functions throughout your body. Other amino acids are distributed to the muscle cells as fuel, while still others are broken down into blood sugar (glucose) or stored as a special fuel molecule called glycogen. When needed, glycogen can be converted into blood sugar to provide fuel for the body.

Carbohydrates are broken down and used immediately as fuel or stored as glycogen (the storage form of blood sugar). However, glycogen storage capacity is limited. Once the glycogen depots are filled, carbohydrate will be converted into fat (your body has an unlimited ability to efficiently store dietary fat).

Your body will turn to burning stored fat only when there is insufficient carbohydrate and protein fuel conveniently available. But what happens if you drastically reduce your consumption of carbohydrates, the primary and preferred source of fuel for your body? Your body will turn to stored fat and start burning it.

In summary, carbohydrates are not stored as fat unless your total caloric intake consistently exceeds the total calories you are burning. So eating carbs per se is not what makes you fat. Eating too many total calories is what makes you gain weight. All you have to do is look at Third World countries where the primary food in the diet is a carbohydrate such as white rice or millet. If carbs make people fat, then people in poor countries would be the fattest people on earth. Instead, they are among the thinnest. They are thinner than Americans because their total caloric intake is much less and they are much more physically active. In short, their dietary caloric intake is balanced with calories expended for energy.

Why Carbohydrates Are Important for Weight Control

Carbohydrates strongly influence your weight management efforts.

Glycemic Index. Some carbohydrate foods, especially refined carbohydrates, have a high glycemic index. A high glycemic index means your blood sugar goes up when you eat that food. When blood sugar is high, insulin is produced in order to store the sugar into the cells. However, if you're always eating high glycemic carbs, your insulin is likely to stay elevated. One of the problems with chronically high insulin is that it encourages fat storage and inhibits fat burning.

A recent study from the University of Massachusetts found an association between body weight and the glycemic index of foods consumed, but not the total carbohydrate intake or the percentage of calories from carbohydrate in the diet.[49] In other words, the type of carbohydrate, not carbohydrates per se, is one reason why carbs may contribute to increased weight. You can find out more about the glycemic index in the *Glycemic Index* chapter.

Caloric Density. Processed, refined carbohydrates have a very high caloric density, meaning that a lot of calories are packed into a relatively small amount of food. High calorie density carbs cause you to consume many more calories than you can use. The excess calories are then stored as fat. To find out more, see the *How Calorie Density Makes You Fat* chapter.

Portion Size. Please keep in mind that the portion size of your meal and the total calories you consume are a critical determinant of your weight. Americans are eating larger meals than ever before.

But even if you cut the carbs, you're going to gain weight if your total calories significantly exceed the calories burned for energy. In other words, if you think you will lose weight by cutting the carbs, but you load up on protein and fat instead, you are defeating yourself. Calorie restriction, reduced calorie density, portion control and exercise are all key components to a successful weight control program.

If you substitute unrefined, whole carbohydrates for refined carbs, the added fiber and essential nutrients will favorably alter your hormonal profile. The hormones that govern your weight will tend to fall into a more normal pattern and thus support your efforts for a lower, stable weight. We review the role of hormones and your weight in the *A Word About Your Weight* section of this book.

A Low-Carb (High-Protein) Diet Helps Save Muscle Mass

People on a calorie-restricted, high carbohydrate diet should be concerned about protein adequacy. Protein is needed to maintain muscle mass. A recent study compared a low calorie/high-carb and a low-calorie/high-protein (or low-carb) diet.[50] Both diets had the same amount of fat. Both groups of dieters lost the same amount of weight, but the high-carb group lost more muscle mass. Loss of muscle mass is not helpful for dealing with insulin resistance. Your goal should be to increase muscle mass, not lose it. Therefore, a diet high in refined carbs is not recommended.

Are Low Carb Diets Healthy?

Low-carb diets are considered "safe" over a period of at least six months. However, they are not appropriate for everyone or for all life stages.

A typical study conducted at Duke University looked at 120 overweight people who were assigned a very low-carb diet or a low-fat diet.[51] Those on the low carb diet lost about twice as much weight over a six-month period. However, they also had a much higher incidence of certain side effects, as shown in the table below:

Side Effect	*Low Carb Diet*	*Low Fat Diet*
Constipation	68%	35%
Headaches	60%	40%
Bad breath	38%	8%
Muscle cramps	35%	7%
Diarrhea	23%	7%
General weakness	25%	8%
Rash	13%	0%

This study did not ask questions that would elicit reports of well-known side effects typical of low fat, low calorie diets, such as low energy, hunger, weakness, dizziness and mood swings.

Increased protein consumption leads to a build up of urea, a toxic metabolic byproduct, in the kidneys that must be excreted in the urine. Therefore, you absolutely must drink more water, even if you don't feel thirsty. In a paper presented at the 2002 Experimental Biology conference,[52] researchers reported that individuals who increased their protein consumption became dehydrated, due to increased urination to get rid of the urea. The problem was that the individuals did not feel thirsty and thus did not drink more water to compensate for their water loss via urination.

High-protein, very-low-carbohydrate weight-loss diets are designed to induce ketosis, a metabolic condition that indicates you are burning body fat (ketones) as fuel. Visit the *Diet and Long-Term Weight Management* chapter for more details.

An excessive increase in circulating ketones can disturb the body's acid-base balance, possibly causing metabolic acidosis. In the long run, even mild acidosis may cause trouble, including low blood phosphorous, loss of calcium from bone and an increased propensity to form kidney stones.[53] Increased risk of colon cancer, heart disease, impaired kidney function, osteoporosis, and possible worsening of diabetic complications are additional concerns.

Critics of the low-carb diet approach are also concerned about the lack of complete nutrition in some of these diets, including an insufficiency of vitamins A, B6, D and E, thiamin (a B vitamin), folate (a B vitamin), calcium, magnesium, iron, potassium and dietary fiber. We have recommended meals and therapeutic supplementation that ensures you will have appropriate amounts of all essential nutrients as you lose fat and build muscle.

Low-Carb Diets and PCOS

Does a low-carb diet help PCOS women lose weight?

Penn State University recently conducted a study of 26 obese PCOS women who wanted to become pregnant.[54] They were put on a calorie-restricted diet for one month and divided into two groups. One group had a high-protein (moderate carb) diet, while the other group was put on a high-carb diet, low-protein diet. The percentage of fat was the same in each diet.

Both groups of women lost an equal amount of weight. Moreover, there was no difference between the two groups in androgen (male hormone) levels, measures of glucose metabolism, or leptin (a fat and reproductive hormone). The most striking result of the study was that both groups had a decline in androgens, better glucose tolerance, and improvements in leptin. Fourteen of the 26 resumed menstruation. The researchers report that the reduction in calories was the variable that caused the favorable outcome, since both the high protein and high carb diets had the same effect.

This study suggests that reduction of calories, not necessarily the reduction of carbohydrates, is a critical variable in losing weight, increasing fertility and reducing other PCOS symptoms.

A similar study of overweight PCOS women was conducted at the University of Adelaide in Australia.[55] The women were divided into two groups: a high-protein, lower carb diet group, and a low protein, higher carb diet group. Both groups were on a calorie-restricted diet and consumed the same amount of calories. The women had improved menstrual cycles and reduced insulin resistance regardless of which diet they were on, although when the calories increased, the high protein diet appeared to be slightly better in controlling androgens.

In addition to the benefits of a low-carb diet, our dietary recommendations are designed to give you healthy protein, carbs and fats in a combination that will nourish and satisfy you without giving you too many calories.

However, your success with any diet — including the diet in this book — will depend to a great extent on how it makes you feel. For example, some women simply feel better if they are on a very high-protein diet whereas others need more complex carbohydrates. We have attempted to strike a balance that will meet the needs of most readers and still provide the benefits of reduced PCOS symptoms, weight loss and increased fertility. However, you may need to adjust our diet a bit according to how well it makes you feel.

2.3 The Other Diets

Besides the "Low Carb" diets, there are dozens of other diet plans available at any bookstore. Let's briefly review some you may have heard of.

Eat Right 4 Your Type

Eat Right 4 Your Type, by Dr. Peter J. D'Adamo, outlines a diet based on your blood type. Dr. D'Adamo's research indicates that certain foods contain certain lectins (Velcro-like substances) that cause clumping of red blood cells and other metabolic problems. By avoiding these reactive foods, you can improve your health.

The *Eat Right 4 Your Type* diet is not specifically a weight-loss diet, although some people on this diet do lose weight. The diet plan for people with blood type O, the most common blood type, emphasizes lean meats and fish, vegetables fruits and some nuts and seeds. It minimizes agricultural products like dairy and grain foods.

Once you know what your blood type is, you can then select the foods that are best for your blood type and eliminate those that are bad for your blood type. When you go on this diet, you will probably find yourself doing without many of the foods you are now eating.

If the family is going to participate in the *Eat Right 4 Your Type* diet, you may have to prepare two or more different meals if their blood type is different from yours.

There is a large body of published research about lectins and their effect on the body, but no large-scale studies have been conducted on Dr. D'Adamo's diet.

Fat Flush Diet

The Fat Flush Plan by Anne Louise Gittleman, is based on a combination of essential fats, balanced proteins and what are called "good" carbs. The author claims this plan aids weight loss by detoxifying the liver, thereby increasing metabolism.

In its final phase, *The Fat Flush Plan* recommends a similar carb-protein-fat ratio to the Zone Diet (40% carbs, 30% protein and 30% fat). But a range of food restrictions applies in Phases 1 and 2.

Phase 1 is a cleansing program to encourage weight loss by giving the liver support and nourishment. Food restrictions include: no herbs or spices except for those fat flushing herbs and spices outlined in *The Fat Flush Plan*. No margarine. No alcohol. No sugar. No oils or fats except those in flaxseed oil. No grains, bread, cereal or starchy vegetables such as beans, potatoes, corn, parsnips, carrots, peas, pumpkin, or acorn or butternut squash. No dairy products.

Phase 2 includes more food choices, including the option of adding back a 'friendly' carb each week while checking for any adverse reaction.

Phase 3 is a maintenance program providing a lifelong eating program aimed at increasing your vitality. Two dairy products can be reintroduced, and a variety of starchier vegetables and grains. These foods are added back one at a time to gauge your body's reaction.

Hunter-Gatherer Paleolithic Diet

The hunter-gatherer Paleolithic diet is based on the concept that our genes have hardly changed at all over the past 10,000 years and therefore we should be eating the same food that we were eating back then. It is well established that foods influence how our genes express themselves. Since our genes tell our cells what to do, it can be said that what we eat strongly influences our function and health.

It is logical that we should be eating according to what our genes are designed for. A Paleolithic diet would exclude all processed foods entirely and it thus represents a huge departure from what you are now eating. Some researchers say that our departure from a hunter-gatherer type of diet to an agricultural diet is the basis for most of our chronic illnesses today.

The hunter-gatherer diet consisted of eating whatever was at hand, including vegetables, fruits, nuts and seeds, seasonal eggs, and animal protein when it was available. The diet was also high in essential fatty acids and other vital nutrients, since the brains, organs and bone marrow were also eaten. Dairy products and cultivated grains and legumes did not exist and therefore are not part of this diet.

Perhaps the most popular of the hunter-gatherer diets is Loren Cordain's *The Paleo Diet*. It describes how you can "hunt and gather" foods in your grocery store and elsewhere. The *Paleo Diet* allows you to approximate what hunter-gatherers actually ate.

The *Paleo Diet* can be characterized as a relatively high protein diet. But it can't be described as a "low-carb" since there is no restriction on the amount of carbs you can have. However, the carbs you eat will be mostly vegetables and fruits. Grain or legume-based carbs are not part of the diet at all.

Ornish (Low-Fat) Diet

The Dean Ornish *Eat More, Weigh Less* diet is a low-fat, mainly vegetarian diet plan. It is 10% fat, 20% protein, and 70% carbohydrates. In contrast, the typical American diet is 45% fat, 25% protein and 30% carbohydrates, with nearly 500 mg of cholesterol per day.

The Ornish diet consists mainly of complex carbohydrates. These are present in fruits, vegetables, grains and beans. All foods containing cholesterol and saturated fats are prohibited from the diet. Meat, poultry or fish foods are not recommended, while only a few dairy products are allowed such as fat-free yogurt, fat-free milk and lower-fat cheese.

The Ornish diet lists "Eat Freely" foods, "Eat Moderately" foods and "Banned" foods. Providing you observe these dietary instructions, you can eat all you want without counting calories or portion sizes. Banned foods include almost all fats and oils, nuts, seeds, avocados, chocolate, olives and coconuts, as well as refined carbs like sugar, white flour and white rice. However, because it is very low in fat, care has to be taken that you are getting the correct amount and balance of essential fatty acids (EFAs).

The Ornish program presumes that you can get an adequate supply of complete proteins from vegetable sources in the diet. This is done by combining rice and beans, tofu and rice, pasta and beans, baked beans and wheat bread, or oatmeal with nonfat yogurt over the course of a day. Egg whites are another source of protein on the Ornish diet.

Weight Watchers

Weight Watchers is not a diet. It is a program is based on calorie-reduction, using the Weight Watchers "points" system. No foods are forbidden, although you are restricted to a certain number of daily points.

Most dieters follow the Weight Watchers program by joining a weekly class, where they meet other dieters, exchange ideas and receive support and advice from the class organizer. Weight Watchers also provides an online at-home program.

Weight Watchers is a useful starting point for some. It provides strong support and common-sense advice.

Sugar Busters Diet

Sugar Busters diet is based on the concept that sugar produces excessive insulin, which prevents weight loss despite strict dieting and exercise. Thus, added sugar is restricted and mostly it recommends foods that are low on the Glycemic Index (GI).

The *Sugar Busters* diet plan is based broadly on 30% protein, 40% fat and 30% carbohydrates. The diet allows red meat, poultry, fish, olive oil, dairy foods, nuts and a selection of fruit and vegetables. Potatoes are banned, as are white bread, pasta, white rice, and most sugar. However, small amounts of whole grain bread, whole wheat pasta and oats are permitted.

The *Sugar Busters* diet also recommends portion control. Success with this diet will probably be derived from the reduction of total calories consumed. The diet is relatively easy to follow.

Metabolic Type Diet

The thesis of this diet is that you should eat according to your "metabolic type." This diet is described in *The Nutrition Solution: A Guide to Your Metabolic Type* by Harold Kristol and James Haig.

Your metabolism is governed by two basic systems, each of which has two divisions:
- Oxidative system - the conversion of food to energy
  - Slow oxidizer - alkaline tendency
  - Fast oxidizer - acid tendency
- Autonomic system - neuroendocrine control of energy
  - Sympathetic nervous system dominance - acid tendency
  - Parasympathetic nervous system dominance - alkaline tendency

The purpose of the diet is to create the optimal acid-alkaline balance in your blood, by eating the foods for your metabolic type that bring you back into balance. For example, if you were a dominant fast oxidizer/parasympathetic, you would eat much more protein and more fat, plus reduce carbohydrates.

Your metabolic type is determined by a glucose tolerance and blood pH test. These tests are inconvenient to administer, so for practical purposes, you're forced to rely on answering a questionnaire in the book to estimate your metabolic type.

Some clinicians advocate this diet but there have been no studies to verify its effectiveness.

Zone Diet

In the book *The Zone*, Barry Sears explains how the right ratio of carbohydrates to proteins and fats can control levels of insulin in the bloodstream. Too much insulin can increase fat storage and inflammation in the body — and lead to obesity, diabetes and heart disease.

You can better regulate your metabolism with a diet of 40% carbohydrates, 30% protein, and 30% fat (now widely known as the 40-30-30 plan).

The diet does not prohibit any foods, but severely restricts those high in fat and carbohydrates such as grains, starches, and pastas. Fruits and vegetables are the favored source of carbs. Protein should be low fat and no bigger and no thicker than the palm of one's hand. As for fat, monounsaturated fats such as olive oil, canola oil, almonds, macadamia nuts and avocados are preferred over other kinds of fats.

For a simple interpretation of *The Zone*, Sears suggests filling one-third of a plate with low-fat protein, and then piling the rest with fruits and vegetables. You may choose to add a monounsaturated source of fat such as olive oil.

The *Zone Diet* is somewhat different from the Low-Carb / High-Protein diets in that it has a mild restriction on fats (30% of calories), whereas low-carb diets may be higher in fat.

The *Zone Diet* could be characterized as a "middle of the road" diet between low carb and low fat diets.

What Most of These Diets Have in Common

Most of these diets have something in common: they all depend on calorie restriction or portion control. In fact, calorie restriction is a key element to their success. Only 5 studies out of 107 lasted over 90 days, so there's not much long-term data.[56] Studies suggest that weight loss is associated with longer diet duration and restriction of calorie intake, but not reduced carbohydrate content.

A calorie is a unit of energy. When you consume calories in food, they are either used immediately for energy or stored for future use. Some calories are stored as glycogen, a complex sugar that can be used immediately by the cells to produce energy. However, your storage capacity for glycogen is somewhat limited. Most of your excess calories are stored as fat, which is a long-term, large-capacity energy storage system.

Whatever type of calorie you consume — carbohydrate, protein, or fat — you will store it as fat if it can't be burned for energy, stored as glycogen or utilized for another essential purpose. An essential way to not gain weight is to avoid eating too many calories. Therefore, most of the diets described above rely on some form of portion control in order to reduce the dietary calories you take in.

Since most of these diets rely on portion control, it's not surprising that you can find one or more studies that support the effectiveness of any particular diet. In other words, whatever diet you are on, there's a good chance you will maintain or lose weight if you restrict the amount of food you eat.

Long-Term Diet Adherence Is Key

Beside portion control and calorie restriction, the weight loss potential of these popular diets depends on how long you stay with them.

A comparison of the Atkins, Zone, Weight Watchers and Ornish programs was recently conducted at the Tufts-New England Medical Center in Boston.[57]

Each popular diet modestly reduced body weight and several cardiac risk factors by the end of one year. Regardless of the diet, those who stayed with their assigned diet the longest had the best results.

On the downside, a high percentage of people could not stay with their diets. The dropout rates were: 47% for Atkins, 35% for Zone, 35% for Weight Watchers, and 50% for Ornish.

The Tufts study showed that a high percentage of people will drop out of any popular weight loss diet. But those who stick it out for a year, regardless of which popular diet they are on, will be successful in losing some weight and reducing cardiac risk.

Our Comments On These Diets

It seems that it doesn't matter very much which popular diet you are on. You will get results if you:
- Control your portion size
- Restrict the number of calories you consume
- Learn how you respond to amounts of carbohydrate and amounts of daily energy expenditure, and make choices accordingly

All of these diets have something good in them. They also have some similarities. But they each take a somewhat different approach. And some of them recommend foods that are clearly not healthy. Few of them carry you beyond the weight loss phase and address transition to a broader, more varied diet that maintains a healthier self. *The key to long term well-being is understanding that weight loss and weight maintenance require two different styles of eating and exercising, both of which are different from the eating style that caused weight gain and compromised your health in the first place.*

The healthy PCOS diet in this book attempts to take the best from each of these diets and exclude those aspects that we have found to be unhealthy. Of all of the diets, the healthy PCOS diet most closely approximates the *Paleo Diet* (hunter-gatherer). Once your desired weight is achieved, you will transition to more choices and less stringent portion control, guided by your close attention to what works for you.

We believe that PCOS women have a genetic predisposition that makes the modern, Standard American Diet a very difficult choice for those who want to reduce their PCOS symptoms, improve fertility, and reduce their risk for diabetes and heart disease. We think that many PCOS women have "thrifty genes" that would respond best to a hunter-gatherer type of diet.

We also think the *Eat Right 4 Your Type* diet deserves some consideration. However, it has complexities that prevent us from proposing it as the primary approach to a healthy PCOS diet. But if the diet in this book does not work for you, consider modifying the diet to accommodate your blood type.

2.4 What Did Your Ancestors Eat?

The genetic makeup of our ancestors is virtually identical to the genes we have today. The foods that they needed for optimal function are the same that we need, since our dietary needs are essentially the same.[58] [59]

Since we know that food is a part of the "environment" that influences what our genes do, it's important to review what foods our ancestors were eating.

For most of human history, we were hunters and gatherers. For millions of years, up to the agricultural revolution 10,000 years ago, people ate what they could get their hands on. We obtained food by going out and getting it from our natural environment. Today, there is no natural environment. We obtain our food indirectly from others who grow and process our foods for us. What is provided to us by others is not what our ancestors hunted and gathered.

What Our Ancestors Ate

Protein. The ancient diet was dominated by wild, lean animal foods. While the muscle meat provided protein and other nutrients, people also ate bone marrow and brains to get essential fatty acids (EFAs) and other specialty nutrients. Compared to how we eat, ancient peoples diets were higher in protein and much lower in carbohydrate.

Carbohydrates. Nonstarchy vegetables and fruits were virtually the sole source of carbohydrates. Cultivated grains and other starchy plants simply did not exist in anywhere near the amounts we consume them in modern times. Our ancestors ate a few handfuls of ripe seeds when the grasses produced these briefly in the fall of the year. As a percentage of dietary calories, their carbohydrate consumption was low and the fiber content was very high.

Fats. Ancient people ate a balance of healthy polyunsaturated, monounsaturated and omega 3 fats, primarily from animal and plant sources. Remember, even though the main feature of their diet was animal flesh, those animals were low in saturated fat because they were wild and active.

What Our Ancestors Did Not Eat

Dairy products. Milk comes from domesticated livestock, which did not exist in any significant numbers before 10,000 years ago. Our ancestors did not consume any dairy at all because they were not yet shepherding cooperative herds of milk-producers.

Grains. Waving fields of wheat or Kellogg's Corn Flakes did not exist in ancient times. It was a wiser expenditure of energy to hunt down a large animal than to go around plucking grain seeds from grasses. Our ancestors did not consume any refined cereal products at all.

Salt. Ancient humans did not salt their food. What sodium they needed was obtained from the mineral content of their whole, unrefined foods.

Sugar. There was no table sugar, no corn syrup. Honey was available, but scarce and difficult to harvest.

Processed Foods. No processed foods were eaten. There was no machinery with which to process foods. Nor was there refrigeration or vacuum packaging to preserve foods.

As you review what your ancestors ate, you'll notice how differently you eat today. For example, you undoubtedly consume grain and dairy products every single day, day in and day out. And, you eat salted, sweetened and highly processed foods every day.

Paleolithic Diet Compared to Modern American Diet

When compared to the present-day typical American diet, the Paleolithic diet contained:
- 2-3 times more fiber
- 1.5 to 2.0 times more polyunsaturated and monounsaturated fats
- 4 times more omega-3 fats (from fish, nuts, vegetation)
- 60-70% less saturated fat
- Monounsaturated fats made up about one-half of fats consumed
- Protein intake 2-3 times higher
- Potassium intake 3-4 times higher
- Sodium intake 4-5 times lower
- No grains
- No sugars except honey
- Abundance of vegetables, fruits and berries in season
  (equivalent to 8 or more daily servings)

Modern Hunter-Gatherers

Researchers have observed the health of "modern" hunter-gatherers in today's few remaining primitive societies. These people appear to be mostly free of cardiovascular disease, high blood pressure, cancer, diabetes, or obesity.

However, they don't all eat exactly the same proportion of wild game, fish, nuts and seeds, non-starchy vegetables and fruits. Among modern hunter-gatherers, carbohydrate consumption can be anywhere from 3% to 64% of the diet. Total protein and fat may range from 36% to 97%.

There is no "one size fits all" diet for ancient man, nor is there a "one size fits all" diet for PCOS and infertility.

However, if you accept the idea that your genes are configured for some proportion of lean animal protein and nonstarchy vegetables and fruits, it's worthwhile to ask yourself why you are not eating those foods, and what the health consequences are.

It is not a big mystery as to why our modern society is beset by a host of chronic health problems. The PCOS diet seeks to emulate the diet of your ancestors.

2.5 The Basis of the PCOS Diet

What you eat influences what your genes do.

Since your genes have predisposed you to have PCOS, you can change your diet and thus cause your genes to change what they do. Altered genetic expression can lead to an improvement in whatever PCOS symptoms you have.

We recommend that you return to your genetic roots and eat like your ancestors did. Since you still have their genes, it makes sense to eat like they did.

Humans and the human genome have slowly evolved over the past 2.6 million years. Our genes changed relatively little until the advent of agriculture about 10,000 years ago, when our diet underwent a rapid, fundamental change.

Moreover, our diet has undergone a complete transformation within the last 100 years with the advent of modern food processing techniques. In fact, most of the food products you see on the supermarket shelf today did not exist 100 years ago.

The mismatch between what we are genetically programmed to eat and what we are actually eating has lead to an explosive increase in health problems. A few examples:
- Two-thirds of Americans are overweight or obese.
- 90% of the population will have high blood pressure at some point in their lives.
- 40% of middle-aged Americans have metabolic syndrome (similar to Syndrome X and PCOS).
- 41% of all fatalities are due to cardiovascular disease.
- 17 million Americans have diabetes and an unknown, much larger number are pre-diabetic.

Since we can't exchange our genes, the best way to get a handle on PCOS and a host of other chronic diseases is to change our diet.

What Agriculture Did to Our Ancestors

Archeological and historical evidence shows ancient hunter-gatherers to be lean, fit and mostly free from signs and symptoms of chronic disease. However, the health of hunter-gatherer societies who ate lean meats, fruits and vegetables deteriorated when they made a transition to a grain-based diet:
- Reduction in average adult height
- Shorter lifespan
- Higher childhood mortality
- Higher incidence of osteoporosis, rickets, other vitamin/mineral deficiencies

A number of studies have also shown that when more recent hunter-gatherers adopted the Western diet and lifestyle, they acquired most of our common diseases, including obesity, diabetes and cardiovascular disease.

Let's Return to Our Dietary Genetic Roots

Because the genetic makeup of our ancestors is virtually identical to the genes we have today, it makes sense that the dietary needs we have for optimum functionality are the same as theirs.

Your ancestors obtained their food by going out and getting it from our natural environment. Today, that natural environment is extinct. So we will have to "hunt and gather" in our local food markets for healthy foods, taking care to avoid all of the unhealthy foods that are presented to us. In this book, we will show you how to "hunt and gather" your food.

Basic Elements of a Healthy PCOS Diet

1. There is no calorie counting or portion control required. Just use your common sense. The PCOS Diet is not a "diet" in the modern sense of the term. It is simply eating food that is helpful for optimal gene expression and avoiding food that is unhelpful.

    (Note: Overweight women who exercise 5 to 6 days a week and eat between 40 to 60 grams of high quality carbohydrate as described in this book will lose weight. But we do not recommend that you go below 40 grams of carbohydrate per day.)

2. There is no "one size fits all" diet. Your genes are different is some ways from anyone else's. So a food that is helpful to someone else may not be helpful to you.

3. Eat the highest quality foods possible. Be aware of and avoid environmental pollutants in your food. Choose organically raised and clean foods as much as possible.

4. You may eat all the freshwater fish, seafood and very lean meat you wish, provided it is as healthy as possible and as free of contamination as possible.

5. You may eat all the nonstarchy vegetables and fruits you wish.

7. Avoid all grains and legumes.

8. Avoid all dairy products.

9. Avoid all processed, fabricated, refined foods.

We'll get into the details in the remainder of this book.

2.6 Healthy PCOS Diet vs. Low-Carb Diet

Is the healthy PCOS diet in this book just a low-carb diet in disguise? The PCOS diet is neither a low-carb diet nor a low-fat diet.

The Atkins and South Beach diets are among the most popular diets. Both are considered "low carb" diets, meaning that they recommend you greatly reduce carbohydrate calories in order to lose weight.

In contrast, the PCOS diet is not specifically designed for weight loss, although weight loss will be one of its primary benefits. It is designed to make you healthier and reduce your PCOS symptoms.

Here are the similarities and differences when the PCOS diet is compared to a low-carb diet:

Food	PCOS Diet	Low-Carb Diet
Protein	Moderately High	Moderate
Carbohydrate	Moderate	Low
Total fat	Moderate	High
Saturated fat	Moderate	High
Monounsaturated fat	High	Moderate
Polyunsaturated fat	Moderate	Moderate
Omega-3 fats	High	Low
Fiber	High	Low
Vegetables & fruits	High	Low
Nuts & seeds	Moderate	Low
Dairy foods	None	High
Gluten grains	None	Low
Salt	Low	High
Refined sugars	None	Low
Glycemic load	Low	Low
Acid-Alkaline balance	Balanced	Acid
Strict portion controls	None	Yes
Processed foods	No	Yes
Artificial food additives	No	Yes
Artificial sweeteners	No	Yes

As you can see, there are quite a few differences between the PCOS diet and a typical low-carb diet.

Type of Carb vs. Carb Restriction

One of the distinguishing characteristics between the PCOS diet and many low-carb diets is in the type of carbohydrates allowed.

We believe the time has come to go beyond the concept of simply reducing carbohydrates in order to lose weight. Increasingly, research is showing that the ***type of carbohydrate*** is as important as controlling total carbohydrate calorie intake.

Johns Hopkins University released a study in 2005 that assessed dietary intake of 572 individuals for a year.[60] The researchers found that body weight correlated with the glycemic index of carbohydrates consumed. The glycemic index is a measure of the glycemic response associated with ingesting different types of carbohydrates. Refined or processed carbohydrates tend to have a higher glycemic index value while unrefined, whole carbohydrates have a lower glycemic index. The higher the glycemic index of carbohydrates consumed, the greater is the tendency to add weight.

The study also showed that there was ***no*** correlation between weight and total daily carbohydrate intake, or percentage of total calories from carbohydrates. In other words, it didn't matter whether the individuals were on a low-carb or high-carb diet.

This study indicates that the type carbohydrate is extremely important for weight control. Of course, the type of carbohydrate you consume is vitally important to your overall health, not just your weight. The diet in this book places great emphasis on eating the best types of carbohydrates — whole carbohydrates in their natural form.

Section 3

A Word About Your Weight

3.1 Diet and Long-Term Weight Management

Changing what you eat should be more than a quick way to lose weight. Your improved diet should be something that you continue for the rest of your life. Here are several important issues to keep in mind:

- How we eat to lose weight is different from a healthy lifelong diet.

- A successful transition from a fat loss diet to a healthy lifelong diet is only beginning to be understood. A successful transition includes a metabolic adjustment period (5 to 10 or more weeks) and the ability to permanently modify eating behavior.

- A successful transition to a lifelong healthy diet is a continuous effort requiring information, self discipline and ongoing support from others.

- Consistent exercise is necessary to maintain muscle strength and tone. Consistent exercise also allows you to eat a larger quantity of highly nutritious food without gaining weight. The higher level of good nutrition builds and maintains your overall health.

- Up to 90% of people who lose weight do not keep it off because they lack the necessary long-term support.

How to Eat to Lose Weight

The most reliable and straightforward way is a "ketogenic" diet. Actually, every successful weight loss diet is a ketogenic diet.

A ketogenic diet is one where you consume fewer calories than body burns in a day. Therefore, your body has to call on stored fat to provide fuel for your muscles. When fat is burned, ketones are produced as a byproduct. This why a fat-burning diet is called a "ketogenic" diet.

The proportion and type of fat, protein and carbohydrate you consume will strongly influence how you feel while on a ketogenic diet as well as the long-term metabolic consequences of your fat loss. We recommend a ketogenic diet in which you limit the amount of carbohydrate so that a significant portion of your fuel for the day has to come from fat.

A ketogenic diet means you do not eat excessive amounts of protein or fat, nor do you completely eliminate carbohydrates. If you avoid these extremes, you can achieve fat burning on a larger number of calories and with more satisfying food choices.

A Lower Carbohydrate Ketogenic Diet Is Safe and Effective for Fat Loss

You can only lose fat by reducing dietary calories to less than the calories used for daily activities. But which calories do you reduce? If you just eat less, without regard to the composition and nutrient quality of your diet, you can have a pretty unpleasant experience, including hunger, fatigue, headaches, muscle spasms, mental fogginess, depression, irritability and insomnia. You also risk losing muscle mass as well as fat.

A lower carbohydrate ketogenic diet involves reducing calories from refined carbohydrates in particular and nourishing yourself with appropriate amounts of water, vegetables, eggs, poultry, fish, meat, nuts and good quality oils. Careful selection of high-quality foods will create fat loss without the usual unpleasant side effects. It also helps to identify "problem foods" so that you will avoid them in the future.

Ketosis and Ketoacidosis

Ketones are a byproduct of fat metabolism and are a source of energy for the body. Ketones are released from stored fat and used for energy when there is insufficient glucose available. Although the brain requires glucose for fuel, the rest of the body will take up ketones as a fuel source instead of glucose.

"Ketosis" simply refers to an increase of ketones in the bloodstream. In contrast, a condition called "ketoacidosis" can occur when diabetics and others who have high levels of glucose (blood sugar) produce dangerously high levels of ketones.

Diabetics do not produce enough insulin from their pancreas, or have a condition called insulin resistance, in which cells have an impaired ability to obey insulin's instructions to store glucose. When cells have a lack of glucose, they will turn to fat as a fuel, and burning fat produces ketones.

The problem with ketones is that they are acids. If the acid level in your blood gets too high, you have a very serious health problem called acidosis. Metabolic ketoacidosis in diabetics is a dangerous condition and should be avoided with strict control and attention to diet and blood sugar levels.

Longer-Term Ketogenic Diet

When a person with normal blood sugar levels is producing ketones by breaking down fat for fuel, and is not eating excess carbohydrates, the blood glucose is delivered elegantly, primarily to the brain, and the rest of the body happily uses ketones to run the show.

Eating carbohydrate foods in amounts that allow for the release of ketones from stored fat is a safe and effective way to reduce body fat while maintaining steady blood sugar levels, having plenty of physical energy, mental alertness and restful sleep.

You could eat this way for the rest of their life and be quite well. You will also be able to diversify your diet after having lost excess fat. Broadening the diet to include fruits and grains can be accomplished without regaining fat. This transition has to be done thoughtfully and with close attention to food choices. Some people will never be able to eat certain foods without negative consequences because of their genetic make up. You'll have to reintroduce foods carefully and maintain exercise levels lifelong, in order not to regain lost fat.

When a Ketogenic Diet is Not Appropriate

A ketogenic diet is not appropriate for pregnancy or breastfeeding, a time when fat stores are very important to mother and baby's well being.

People with kidney damage should not use this diet. People with diabetes, epilepsy, and gall bladder problems need special care and support to use a ketogenic diet successfully.

Women lose weight somewhat slower than men since feminine hormones effect how women hold onto water and fat. Men in general have greater muscle mass and androgenic hormones to help them burn fat somewhat more efficiently than women. Regular exercise is absolutely necessary for everyone's health.

Transitioning to Long-Term Success

How we transition from fat loss to a long-term healthy diet determines our success.

When you let go of stored energy by reducing caloric intake, primitive protective mechanisms kick in. Your basic metabolic rate starts to slow down to protect you from what your ancient brain thinks is a famine. For ancient humans, an unreliable food supply made this mechanism essential for survival. For those of us whose caloric restriction is a matter of choice, and whose work and family demands are usually complex and can make an exercise routine hard to establish, there has been a pattern of steady weight gain or yo-yo weight fluctuations.

However, some people do not regain their weight. In a nutshell, what these people do differently is to be acutely aware of small amounts regained, and they return to their weight loss behaviors for brief periods of time to correct the small regains. Eventually, as long as they maintain healthy food choices and exercise levels, the episodes of regain stop and they stabilize at their new weight.

This means there is one way to eat to lose fat and then another, more generous and complex way to eat once your goal is attained.

Although essential for success, it's uncommon for people to make a thoughtful transition between these two ways of eating. The ability to lose weight, move to a more varied diet, and then return as needed to the weight loss diet for brief periods is not something people naturally tend to do.

Thus long-term guidance and support seems crucial. A number of studies with weight loss for diabetics have demonstrated that knowledgeable support helps people to remember the basic straightforward steps of the diet cha-cha and to deal with the stresses involved with weight loss.

We have many behaviors and beliefs that affect our sense of self and our ability to pursue loving self-discipline over a long term. It is clear that ongoing and specific support, such as individual counseling or a support group, increases success. We encourage you to use both the weight loss and maintenance aspects of the diet in this book — and be sure to consistently exercise and get all the support you need.

3.2 Thrifty Genes and Your 'Set Point'

There are many possible reasons why people are overweight. A few of them are:
- Genetic predisposition
- Endocrine disorders
- Overeating
- Sedentary lifestyle and lack of exercise
- Chronic stress
- Sodium retention
- Hidden food allergies
- Chronic illness
- Medications
- Pregnancy
- Cultural factors
- Food choices

Most people have some combination of the above factors that are actively causing them to gain weight, or have difficulty losing weight.

We've heard lots of stories about PCOS women who are very disciplined in what they eat, yet they still gain weight or can't lose weight. Meanwhile, their family or friends can eat more and stay thin.

This is borne out by a study at the University of Pittsburgh where the diet of PCOS women was compared with non-PCOS women.[61] The study found that although PCOS women tended to be more overweight, there was virtually no difference in their dietary intake. However, when lean PCOS women were compared to lean normals, the investigators found that the lean PCOS women consumed fewer calories than the lean non-PCOS women. In other words, the lean PCOS women eat fewer calories to maintain their weight compared to normal lean women.

This study suggests that PCOS women tend to gain more weight with the same amount of calories when compared to non-PCOS women.

What would cause PCOS women to be so efficient at converting calories into fat?   Or to maintain their weight with fewer calories than normal women? In this chapter, we'll review one of the factors that may be responsible: your genetic predisposition.

Thrifty Genes

Recent genetic research suggests that PCOS is the result of "thrifty" genes, providing advantages in times of shortage of nutrition such as muscular strength, moderate abdominal fatness and decreased insulin sensitivity, i.e. an anabolic (body building), energy saving constitution.[62] [63]

In certain ancient nomadic populations, hormones were released during seasons when food supplies were traditionally low, which resulted in resistance to insulin and efficiently increased fat storage.

These thrifty genes were a means to survival for ancient humans. A powerful mechanism to increase appetite and decrease metabolism when weight loss occurs is likely to have evolved because our species was subjected to periods of famine, and the threat to survival came from starvation, not over-nutrition.

People with an array of genes that promoted gluttonous consumption in times of plenty and efficient storage of fat might survive and pass on those genes, while the finicky eaters would die. But in the developed world, where we have continuous access to highly caloric, highly palatable food, those genes do us a disservice.

When this thrifty gene constitution is exposed to unlimited food supplies and modern sedentary life style, a full-blown polycystic ovary syndrome with insulin resistance and infertility is triggered, presumably via several mechanisms, which are a consequence of interaction between two basic anabolic hormones: insulin and testosterone.

Of course, not everyone has PCOS, insulin resistance, or weight problems. It's speculated that the ancestors of leaner people among us may have lost their thrifty genes several generations back.

Set Point Theory

Another genetic predisposition you may have is a certain "set point" for your weight.[64]

The regulation of food intake and output (activity and metabolism) is tremendously complex, intricate, and finely tuned. Although we take in close to 10 million calories over the course of a decade, body weight for most of us varies very little. We may take in a little more one day, have an increase in activity on another — and yet, without much thought, most people naturally adjust and weight stays fairly stable. This point of weight stability is called a "set point."

Your set point is genetically determined. Some people are able to eat anything they desire, exercise little and still remain slim. In contrast, others struggle with rigid diets and exercise to lose weight. The lost weight is usually a combination of water, fat and muscle. Inevitably, though, the diet and exercise program cannot be maintained and all of the lost weight is regained, plus a little bit more. The regained weight is mostly fat.

What causes your set point to sabotage your best intentions?

Body fat is regulated by processes in your hypothalamus (a master gland in your brain). Your hypothalamus chooses the amount of body fat it considers ideal for your needs and then works ceaselessly to maintain that level. If you are losing weight below your set point, it will create hunger signals that cause you to eat. It may also cause you to conserve energy by slowing down metabolism in order to protect your remaining fat stores. In this case, you need fewer and fewer calories to maintain your weight.

If you have "thrifty genes" and a high weight "set point," you will find it quite challenging to lose a significant amount of weight. But, it is entirely possible that *you can lose weight*. However, just losing your weight is not the main problem.

The main problem is keeping the weight off. Most people are very resistant to maintaining a body weight that is below their set point. That's partly because your hypothalamus is putting out hormones that are telling your body to get back to its weight set point. Bariatric medicine (the medical specialty that studies body fat) has recently been focusing on how to readjust the hypothalamic set point in order to maintain weight loss.[65]

Interplay Between Genes and Environment

There are many hundreds, if not thousands, of genes that directly or indirectly influence fat metabolism and your weight. Many of them have not yet been identified. Regardless, we do know that environmental factors can change the behavior of genes.

Based on what we know at this point in time, we think it is possible to influence your genes to do a better job in helping you to control your weight. One way to do that is to optimize the quality and components of your diet.

3.3 Hormones, Inflammation and Your Weight

Many believe that the insulin hormone is responsible for PCOS and weight problems. This is an oversimplification.

There are dozens of hormones and other signaling molecules in your body that influence your weight by regulating your appetite and metabolism. In addition, chronic inflammation is a common characteristic of PCOS and is closely associated with excessive weight and hormone dysregulation.

There is no single factor that governs your weight, your fat metabolism or your hunger. It is a bewildering combination of factors, all interacting or influencing one another. An imbalance or disturbance of one signaling molecule will affect others, which in turn will affect still others.

No one, including research scientists and doctors, fully understands the functions and relationships of all these various signaling molecules, particularly as they exist in each unique woman. And, there are probably additional signaling molecules that haven't yet been discovered.

Nevertheless, some readers will want to know as much as possible about the factors that contribute to PCOS and its varied symptoms, including weight problems. If you are one of these readers, please take a look at Section 16 (*More about Hormones, Weight and Inflammation*). This section is more complex, but most readers with interest in some of the technical aspects of the physiology of PCOS will gain important information from it.

Section 16 contains these chapters:

- **Chapter 16.1: What Makes You Hungry?** Women with PCOS tend to have a bigger appetite (than non-PCOS women) and they feel hungrier. Numerous hormones are involved in this appetite problem. In this chapter, we describe how the hunger process works and three hormones that are involved in this process.

- **Chapter 16.2: 'Evil Twins': Insulin Resistance and Leptin Resistance.** Resistance to the actions of these two hormones is a big reason why you have PCOS, infertility problems, and weight/appetite problems.

- **Chapter 16.3: Inflammation and Your Weight.** Chronic inflammation plays an important but under-recognized role in PCOS. It is involved in obesity, insulin resistance and leptin resistance, which are common problems in PCOS.

3.4 How Calorie Density Makes You Fat

A calorie is a unit of energy. The more calories you consume, the more energy you take in. If you take in more energy than you burn off, you will gain weight.

A steady stream of research is showing that we consume a lot more calories than we think, for two reasons:

- Processed foods are "calorie-dense," meaning that there are a high number of calories in a given weight of food.
- We are eating much larger food portions than in the past.

If you're having a problem with weight, you can help yourself by avoiding calorie-dense foods and eating smaller portions. "Calorie density" refers to the number of calories in an ounce of food.

To better understand the challenge of calorie density, let's review some of the latest research.

Calorie Density, Not Fat Content, Affects Intake

The calorie density of foods, rather than the fat content, affects how many total calories you will eat in a meal.[66] [67] In a recent study, women ate various types of meals and were allowed to eat as much as they wanted.

In one part of the study, low-calorie-dense meals were compared to high-calorie-dense meals. Both meals were "low fat." The low-density foods contained 31 calories per ounce, while the high-density foods contained 45 calories per ounce. Women consumed 16% fewer total calories when they ate the low-calorie-dense meal.

In another part of the study, high-calorie-dense, high-fat foods containing 36% fat were substituted for high-calorie-dense, low-fat foods containing 16% fat. You would expect the total calories consumed in the high-fat meal to be more than with the low-fat meal. That was not the case. The total calories consumed during the meal were the same for both meals.

These results indicate that when a portion of the diet was manipulated, the calorie density, but not the fat content itself, of the foods affected total calorie intake of meals consumed by women.

Perceptions May Trick You into Eating More Calories

A study at Penn State University demonstrated that information about the fat content of a food can influence total calorie intake of meals.[68] In this study, women were given a fixed amount of three different yogurts (low-fat and low-calorie; low-fat and high-calorie; high-fat and high-calorie), or no yogurt, followed by lunch and then dinner. Half of the women received information, in the form of a label, about the fat content of the yogurts; the other half received no information.

Women who received the information consumed more calories at lunch after eating yogurt labeled "low-fat" than after eating a yogurt labeled as "high-fat." The opposite response was seen in women who did not receive information.

When calories consumed at dinner were included in the analyses, overall intake was still significantly greater in the women who received information and ate a "low-fat" yogurt before meals.

Except for the yogurt labeling, the contents of the meals were essentially the same. We can speculate that the perception of eating a "low-fat" food provided a rationale for the women to eat more of other foods at the meals.

Soup or Salad - Two Ways to Cut Calories Out of Your Meals

Reducing the number of calories per ounce of food is an easy way to cut calories without feeling deprived or hungry.

Penn State researchers have discovered a couple of ways to do this.

To Eat Less, Start a Meal with a Low-Calorie Salad

Eating a salad at the beginning of a meal may cause you to eat less food and thus cut calories without feeling deprived.[69]

In a recent study, women were given different salads as a first course to a meal. The salads came in two sizes, 3 cups and 1-1/2 cups. Each size salad had 3 different amounts of cheese and salad dressing, so that each size salad had a low, medium, and high calorie version.

As compared to women who had no salad at all before a meal, the women who first had a large "low calorie" salad ended up consuming 12% fewer calories for the whole meal. Women who first ate a small "low calorie" salad consumed 7% fewer calories for the entire meal.

In contrast, those women who had a large high-calorie salad (lots of cheese and salad dressing) actually ended up eating 17% more calories in the meal than the women who ate no salad at all.

This study suggests that if you have a good-sized low-calorie garden salad before a meal, you will consume substantially fewer calories for the total meal.

If you find yourself eating more at a meal than you like, we recommend that you have a sizeable mixed garden salad first. Use only a small amount of dressing, or a dressing that is low in calories. Also, don't add cheese, ham, luncheon meats or other fatty animal foods. Some avocado is OK. Eat at least 2-3 cups of garden salad before starting the rest of your meal.

You may be pleasantly surprised to find that even though it feels like you're eating a lot of food, you'll actually be reducing your total calorie intake. The study suggests a 12% reduction in calories is possible, which is quite significant. Calorie reduction is a proven way to improve symptoms of PCOS.

Soup Makes You Feel Fuller

It's known that adding water to a meal reduces its calorie density and makes you feel full sooner. But should you drink water with the meal or should you add the water to the food itself?

You're probably thinking it doesn't make any difference. After all, water is water. However, a study investigated how water should be taken with a meal.[70]

Twenty-four lean women consumed three test lunches. At the beginning of the lunches, the women were given a serving of either chicken rice casserole with a glass of water, or chicken rice soup. The soup contained the same ingredients, number of calories, and amount of water as the casserole and glass of water.

When the women had soup at the beginning of lunch, they consumed only about 1,209 calories at lunchtime, whereas they consumed about 1,657 calories when they ate the casserole and a glass of water.

The authors of the study concluded that consuming foods with high water content is more effective at reducing subsequent calorie intake than drinking water with food. For some reason, water in the food itself made the women less hungry and they simply ate less food. In contrast, drinking water separately does not seem to trigger signals of satiety.

The same principle applies to whole vegetables and fruits, which have high water content.[71] The whole vegetable or fruit is more filling than a processed or dried version and some water. For example, you would feel more satisfied if you ate 20 grapes as opposed to 20 raisins and a swallow of water.

Feeling full depends on eating a satisfying amount of food. Tiny portions of food won't make you feel satisfied no matter how much water you drink on the side. The calorie density of food (the ratio of calories to the weight of food) is what counts. The lower the calorie density, the better.

3.5 Portion Control

If you're trying to lose weight, portion control will be a key element in your success. However, it seems that almost no one can stop eating if their plate has extra food, according to recent trends and studies.

The increasing size of American's waistlines over the past 30 years has coincided with a sharp increase in food portion sizes inside and outside the home.

In a recent study, data was analyzed from national surveys conducted between 1977 and 1998 and including more than 63,000 people.[72] It was found that portion sizes and caloric intake for specific food types have increased markedly with greatest increases in food consumed at fast food establishments and in the home.

The serving size of an average soft drink, for instance, increased from 13 ounces and 144 calories to nearly 20 fluid ounces and 193 calories. The average cheeseburger grew from 5.8 ounces to 7.3 ounces, swelling from 397 to 533 calories.

Since an additional 100 calories a day can translate into 10 extra pounds a year, the study underscores the need to control portion size as a way to control weight.

People Prefer Larger Portions — and Will Eat Them

We hope that you're not among the typical American who seems to prefer eating larger portions of food.

When people have larger meal portions before them, they tend to eat more food and thus ingest many more calories than they need, according to studies at Penn State University.[73] Even worse, they don't feel fuller or more satisfied than people who eat smaller portions.

Each week, the participants in this study were served macaroni and cheese in one of four portions ranging from two and a half to five cups. The participants were required to eat all of the carrots and a chocolate bar that were also included in the meal, but could eat as little or as much of the macaroni and cheese as they wanted.

One group received different amounts of macaroni and cheese, pre-portioned on a dinner plate from which they ate. Another group received different portions in a serving dish and could scoop as much of the entrée as they liked onto their plates.

In both cases, the participants ate more when more food was available but didn't report feeling any fuller after eating. The bigger the portion, the more the participants ate. On average, they ate 30% more from a five-cup portion of macaroni and cheese than from one half its size.

Large Portion Plus High Calorie Density - A Double Whammy

What happens when you combine large food portions with high-density foods?   According to another study from Penn State University, the calorie density and the portion size act independently to increase total calorie intake.[74]

In this study, a group of women ate breakfasts and dinners that were standardized. But the main entree at lunch was formulated to vary in calorie density as well as portion size. The lunch entree was a pasta bake made from medium shells, zucchini, broccoli, carrots, onions, tomato sauce and parmesan, mozzarella and ricotta cheese. The calorie density was changed by varying the proportions of ingredients. The amount served was also varied from 2 cups up to 3-1/2 cups.

Large portion size alone increased calorie intake by 20%. High calorie density alone increased intake by 26%. Together, large portion size and high calorie density increased calorie intake by a whopping 56%!

When the women ate a smaller meal of lower calorie density, they consumed 221 fewer calories, and they felt just as full and satisfied as when they had consumed a larger meal of higher calorie density.

If you have a challenge with weight, we recommend that you not expose yourself to large portions of food at a time. Have a smaller portion. Then wait and see how you feel before deciding to get more food. Chances are, you'll be satisfied with the more moderate-sized portion.

Binge Eating and PCOS

Some women with PCOS have reported to us that they are binge eaters, eating until their stomachs hurt and they cannot eat another thing.

In one study, an association between binge eating and the presence of polycystic ovaries was found in 33% of those with PCOS.[75] Some researchers suspect that polycystic ovaries and menstrual irregularities are characteristics of women who maintain normal body weight, yet fluctuate between starvation and binge eating.

Insulin resistance due to huge fluctuations in calorie ingestion, especially carbohydrates, may contribute to the development of polycystic ovaries and PCOS.

Portion control and meals on a regular schedule is one way to reduce chaotic eating patterns.

3.6 Is Calorie Restriction a Good Idea?

A calorie is the amount of energy necessary to raise the temperature of 1,000 grams (2.2 pounds) of water by one degree Celsius (1.8° F).

Dietary calories come from proteins, carbohydrates, fats and alcohol.

Calories are used to provide energy to your cells so they can function and to provide heat so you can stay warm.

If you consume more calories than you burn, the remainder is stored as glycogen or fat. One gram of fat contains 9 calories. Therefore, a pound of body fat holds about 4,100 stored calories.

A woman might consume anywhere from 900 to 2,500 calories per day, although some women consume more than 2,500 calories.

Whether she can burn off all those calories depends on a number of factors:
- "Thrifty genes" - genetic tendencies that inhibit burning of fat calories
- Low (sluggish) metabolic "set point"
- Activity level and exercise
- Temperature of the environment
- Organ or glandular disorders (e.g., hypothalamus, liver, underactive thyroid)
- Hormonal disorders (e.g., high insulin levels)
- Health status
- Dietary deficiencies (nutrient co-factors that aid energy metabolism)
- Disturbed hormonal signaling due to environmental toxins
- Other possible factors

How many calories can a woman with PCOS burn? We honestly don't know, because there is so much variability among individuals, according to the factors listed above. For example, if a woman has chronically high insulin levels and insulin resistance, she will have a tougher time burning calories, especially calories stored as fat.

You may be thinking that if you have trouble burning calories, perhaps the answer is to restrict the intake of calories.

Is Calorie Restriction Effective?

Calorie restriction is simply consuming a limited number of calories, probably fewer than you have been consuming in the past. A good example of calorie restriction is the Weight Watchers program, where your goal is not to exceed a certain number of calories in your diet.

How does calorie restriction (Weight Watchers) compare with other dietary approaches? A study conducted at the Tufts-New England Medical Center in Boston was just released in January 2005, comparing people who went on one these popular diets for one year: Atkins, Zone, Weight Watchers, and Ornish.[76]

After one year, here's what happened:
- Atkins (carbohydrate restriction - "low carb" diet): 10.5 lbs. lost
- Zone (macronutrient balance diet): 7 lbs. lost
- Weight Watchers (calorie restriction): 6.6 lbs. lost
- Ornish (fat restricted diet): 7.3 lbs. lost

As you can see, the amount of weight that was lost over one year was nearly the same with all of the diets. Those individuals on Weight Watchers, the calorie restriction diet, did not experience weight loss any greater than people on diets whose focus was not on calorie restriction.

In other words, simply cutting calories is, by itself, helpful if you are overweight; but it is certainly not the entire answer to weight loss. We think it may be more important to **improve the quality** of your calories. For example, our view is that it is better to consume 100 calories of an apple than 100 calories of table sugar. Why? Because, in comparison to table sugar, the apple has fiber and multiple nutrients you need to normalize your body and regain your health.

Very Low Calorie Diets

We need to say a brief word about "crash diets," also known as "very low calorie diets." On this kind of diet, you are nearly starving the body in order to force it to lose weight. The premise is that you will be consuming many fewer calories than you are burning and consequently, you will lose weight. That is not always what happens. Below a certain point, calorie restriction may trigger a "starvation-survival response," where your body will slow down its metabolism in order to prevent the further loss of stored calories.

In addition, depending on the nature of your severely restricted diet, your body may "cannibalize" itself in order to get protein. Crash diets may be so low in dietary protein that the body cannot sustain itself. It will then rob protein from your muscles and organs in order to get protein needed to maintain vital functions. In addition, as you lose muscle, you lose your ability to burn fat because fat is burned mostly in muscle cells.

At some point, you will find yourself compelled to start eating again. When you do, you may overeat and the excess calories will be stored as fat. However, since you have lowered your metabolic rate, and since you have probably lost some of your muscle cells where fat is burned, you will store more and more fat and have real difficulty burning it off.

Calorie restriction is a tool for weight loss. But you must be very discerning in terms of what type of calories you are restricting. Also, you don't want to severely restrict calories unless you are under the guidance of a physician.

Calorie Restrictions and PCOS

There is some evidence that calorie restriction may help PCOS and infertility.[77]

A very interesting study conducted with at the University of Adelaide (Australia) with 28 mildly overweight women with PCOS.[78] Half the women were put on a high-protein diet for 12 weeks. The other half was put on a high-carbohydrate diet. On either diet, they were restricted to 1,433 calories a day. After the 12 weeks, they were put on a 4-week "maintenance" diet that allowed them to eat more calories from their diets.

At the end of the trial, the high-protein group had lost 18.7 lbs, while the high-carbohydrate group had lost 15.2 lbs — not a significant difference between the two groups.

However, even this minor loss of weight resulted in significant reproductive, endocrine and metabolic improvements in both groups of women. They had an improvement in menstrual cycling, including ovulation in some cases. Three women became pregnant.

The most striking difference between the women who had restored menstrual cycling and those who did not was a change in insulin. In the women with restored cycles, the calorie restriction caused a 35% decrease in insulin, and a 21% decrease in insulin resistance, which continued during the maintenance phase of the diet. The better insulin control apparently caused these women to regain their menstrual cycles.

A very similar study was done at Pennsylvania State University with 35 obese women with PCOS.[79] Regardless of diet composition (high protein or not), the calorie restriction reduced androgens (male hormones), insulin and leptin. The women also lost a modest amount of weight. Nearly half the women resumed their menstrual cycles.

In a third study conducted in Finland, calorie restriction in overweight, infertile women for six weeks caused a reduction in luteinizing hormone (LH) and a reduction in the LH/FSH ratio.[80] Chronically high LH is a primary reason why PCOS women do not ovulate. The reason for the reduction in LH appeared to be a reduction in insulin resistance.

In summary, if you are overweight and infertile, a diet that is very moderate in calories and which promotes weight loss would be advisable for regaining normal menstrual cycling.

3.7 Weight vs. Body Composition

Body fat and its distribution is a better indicator of health and fitness than weight.

A growing collection of data clearly shows a relationship between excess body fat and an increased risk of heart attack, hypertension, high cholesterol, diabetes, gall bladder disease, and some cancers. Most people, however, believe that weight and fat are the same things. This is an oversimplification.

In our view, it's more important to lose inches than weight.

Women with PCOS who are also overweight appear to have a genetic predisposition that makes it more difficult for them to lose weight. So you need to be patient and very persistent with your physical activity program. There's no need for you to get discouraged if you don't lose 30 pounds in 30 days. (In fact, we discourage such extreme measures).

A better indicator of progress is your percentage of body fat, which is the ratio of fat to lean body mass. For example, if you compare two women of the same height and weight, but one has a body fat percentage of 25% and the other has 50%, you will notice how different they look.

The woman with the lower body fat percentage will be noticeably smaller, even though she is the same weight. She will be a more muscularly fit person, and muscle is heavier than fat. The other reason is that muscle cells are smaller than fat cells. Therefore, the woman with a lower body fat percentage will have heavier, but smaller cells.

Regular exercise causes your muscles cells to multiply and they get more efficient at burning fat. So building muscle mass actually adds to your weight. On the other hand, you are burning more stored fat, thus causing your fat cells to lose their weight and shrink in size.

In other words, consistent exercise helps you to gain muscle weight and lose fat weight. So long as you are doing that, you are heading in the right direction — a lower body fat percentage.

How to Measure Fat

There are several ways to estimate how much fat you are carrying.
- Body Mass Index (BMI)
- Body fat percentage (BFP)
- Waist circumference

We think that a body fat percentage test is the best way to estimate the amount of fat you are carrying relative to your total weight.

We recommend that you get a periodic body fat percentage test from your health practitioner or health club.

Body Mass Index

First, let's review the body mass index. The body mass index is an estimate of your obesity level according to the ratio of your weight to your height. Health professionals often use the BMI as a simple screening tool for the possible risk of chronic health problems such as obesity, diabetes or cardiovascular disease.

The body mass index is a table of numbers for every weight and height level. By looking at the table, you can determine the body mass index number for your height and weight. For example, a person weighing 120 lbs who is 5'5" tall would have a BMI of 20. A 5'5" person weighing 180 lbs. would have a BMI of 30.

BMI Categories:
- Underweight = <18.5
- Normal weight = 18.5-24.9
- Overweight = 25-29.9
- Obesity = BMI of 30 or greater

In our example, the 120 lb. person is a "normal weight" while the 180 lb. person is "obese."

The BMI is a very rough indicator of body fatness. For example, if our 5'5," 180 lb. person is a champion weight lifter, she is a muscular — but not obese — individual. On the other hand, if she is totally sedentary, she is considered obese because much of her total weight is fat, not muscle.

If you wish to view a body mass index table, go to this web page: www.ovarian-cysts-pcos.com/bmi

The BMI is a very approximate estimate of your level of fatness. A body fat percentage test is a lot more accurate.

Body Fat Percentage

Body fat percentage is the amount of fat tissue in your body as a percentage of total body weight. If your total body weight is 140 pounds and you have 40 pounds of fat, your body fat percentage is 29%.

A body fat percentage measurement does something a BMI or wait-hip measurement cannot do, if the appropriate measuring device is used. A body fat percentage test can measure the amount of fat that is "hidden" inside your muscles and your body. If you are someone who does not exercise, chances are that fat has infiltrated into your muscles. Your muscles may be the same size, but you are carrying more fat in them.

Have you ever noticed the marbled fat in the middle of a prime steak? That steak is a cut of muscle from a steer that has not exercised. They cannot exercise because they are kept in pens and fed an unlimited diet of fattening foods such as grains. In contrast, a steak from a free-range steer is mostly muscle and very little fat, simply because the free-range steer got a lot more exercise and ate a healthier diet of vegetation.

A body fat percentage test can detect your "hidden" fat in addition to the obvious fat on the outside of your body. The two body fat tests that can measure hidden body fat are the "bio impedance" (electrical resistance) and "near-infra red" (Futrex) methods. Skin fold calipers are often used to measure body fat percentage, but they do not measure hidden fat.

Why Body Fat Percentage Is Important

There are two reasons why the percentage of body fat is important with regard to weight.

First, the higher your percentage of fat above normal, the higher your risk for weight-related illness such as heart disease, high blood pressure, gallstones, type 2 diabetes, osteoarthritis, and certain cancers.

Second, the more fat you have in your body (and thus the less lean body tissue or muscle you have), the fewer calories you need to maintain your weight. That's because you don't burn any calories in fat cells. You burn calories in muscle cells. So if you don't have much muscle, you don't need many calories before you start gaining weight. If you compare two people eating the same number of calories, the person with the higher body fat percentage is more likely to gain weight.

Body Fat Percentage, Weight Loss Diet, and Exercise

In general, weight loss is a combined loss of fat, muscle mass and water. However, if you regularly exercise during a weight loss diet, you can accelerate fat weight loss and minimize muscle loss. Exercise builds muscle and it burns fat.

Even if you lose very little weight, you're on the right track so long as your body fat percentage continues to decline.

Healthy Body Fat Percentage

A certain amount of fat is essential. Fat regulates body temperature, cushions and insulates organs and tissues and is the main form of the body's energy storage. But there is no clear consensus on what is a healthy body fat percentage. Below are body fat percentage guidelines from two sources.

Body Fat Percentage - Guidelines

Body Fat Guidelines from American Council on Exercise:

Classification	Women (% Fat)
Essential Fat	10-12%
Athletes	14-20%
Fitness	21-24%
Acceptable	25-31%

Body Fat Guidelines from American Dietetics Association:

Classification	Women (% Fat)
Normal	15-25%
Overweight	25.1-29.9%
Obese	Over 30%

Where Is Your Body Fat Located?

Where your excess fat is located is almost as important as the amount of body fat you have. Recent studies have shown that if you carry your extra fat around your waist, you are at a higher risk for developing chronic diseases than if you carry the same amount of extra fat around your thighs and buttocks.

Waist Circumference Measurement

In addition to body fat percentage measurements or your BMI, you should also take sequential measurements of your waist circumference. As you lose fat weight, your waist will get smaller, which goes a long way toward reducing your risk of chronic disease.

In fact, a diminishing waist size is a very important indicator of your progress, just as important as body fat percentage or total body weight. That's because PCOS and infertile women tend to have fat around their abdomen. Abdominal belly fat has been linked to insulin resistance, elevated cortisol, and other PCOS-related disorders. A shrinking waist may be a "leading indicator" that your other PCOS symptoms will also start to diminish.

Women are least likely to be at risk for heart disease and diabetes with their waist-to-hip ratio is less than 0.85. (Example: if your waist is 35" and hips are 42," 35/42 = 0.83). A waist measurement greater that 39," or a waist-to-hip ratio greater than 0.85, suggests that you are carrying excessive fat around your abdomen, vital organs like the liver, and the whole digestive tract.

3.8 What If You're NOT Overweight?

You may be getting the impression that this book is only for women who are overweight. If you are at a healthy weight but have PCOS, rest assured this book is also for you.

We appear to focus on women who are overweight because they generally have the most severe metabolic and hormonal problems. They are the ones who are at highest risk for chronic diseases associated with PCOS and for whom effective help with diet and exercise is essential for disease prevention and recovery. So we designed the Recommended Level of our diet for the "worst case" scenario, i.e., women who have serious PCOS symptoms and weight issues.

But if you don't need to lose weight or if your PCOS symptoms are mild, you don't have to start with the Recommended Level of the diet. You can start at the Maintenance Level, which includes everything at the Recommended Level plus selected starchy vegetables, whole legumes and whole grains. In addition, we do not restrict your meal portions. A person who is not overweight can eat as much as she likes, provided she maintains a healthy weight level and PCOS symptoms do not get worse.

Please bear in mind that regardless of your body dimensions, the foundation of our diet is healthy, unrefined food. A diet laden with refined carbohydrates and fabricated "convenience" foods is unhealthy for anyone, no matter what your shape.

Our diet is a set of guidelines and recommendations, not a set of rigid rules that you must slavishly follow. You know your body better than we do. Please use your own good judgment, based on what your body is telling you and the huge amount of information provided in this book.

Ideally, each woman would be on a diet that is uniquely most beneficial to her, a diet based on her unique medical history, present health status, genetic predisposition and desired health goals. Unfortunately, that is not possible to do in a book. So if you're not overweight but do have PCOS symptoms, consider experimenting a little to find out what foods work best for you.

Section 4

Carbohydrates

4.1 What's a Carbohydrate?

Carbohydrates are organic compounds that consist of carbon, hydrogen and oxygen. They are a major source of energy in the diet and are found primarily in plant foods such as fruits, vegetables, legumes, grains, nuts and seeds, and to a much lesser extent in dairy products.

We read and hear so much about carbohydrates these days that it can be very confusing. Are carbs bad for us? Should we cut them out altogether? Are the 'low carb' foods that are suddenly showing up on grocery store shelves chemically altered? Why do runners load up on carbs? Well, there's a lot to understand, so in this section of the book we'll take a closer look.

Dietary carbohydrates consist of one or more of these elements:
- Starches
- Sugars
- Fiber

Starches

Starches are carbohydrates consisting of huge numbers of glucose molecules stitched together in long chains. These stitches are digestible, allowing the long chain to be broken down into glucose fragments, which are absorbed into the bloodstream. These long chains can have many different structures.

Sugars

Sugars are the building blocks of carbohydrates, just like amino acids are building blocks of protein.

A "sugar" is the name given to a group of small molecules characterized by a formula equivalent of 1 molecule of water per 1 molecule of carbon.

Single Sugars
Glucose and fructose are called single sugars and have identical chemical formulas. However, the structure of their molecules is slightly different. Fructose is much sweeter than glucose.

In the market, the most common form of glucose is old fashioned corn syrup.

Double Sugars
Sucrose consists of two single sugars stitched together from one glucose and one fructose molecule. Sucrose is common in plants. We process these plants (such as sugar cane and

sugar beets) to create a pure chemical that we call table sugar.

Lactose is made from two single sugars, glucose and galactose. Galactose is very similar in structure to glucose. Lactose is produced by mammals and is found in milk products.

Maltose is another double sugar, consisting of two molecules of glucose stitched together. Maltose occurs naturally in some malt products and is not especially sweet tasting. It is also an ingredient of corn syrup.

Fructose (Fruit Sugar)

Fructose, a simple sugar also known as levulose or fruit sugar, is the sweetest of the simple sugars. Fruits contain between 1 and 7% fructose, although some fruits have higher amounts. Fructose is also found in other plants, such as corn.

Fructose makes up about 40% of the dry weight of honey. Fructose is also available in crystalline form; its sweetness rapidly declines when dissolved in water.

Until about 40 years ago, fructose was not commercially available on a wide scale as a sweetener.   In 1910, it's estimated that the annual per capita consumption of fructose from all food sources was only 15 lbs.

Today, modern processing methods can create an endless supply of cheap fructose from corn. Due to the pervasiveness of high fructose corn syrup in foods and beverages, consumption of fructose from all sources is estimated at 70 lbs. per person per year. Combined with all other sugars, we're talking about an unbelievable 150-170 lbs. of refined sugar annually per person, or nearly a half pound per day!

We have to question how well the human body is adapting to this enormous increase. It's hard to imagine how the body can cope with this load.

Many people have the misconception that fructose is healthier for you than table sugar since it presumably comes from fruit and is therefore more "natural." This is simply not the case. Most fructose is extracted from corn, not from fruit. When you see a food that is "naturally sweetened" with fructose, it's a marketing ploy to get you to buy the product.

You may also have also heard that fructose has a much lower "Glycemic Index" than glucose, table sugar or many refined starches. What that means is that after you eat fructose, your blood sugar rises less than if you were to eat table sugar or glucose (old fashioned corn syrup). A lower glycemic sugar is presumably better than a higher glycemic sugar for those who have trouble controlling their blood sugar, such as diabetics. If your blood sugar is kept within bounds, you don't need as much insulin to store it into the cells. Since insulin is commonly regarded as the villain responsible for obesity, you would think the lower your insulin, the better.

This paradigm overlooks the importance of insulin in the ***long-term*** management of your weight and fat stores. (By "long-term," we mean days, weeks, years, not hours). There are at least three major hormones involved in maintaining long-term energy balance: insulin, leptin, and ghrelin. Although these hormones fluctuate in response to food intake or absence of food intake, their main role may be to work together to try to keep a balance between calories consumed and calories expended. Without some increase in insulin, you cannot keep your weight management hormones in balance.

This is where fructose enters the picture. We all know that glucose produces an insulin response. That's what the Glycemic Index[81] [82] is all about — the ability of food to increase blood glucose and thus raise insulin. But what about fructose?

Unlike glucose, fructose does ***not*** increase insulin levels. Therefore, by consuming fructose, you are adding calories but not alerting your body to produce insulin, which is one of your long-term hormonal weight managers.[83] Without appropriate insulin levels and insulin signaling, your body has an impaired ability to manage weight over the long term.

Moreover, in contrast to glucose, the liver appears to have a tendency to convert fructose into triglycerides (blood fats). This appears to be especially true for people with insulin resistance or diabetes. A large number of animal and human studies have demonstrated that high levels of fructose feeding result in weight gain.[84]

A number of recent studies suggest that excessive intake of fructose actually worsens insulin resistance, impairs glucose tolerance, and leads to hyperinsulinism (high insulin levels), high triglycerides (blood fats), high blood pressure and weight gain.[85] [86]

Contrary Opinion about Fructose

Some researchers argue that fructose itself is not the cause of gaining weight. They propose two other factors for the increases in overweight problems.

One factor is that we simply consume way too many total calories, of which fructose is only a portion.

Secondly, consumption of any carbohydrate will reduce the amount of fat that is burned, simply because the body prefers to burn glucose from carbohydrate rather than fat. In other words, the problem is not that we are gaining fat. The problem is that we are not ***burning*** fat. The presumed solution is to reduce total carbohydrate consumption and thus force the body to burn more fat.

Whatever viewpoint you choose, it's undeniable that we consume much too much fructose. We recommend that you not consume any added fructose, such as products containing high-fructose corn syrup.

Fiber

Fiber consists of glucose and other sugars hooked together with a **non**-digestible stitch to form the "hard" parts of plants, including the cell walls that give the plant its structure and form. Fiber is generally not digestible by humans. A few of the common dietary fibers are pectin, agar, carrageenan, guar gum, and various forms of cellulose.

To learn more about fiber, visit our *What Is Fiber?* chapter.

Refined vs. Unrefined Carbohydrates

So what is best for you? Sugar, starch, or fiber? The best carbohydrate is an unrefined, unprocessed one, such as whole vegetables, whole fruits, legumes, whole grains, whole nuts, and whole seeds.[87] Whole, unrefined, natural carbohydrate foods contain a combination of starch and fiber as well as protein, fat and other essential nutrients.

In contrast, refined carbohydrates are usually devoid of beneficial fiber and are found in foods such as sugared cereals, white rice, white flour, soft drinks, fruit drinks, baked products, pies, ice cream, candy and other "convenience" foods. Besides being nearly devoid of essential nutrients, refined carbs promote an excessively large blood sugar surge, which causes hormonal fluctuations that may lead to overeating, weight gain, and worsening PCOS symptoms.

Carbohydrates Are "Brain Food"

Carbohydrates are the preferred form of energy for the body. The energy from carbohydrates is broken down relatively easily in the body and used as fuel for the brain and muscle activity. The energy going to the brain utilizes about 25% of all the energy circulating in the body at any time. The brain has a huge appetite for fuel and no storage capacity, so it must receive a regular supply of energy, primarily in the form of glucose from carbohydrates.

Definition of "Net Carbs"

A number of food products have appeared in the commercial market to address the increasing popularity of low-carbohydrate diets for weight loss. Some products are claiming or implying that they are "low-carb," "reduced carb" or "carb-free." A seal describing a specific amount of "net carbs" is sometimes displayed on the package. In this context, the term "net carbs" refers to the amount of carbohydrate remaining after subtracting other carbohydrates that are claimed to have "minimal impact on blood glucose compared to sugar," such as fiber and low-calorie polyol sweeteners (sorbitol, maltitol, xylitol and others).

Essentially, the perception conveyed is that net carb counting classifies carbohydrates into those that pass quickly into the bloodstream ("bad"), and those that do not ("good"). The net carb approach suggests that these products may assist with weight loss since they have a low proportion of carbs that could raise your blood sugar level.

Carbohydrate Regulation

Net carb labeling is not regulated by the U.S. Food and Drug Administration (FDA) so there is no legal definition of a 'net carb.' Our position is that this term can be misleading. The most effective strategy for optimum health is a balanced diet that includes the complex carbohydrates listed here and included in our PCOS recipes.

4.2 Glycemic Index

The Glycemic Index is a ranking of foods by how much they increase your blood sugar levels 2-3 hours after you eat them. Foods high in carbohydrates (starches and sugars) are the ones you'll find in the index, because they're most likely to increase your blood sugar.

An increase in blood sugar (blood glucose) usually causes an increase in insulin levels. Insulin is a hormone that performs a number of functions in your body, one of which is to lower your blood sugar if it is too high. The more sudden the increase in blood sugar, the more likely it is that insulin will be increased in response.

Chronically high insulin is a problem for women with PCOS, because insulin profoundly alters overall hormone balance, and causes your metabolism to go awry. For example, hyperinsulinism (excessive insulin) contributes to obesity, diabetes, heart disease, and some cancers. It is highly desirable to regulate your diet to avoid chronically elevated insulin levels. A number of studies indicate that consumption of foods with a low glycemic index or low glycemic load reduces the risk of PCOS complications such as diabetes, insulin resistance, cardiovascular disease and chronic inflammation.[88] [89] [90] [91] [92]

You can control your insulin to a great extent by avoiding upward spikes in your blood sugar from eating the wrong kinds of food.

The ranking of foods according their glycemic index value has led to the popular terms such as "high glycemic foods," "low glycemic foods," and "glycemic load."

In this chapter, we'll explain these terms and describe what the glycemic index is. From here on, things get pretty complex. But if you can understand and implement the glycemic index concept, you will progress towards better management of your PCOS symptoms.

Complex vs. Simple Carbohydrates

Before the glycemic index came along, the primary distinction between a "good" carbohydrate and a "bad" carbohydrate was whether it was a "complex" or "simple" carbohydrate food.

A complex carbohydrate:
- consists of a huge number of glucose (sugar) molecules stitched together in long chains;
- is usually less processed than a simple carbohydrate;
- tends to be digested more slowly, and thus is less likely to raise your blood sugar;
- is often referred to as "starch" or "fiber." A starch is a complex carbohydrate held together by digestible stitches. Fiber is held together by indigestible stitches.

Two examples of complex carbohydrates: corn on the cob, sugar cane.

In contrast, a simple carbohydrate:
- is a much smaller number of glucose molecules stitched together into short chains;
- is frequently more processed than a complex carbohydrate;
- is digested more quickly, and thus raises blood sugar more quickly;
- is often referred to as a "sugar."

Two examples of simple carbohydrates: corn syrup, table sugar.

Humans have been consuming unrefined complex carbohydrates for hundreds of thousands of years with no apparent ill effects. But as soon as we started refining and processing natural, complex carbohydrates into fabricated convenience foods, the rate of chronic disease began to increase dramatically. A large number of studies have shown a correlation between consumption of refined carbohydrates and chronic health disorders, including polycystic ovary syndrome.

Therefore, you are generally better off eating complex carbohydrates instead of simple ones. Complex carbohydrates are most commonly found in whole vegetables, whole fruit, whole legumes and whole grains. These whole foods have a much lower glycemic index than processed foods.

What Is the Glycemic Index?

Recent research has revealed another very important distinction among carbohydrates: the ability of different carbohydrates to increase your blood sugar level.

The glycemic index consists of a scale from 1 to 100, indicating the rate at which 50 grams of carbohydrate in a particular food is absorbed into the bloodstream as blood sugar (glucose). Glucose itself is used as the main reference point and is rated 100. All foods containing carbohydrate are compared to glucose, and ranked accordingly.

However, white bread has been used as the reference instead of glucose in some glycemic index tests, which yields different index values. However, the relative ranking of various foods remains the same. In our discussion, we use glucose as the reference value.

How to Interpret the Glycemic Index
70 or higher = High glycemic index food
56-69 = Medium glycemic index food
0-55 = Low glycemic food

Take a look at the table below. Columns 1 and 2 list the food and its glycemic index. (Don't worry about the last 3 columns. We'll explain them in a moment.)

Glycemic Index of Selected Foods

Food Description (Col. 1)	Glycemic Index (GI) (Col. 2)	Nominal Serving Size (grams) (Col. 3)	Available Carbohydrate Per Serving (Col. 4)	Glycemic Load Per Serving (Col. 5)
Glucose	100	10	10	10
Mashed potato *	92	150	20	18
Corn flakes *	81	30	26	21
Rice cakes *	78	25	21	17
French fries	75	150	29	22
White bread *	70	30	14	10
Macaroni and cheese (Kraft)	64	180	51	32
Coca Cola	63	250	26	16
Sucrose (table sugar) *	61	10	10	6
Sweet potato *	61	150	28	17
Bran muffins	60	57	24	15
PowerBar *	56	65	42	24
Snicker's bar *	55	60	35	19
Brown rice *	55	150	33	18
Honey *	55	25	18	10
Sweet corn *	54	80	17	9
Banana *	52	120	24	12
Carrots, raw *	47	80	6	3
L.E.A.N. Fibergy Bar, Harvest Oat	45	50	29	13
Apple juice *	40	250	30	12
Apple *	38	120	15	6
Lentils *	29	150	18	5

Notes: (1) The asterisk indicates that the glycemic index value is the mean value of more than one study. (2) Serving size is in grams. 100 grams = 3.5 ounces. (3) "GI" is an abbreviation for glycemic index.

As you look at the first two columns, there are several things worth noting.
- Mashed potatoes (GI = 92) increase your blood sugar almost as much as pure glucose does (GI = 100). So mashed potatoes are classified as a "high glycemic" food. In contrast, lentils have an index value of only 28, so lentils are a "low glycemic" food. In general, low-glycemic foods are better at controlling your blood sugar than high-glycemic foods. Thus, lentils are obviously much better for controlling your blood sugar than mashed potatoes.

- Refined or processed foods generally have a higher glycemic index. For example, the glycemic index for rice cakes is 78 vs. 55 for brown rice. Corn flakes are high at 81 vs. sweet corn at 54. In general, the less refined or processed the food is, the lower its glycemic index will be. So consuming foods in their natural form is very much to your advantage.
- You can make intelligent food substitutions that will lower the glycemic index of a snack or a meal. For example, some people consider a bran muffin or PowerBar as a healthy snack. However, an apple (GI = 38) is a much better choice than a bran muffin (GI = 60) or PowerBar (GI = 56). Or, if you're having a carbohydrate food as part of a main meal, sweet potatoes (GI = 61) are a better choice than mashed potatoes (GI = 92).
- Some whole foods, such as carrots and bananas, have received a bum rap. There's a widespread but mistaken belief that carrots and bananas have a high glycemic index and must be avoided. In fact, both are classified as "low glycemic" foods, because they have beneficial fiber in addition to their carbohydrates. (However, the cooking of any starchy carbohydrate will increase its glycemic index somewhat.).

To see a much more complete list of the glycemic index for foods, we suggest that you read *The New Glucose Revolution*, by Jennie Brand-Miller and Thomas Wolever.

OK. Now that we're familiar with the glycemic index for our list of selected foods, let's move on to columns 3 and 4 in the table: "nominal serving size," and "available carbohydrate per serving."

Serving Size for Glycemic Index

The "nominal serving size" refers to the amount of food, in grams, that was used during the test to determine the glycemic index for that food. For example, in the studies for mashed potatoes, people consumed 150 grams, which produced a glycemic response of 92, which is only slightly below the reference food, which is pure glucose (GI = 100),

So if you're interested in knowing how much of a food was consumed to produce the glycemic response in the test, the "serving size" column in a food table will tell you.

Now let's turn our attention to column 4 in the GI table, "available carbohydrate."

Fiber and "Available Carbohydrate"

When the glycemic index study is conducted for a specific food, ten people consume 50 grams of "available carbohydrate." This is the standard amount for all foods. It allows a direct comparison between different types of foods, such as corn flakes vs. an apple. All we care about for glycemic control purposes is the amount of "available carbohydrate" that can actually raise your blood sugar.

What do we mean when we say "available carbohydrate," as shown in column 4 of our food table?

The carbohydrate in any food consists to two types: digestible and indigestible. The digestible part is "available" to be absorbed into your body to provide energy. The indigestible is called "fiber," and is excreted.

Total carbohydrate = digestible (available) carbohydrate + fiber

In other words, it's helpful to know how much of the carbohydrate that you're eating will be digested, because the indigestible part will not increase your blood sugar. In fact, certain kinds of fiber will actually help you slow down the absorption of digestible carbohydrates, and thus avoid spikes in blood sugar and insulin.

Let's look at an example from our food table. You'll notice that a 30-gram serving of corn flakes contains 26 grams of available carbohydrate. In other words, most of the corn flakes you eat are carbohydrates that are capable of increasing your blood sugar. In contrast, an 80-gram serving of sweet corn only contains 17 grams of available carbohydrate. You can eat more than twice as much sweet corn (by weight) as corn flakes, while consuming 35% fewer digestible (available) carbohydrates.

So what's the take-away from this knowledge? By using the glycemic index table as a guide, you can actually eat a larger quantity (by weight) of carbohydrate foods while exposing yourself to fewer carbohydrates that can increase your blood sugar.

So far, so good...the last column in our glycemic index table is a listing of the "glycemic load" for each food.

Glycemic Load

The "glycemic load" is an index number you get when you multiply the glycemic index and "available" carbohydrate in a serving of food, and then divide by 100.

Glycemic Load = Glycemic Index x Available Carbohydrate / 100

Why should you care about the glycemic load? Let's look at each component of the glycemic load: glycemic index and available carbohydrate.

Remember that the glycemic index value for a food only tells you how quickly the available carbohydrate is converted into blood sugar. You can think of the glycemic index in column 2 as indicating the glycemic "quality" of the food.

The "available carbohydrate" number in column 4 tells you the "quantity" of potential glycemic increase.

The glycemic load in column 5 takes into account both the "quality" and the "quantity" of the carbohydrate food you are eating.

Take carrots, for example. According to our table, the glycemic index for carrots is 47. The available carbohydrate in 80 grams of carrots is 6 grams. (One medium carrot weighs about 80 grams.) So let's calculate the glycemic load of eating a medium carrot:

Glycemic load of 1 medium carrot = 47 x 6 / 100
Glycemic load of 1 medium carrot = 2.82 (which is then rounded off to 3)

If you check our table for the glycemic load for carrots, you'll see that it is 3. To summarize, here's the relevant data for our medium carrot:
- Glycemic index = 47 (indicates high "quality," because the lower the GI, the better for blood sugar control)
- Glycemic load = 3 (indicates low "quantity" of carbohydrates that could raise your blood sugar)

So you have the best of both worlds. The quality is good (low glycemic index), and the quantity is low (low glycemic load).

But what would happen if you had ten servings of carrots, instead of just one? Your glycemic index would remain the same at 47. However, the glycemic load would increase from 6 to 60.

The reason your glycemic load increased is that you are eating more servings. Of course, that's no problem with carrots. It's unlikely you would want to eat ten carrots at one sitting! After eating five or six, you would probably lose your appetite altogether. By the way, that's a big advantage of low glycemic index foods: they fill you up before you can eat too many "available" carbohydrates.

On the other hand, it's a different story with French fries:
- Glycemic index = 75 (indicates low "quality," because the higher the GI, the worse for blood sugar control)
- Glycemic load = 22 (indicates high "quantity" of carbohydrates that could raise your blood sugar)

So you have the worst of both worlds. The quality is poor, and the quantity is high. Worst of all, French fries taste good! It's tempting to have a few extra fries instead of a serving of carrots.

A serving of fries is listed in our table at 150 grams, or about 1/3 pound. If you get the "hungrys" and have an extra serving, you would double your glycemic load from 22 to 44. Although French fries are clearly bad for you because they contain altered fats, how bad is it when you double your glycemic load to 44 by having that second serving of fries?

Whether a glycemic load of 44 is "too much" depends on the amount of other carbohydrate you're consuming throughout the day, your activity level, and your body size. Fries and a Big Mac would have a higher total glycemic load than fries and a salad. If you are a large person who is physically active, a higher glycemic load may be OK. But regardless of the glycemic load, French fries are not good for you!

Women with PCOS are very likely to have insulin resistance and blood sugar abnormalities. Therefore, we recommend that you be cautious about the total glycemic load in any one meal.

Don't forget – the rise in your blood sugar depends on both the quality (glycemic index) and the quantity (glycemic load) of carbohydrate in your meal.

Other Tips for Lowering Your Glycemic Index

1. Don't overcook carbohydrates. Extensive cooking causes the starch fibers to break down, thus making them easier and faster to digest. This is especially true for starchy foods like grains.

2. Use whole foods. By "whole," we mean the hull or skin is still attached. This fibrous coat slows down the assimilation of the carbohydrates inside.

3. Minimize products that contain finely milled carbohydrates, especially flours. Small particle sizes are more quickly digested and absorbed. When you look at any glycemic index table, you'll notice that bread made with white flour has a value of 73 while bread made with whole wheat flour has glycemic index of 71, nearly the same. You would think that whole wheat bread would be have a much lower glycemic value because it has a lot more fiber. However, the fine milling nullifies the anti-glycemic effect of this fiber.

4. The type of fiber in the carbohydrate is important. There are two types of fiber: soluble and insoluble. Insoluble fiber does not absorb water, whereas soluble fiber does. As soluble fiber absorbs water, it becomes viscous and slows down the digestion of starches, which reduces your glycemic response. Apples, lentils, beans, and rolled oats have soluble fiber. Psyllium seed powder is a popular soluble fiber supplement.

Special Note

Many of the foods listed in the glycemic index table in this chapter and in other books are **not** included in the healthy PCOS diet. The purpose of this chapter is only to explain what the glycemic index is. You will frequently see the term "glycemic index" in books and articles. So it's important that you understand what it is and how it applies to you.

The glycemic index is especially useful for those people who consume processed foods, since much of the index is a listing of processed foods.

Even though you will not be consuming refined foods on our diet, you can use the glycemic index to compare one whole food to another. For example, you could compare an apple to a sweet potato to see which has the lower glycemic index value.

The diet plan in this book has removed nearly all processed foods and nearly all high-glycemic foods, so you don't need to be terribly concerned about the glycemic index if you're on this diet.

4.3 Anti-Nutrients in Grains and Legumes

Since homo erectus came upon the scene 1.7 million years ago, humans have rarely (if ever) consumed cereal grains. Humans are primates. Primates evolved in the tropical forest where cereal grasses were not the predominant source of plant foods. It has only been within the last 10,000 years…less than 500 generations…that we have started to eat and adapt to eating a significant amount of cereal grains. Yet the human genome appears to have changed very little over the past 40,000 years. Our human genetic makeup, therefore, has not yet had a chance to fully adapt to the consumption of grains, which are, in fact, the seeds of grasses.

The story of adaptation is a long and interesting one, and plants have their version of it as well.

In order to survive over the eons, grasses, grains, legumes and other plants have developed substances to protect themselves from microorganisms and creatures that want to eat them. These substances, called antinutrients, are toxic or otherwise interfere with the predator's physiology so that the predator is discouraged from eating the plant. In essence, they oppose or neutralize the nutritional benefits of the food. Although much is not yet known, the available evidence suggests that some plant antinutrients may adversely affect human health.[93]

Antinutrients are not something to be alarmed about since most foods typically have one or more antinutrients. The issue is the ***concentration*** **and** ***type*** of antinutrient, and whether that specific antinutrient profile will adversely affect your health. Let's take a closer look at antinutrients so you will better understand what they do in the human body.

Alkylresorcinols

Alkylresorcinols are compounds found in high amounts in rye and wheat, and to a lesser extent in oats, barley, millet and corn. They are found in the bran, or outer layer of the grain. Studies suggest that large amounts of these compounds appear to retard growth in livestock. They appear to act as both an appetite suppressant and as a toxin. As a toxin, they are implicated in many pathological processes, including death of red blood cells, as well as liver and kidney damage. They also stimulate a powerful inflammatory compound called thromboxane. On the other hand, low levels of alkylresorcinols may have anticancer and antioxidant properties.

Alpha-Amylase Inhibitors

Alpha amylase is a digestive enzyme that is present in your saliva and your pancreas. It helps you to begin the digestion of starches in your food. Alpha amylase inhibitors are compounds that inhibit alpha amylase from doing its job. Alpha amylase inhibitors are found in wheat, rye, barley, oats, rice and sorghum. They survive the baking process and are found in bread and baked products.

There isn't much information about how these inhibitors affect human health, although some people are allergic to amylase inhibitors.

Protease Inhibitors

Proteases are enzymes in human gastric juices that break down protein. Two examples of proteases are trypsin and chymotrypsin. Many plants, especially legumes, have protease inhibitors.

Trypsin helps to regulate secretions from the pancreas. When trypsin is inhibited by protease inhibitors, the pancreas does not receive the signals it needs to slow down. In animal experiments, the failure to get proper signals to the pancreas caused pancreatic enlargement and increased the risk of eventual cancer.[94] Feeding of rice bran, rye or barley to chicks resulted in enlargement of the pancreas.

Protease inhibitors are found in nearly all cereal grains and legumes. However, there is a lot of variability. For example, the amount of trypsin inhibitory activity in wheat is only 1.5% of the inhibitory activity found in soybeans.

The effect of long-term, low-level exposure to protease inhibitors in humans is not yet known.

Lectins

Lectins are proteins in foods (both plant and animal) that bind themselves to carbohydrate molecules, especially the sugar part of the molecule. Lectins are especially abundant in plant foods.

Because of their ability to cause red blood cells to clump together, lectins were originally used to create the blood typing system. The red blood cells of different people have slightly different cell membranes with different "docking sites" for external proteins such as hormones. If the shape of a lectin protein fits into a cell's docking site, it becomes attached to that cell. Lectins act like miniature Velcro strips, causing red blood cells to form into masses or clumps. Here's how it works: If you are blood type A and you eat a dish of lima beans (which contain lima bean lectins), your red blood cells will clump. On the other hand, if you have type O blood, or type B blood, and you eat lima beans, your red blood cells will not clump.

Lectins can attach themselves to other cells in your body, not just red blood cells. The result of lectin attachment to your body's cells can have a toxic effect, or influence your physiology in other ways.[95] [96]   Reactions to lectins can occur in your gut, blood vessels, muscles, brain, or any gland or organ.[97] [98] The reaction can be severe.   One example is that ingesting even a small amount of castor bean lectin can kill you. However, most plant lectins have a much milder effect!

Lectins are the most important antinutrients in your food. Lectins have been found in wheat, rye, barley, oats, corn and rice, but not in sorghum or millet. The lectins in grains appear to have somewhat similar biological activity.

The most-studied lectin is a wheat lectin called "wheat germ agglutinin" or WGA. WGA appears to have widespread effects in the body.[99] Almost every cell in the body can be bound by WGA, including mouth, stomach, intestines, pancreas, musculoskeletal system, kidney, skin, nervous system tissues, reproductive organs, blood platelets, and proteins floating in the blood. The effect of this binding activity is not fully known, although it is suspected to be unhealthy for many individuals. Moreover, WGA is persistent — it is not destroyed in the baking or heating process; nor is it destroyed by your digestive juices.

WGA and other lectins can activate your immune system, which leads to inflammatory problems. Significant amounts of lectin enter the bloodstream where the immune system may identify them as "foreign" and cause an allergic-inflammatory reaction. Lectins may increase the permeability of the gut wall and thus facilitate the passage of other incompletely digested dietary particles into the bloodstream. When undigested particles enter the bloodstream, an allergic reaction is likely to occur.

Lectins and Immunity

Lectins are also implicated in autoimmunity. Autoimmune disease is a condition where the immune system has difficulty distinguishing "self" from "not self," resulting in immune cells attacking the body's own tissues by mistake.

The cause of autoimmunity is not entirely clear, but it appears to be triggered in part by the foods we eat. Certain dietary particles, such as lectins, enter the bloodstream after a meal. Some of these particles are similar in structure to molecules in your own tissues. When these food particles are detected by the immune system, white blood cells are dispatched to destroy the particles — or anything that looks very similar to the particles. In a case of mistaken identity, the white blood cells attack tissues that appear similar to the "foreign" food particles. The result is inflammation and cell damage.

Autoimmune disease is not the direct cause of PCOS, but it exacerbates the problem. For example, if you have autoimmune thyroiditis (Hashimoto's Disease), your thyroid will be underactive and thus adversely affect your fertility, weight, energy, and hair.

Lectins and Hormones

Lectins may possibly contribute to hormonal imbalances.[100] For example, at least one clinician has suggested that WGA appears to interfere with proper insulin signaling by binding to insulin receptors and mimicking insulin.[101] However, unlike insulin, WGA is not subject to any endocrine or metabolic controls. Therefore, WGA would have a more persistent effect than insulin itself. However, we haven't seen any published studies that address this issue.

Lectins or other substances in plants may affect insulin and blood sugar levels. For example, certain mushrooms stimulate release of insulin from the pancreas.[102] [103]

The effects of lectins upon health vary greatly with the specific lectin and the specific individual. There are many hundreds of lectins, most of which have not been studied regarding the health effects.

Phytates

Phytates are phosphorus compounds found mainly in cereal grains, legumes, and nuts. They bind with minerals such as iron, calcium, and zinc and thus could interfere with mineral absorption in the body. Baking and food processing will destroy phytates in grains and most legumes.

The mineral-binding capacity of phytates is a mixed bag. On the one hand, it may prevent absorption of minerals that you need. On the other hand, it may prevent absorption of minerals that you don't need. For example, if you already have a high level of iron, the iron-binding capacity of phytates is a benefit because too much iron leads to serious free radical damage to your cells. Excessive free radical damage increases your risk of cancer and other degenerative disorders. Phytates may have additional anti-cancer activity since they appear to increase the activity of natural killer cells that attack and destroy cancer cells and tumors.

Phytates are generally found in foods high in fiber. Since fiber-rich foods protect against colon and breast cancers, it is now thought that phytates may be the protective agent in the fiber.

Phytates, in combination with fiber, slow down the absorption of glucose from starch, thus helping you to balance blood sugar and insulin.

Risks of Excess Phytates

Soybeans contain high levels of phytates, perhaps more than other beans. Soy phytates are very stable and many survive phytate-reducing techniques such as cooking whereas the phytates in whole grains and some legumes can be deactivated simply by soaking or fermenting.

It is possible that only long periods of soaking and fermenting of soyfoods significantly reduces their phytate content. In contrast, unfermented soy products may retain higher levels of phytates. Examples of fermented soyfoods are miso, natto, shoyu, tamari, and tempeh. Unfermented soyfoods include tofu, soymilk, texturized soy protein, or soy protein isolate. Eating a lot of unfermented soy (high in phytates) could conceivably lead to a shortage of crucial minerals. If you intend to eat a lot of soy products and other legumes, you may wish to add a multi-mineral supplement to your diet.

Gluten and Gliadin

"Gluten" refers to a group of proteins in cereal grains such as wheat, rye and barley. A component of gluten is gliadin, which is thought to be the cause of "gluten intolerance." Gluten intolerance means that when you consume gluten, the cells in your gastrointestinal system are damaged. Moreover, gliadin can enter the bloodstream where it may cause an allergic response.

Gliadin appears to be involved in celiac disease, type 1 diabetes, dermatitis herpetiformis, schizophrenia, osteoporosis and other disorders.[104] [105]

The issue of gluten or gliadin damage to the intestinal tract is a serious one. Once your GI tract starts to seriously malfunction, it is impossible to properly nourish your body. Therefore, if you are not tolerant of gluten and have PCOS, you greatly reduce your odds of ever becoming healthy if you continue to consume gluten. The main dietary source is wheat and products made from wheat. The reason that bread has the nice chewy texture we enjoy so much is because of gluten. So if you eat bread or any baked product made from wheat, or similar grains like rye and oats, you are getting a lot of gluten and gliadin.

Summary

As we've said, antinutrients have not been extensively studied so you will have to experiment to find out what works for you and what doesn't. Since you have PCOS, we suggest that you consider changing your diet and notice what happens. For example, you could remove wheat and all foods containing wheat from your diet for at least six months and see if your symptoms diminish.

In general, however, in light of your probable genetic tendencies, we recommend avoidance of all grains and most legumes.

4.4 To Soy or Not to Soy

There is some controversy about whether soy is good or bad for you.

Soybean producers, soyfood manufacturers, supplement companies and the FDA say soy is good for you. On the other hand, some health consumer groups say soy may be bad for you. The scientific community is divided on the issue, with the preponderance leaning toward the concept that soy is good for you.

So who's right?

Sorting Through the Data on Soy

There's a flood of new research on soy, and it's a challenge for scientists to evaluate the information and come to a solid consensus on soy's role in human health. Many different types of studies are performed using a variety of methods as well as all of the many different kinds of soy products. Conclusions from only one or a few studies on specific soy preparations cannot be applied across the board to all types of soy products available in the marketplace. As a result, there's a great deal of confusion regarding the health effects of soy.

Much of the published soy research to date consists of epidemiological studies in which the relationship between soy intake and health outcomes in Asian populations is examined. (Epidemiology is a branch of medical science that deals with the incidence, distribution, and control of disease in a specific group, like the population of a country). These studies are based primarily on the intake of traditional soy foods derived from soybeans, such as tofu, fermented soy cakes (tempeh) or soy paste (miso). Highly processed or manufactured soy products, such as soymilk or soy protein added to foods, may not yield the same nutritional results as traditional soy foods.

Much of the confusion about soy relates to the difference between observed health outcomes from epidemiological studies on soy food intake vs. the data obtained using specific isolated and concentrated fractions of soy. In contrast to epidemiological studies that look at soy food consumption, research data from animal or human intervention studies use fractions of soy (e.g., refined soy concentrates or isolates, isolated isoflavone mixtures, or pure genistein).

We do not have a systematic method for comparing results of studies that analyze different types or forms of soy. It's like comparing apples to oranges. Therefore it's difficult to draw general conclusions about soy.

The History of Soy

The soybean is noted in the historical artifacts of the Chou Dynasty (1134-246 BC). However, the pictograph for the soybean, which dates from earlier times, indicates that it was not first used as a food. While the pictographs for other grains show the seed and stem structure of the plant, the pictograph for the soybean emphasizes the root structure. Agricultural literature of the period speaks of the soybean and its use in crop rotation. Apparently, the soy plant was initially used as a method of fixing nitrogen and thus improving the fertility of the soil.

The soybean did not serve as a food until the discovery of fermentation techniques, some time during the Chou Dynasty. The first soy foods were fermented products like tempeh, natto, miso and soy sauce.

At a later date, possibly around 2 BC, Chinese scientists discovered that a purée of cooked soybeans could be precipitated with calcium sulfate or magnesium sulfate to make a tofu. The use of fermented and precipitated soy products soon spread to Japan and parts of Southeast Asia.

However, soy was not the main feature of their diets. The Japanese traditionally ate a small amount of tofu or miso as part of a mineral-rich fish broth, followed by a serving of meat or fish. The Chinese ate lentils and other legumes, but apparently not unfermented soybeans, possibly because of the antinutrients found in soybeans.

The soybean of ancient China is a far cry from the genetically modified soybean of today. *Glycine soja*, the wild soybean, is found in China, Korea, Taiwan and Japan. *Glycine soja* is the species of soybean that was consumed traditionally and is the ancestor of the modern cultivar, *Glycine max*. In contrast, the genetically modified soybean that composes about 95% of the total soybean acreage today simply did not exist a few decades ago.

By the 20th century, soybeans were a minor crop that was listed in the 1913 US Department of Agriculture (USDA) handbook as an industrial product, not as a food. Today, over 72 million acres are under cultivation for soybeans. Within the past half century, soy has found its way into hundreds of food products that we eat every day. In fact, you could argue that besides wheat and dairy, soy is the most widespread ingredient in our processed foods today.

We can conclude the following:
- Originally, soybeans were not used as a food.
- Soybeans were not a primary staple of any ancient culture.
- Today's genetically modified soybean is vastly different from the ancient wild soybean.
- Soybeans were not widely consumed in the U.S. until the mid-20th century.
- We are consuming more soy than ever before.
- The soy we are consuming now is not identical to the soy eaten by older cultures, so the benefits that accrued to them may not accrue to us to the same extent.

- The nutritional makeup of any particular crop of soy beans will differ according to variety of bean used, growing environment, time of harvest, storage conditions and processing techniques.

The health long-term effects of this rapid increase in consumption of modern soybeans are unknown.

Soy and Your Thyroid

Soy foods interfere with thyroid function. Perhaps the primary concern of PCOS women is that soy may have a depressing effect on the thyroid. A fully functioning thyroid is crucial to management and reduction of PCOS symptoms.

The problem with soy is that two of the primary isoflavones, genistein and daidzein, inhibit certain chemical reactions essential to thyroid hormone synthesis.[106] The soybean has been implicated in diet-induced goiter and depressed thyroid function in many studies. The extensive and growing consumption of soy products in infant formulas and in vegetarian diets should be considered when looking into the factors that may contribute to the hormone dysregulation that is associated with PCOS.

The suggestion in the popular press that some soy products — such as fermented miso, natto or tempeh — do not interfere with thyroid hormone production has not been supported by research. For example, one study showed that the level of genistein in the fermented soybean products was higher than in soybeans and soybean products such as soy milk and tofu.[107] The highest levels of genistein and daidzein (other than in dietary supplements or high isoflavone soy protein powders) are found in tofu.

There is also a strong relationship between soy intake and later development of autoimmune thyroid disorders such as Hashimoto's thyroiditis or Grave's disease. These conditions are also associated with excessive intake of iodine (as in supplements or sea vegetables).

One small study in Japan reported that women consuming 30 grams of soybeans for 3 months had symptoms of hypothyroidism — malaise, constipation, and sleepiness.[108] Even after one month, the women had a beginning sign of hypothyroidism as shown by rising TSH levels. TSH (thyroid stimulating hormone) is a hormone that rises when thyroid hormones drop. TSH signals the thyroid to start producing more hormones.

Hypothyroidism & Pregnancy

Fertility problems are a primary concern of women with PCOS. Normal thyroid function is essential for successful pregnancy.[109] [110] Interference with optimal thyroid function because of soy foods in the diet may add an extra burden on a woman whose ability to achieve pregnancy and carry to term is already impaired by PCOS.

The following statistics profile the importance of optimal thyroid function[111].
- Nearly 1 out of 50 women in the U.S. is diagnosed with hypothyroidism during pregnancy.
- Six out of every 100 miscarriages can be attributed to thyroid deficiency during pregnancy.
- 5%-18% of women are diagnosed with postpartum thyroiditis.
- Approximately 25% of women will develop permanent hypothyroidism.

Although soy foods have real nutritional benefits and can be used to enhance our diets, women with PCOS have special reason to be cautious with soy.

Soy and Other Hormones

Soy contains compounds called "isoflavones." Some women are under the misconception that soy isoflavones are the same thing as estrogen, or act the same as estrogen. That is not quite the case.

The biological effects of isoflavones differ substantially from estrogen. For one thing, the biological effect of estrogen is 400-1,000 times stronger than that of isoflavones. Another difference is the ability of isoflavones to preferentially bind one of the two estrogen receptors, whereas estrogen binds robustly to both receptors. More research is needed to establish which tissues respond to isoflavones through these different estrogen-receptors, as well as the indirect effects of isoflavones on various tissues.

In a small study in England, six premenopausal women were given 60 grams of soy protein (containing 45 mg of isoflavones) daily for one month.[112] The women experienced an increased follicular phase of their menstrual cycle (delayed menstruation). Mid-cycle surges of LH (luteinizing hormone) and FSH (follicle stimulating hormone) were significantly suppressed while the soy protein was being consumed. The effects continued for three months after the soy was stopped.

This was a very small study for a very short period of time. However, many PCOS women do not have a LH surge in mid cycle. Without a mid cycle surge of LH, ovulation cannot occur. It's an open question as to whether a woman who is seeking an increased LH surge would want to eat something that might suppress that surge.

On the other hand, some research indicates that soy foods have a number of benefits potentially important for women with PCOS. With one daily serving, it can reduce serum estradiol (a form of estrogen). When eaten regularly from childhood, soy food is associated with a lower risk for breast cancer. Studies suggest soy may be associated with lowering the rate endometrial cancer. Soy lowers cholesterol and thus may help to reduce the cardiovascular risk that many PCOS women face.[113] Whole soy foods are a good source of fiber and plant protein.

However, if you need to lose 10% or more of your body weight as part of your PCOS treatment plan, we recommend a lower carbohydrate, ketogenic diet. It is difficult to include carbohydrate-rich soy foods into a ketogenic diet, without sacrificing other essential metabolic features of the diet.

Once weight loss has been achieved and you are transitioning into a broader-based, more varied lifelong maintenance eating style, soy foods can be incorporated into your diet.

Soy and Food Additives

Some soy products contain food additives in order to improve mouth feel, taste or shelf life.

Carrageenan is a thickening and stabilizing agent used in a variety of soy products, including soy milk and soy ice cream. Although the FDA has approved it as "safe" in foods, carrageenan contains various forms of galactose. There is clinical and experimental evidence to suggest that galactose may be detrimental to ovarian function and to ovarian germ cells, which are necessary for reproduction.[114] [115] In addition, there is at least one report of a possible link between carrageenan consumption and cancer.[116]

Genetically Modified Soy

Most of today's soybeans are genetically modified. Genetically modified foods are created by splicing lectins from one plant family into another, thus creating a plant that looks the same but is functionally quite different. The health consequences of this technique are unknown. If you know you react to a particular plant family but that lectin has been put in a plant not of that family, you may unknowingly consume the "toxic to you" lectin, thus causing an allergic reaction or other health problem.

Summary

Soy is beneficial for some of the diseases for which PCOS women have an increased risk such as heart disease and certain cancers. However, soy can interfere with thyroid function. Low thyroid function can contribute to pregnancy problems as well as obesity.

The high carbohydrate content of soy foods also interferes with the essential effort overweight PCOS women must make to reduce body weight by at least 7% to 10%. Therefore, we do not recommend soy foods or include them in the menu plans featured in this book.

In summary, soy is not recommended for women with symptomatic PCOS.

4.5 What Is Fiber?

Fiber is the part of a plant food that is not digested by humans. Fiber is necessary for good health, and a diet high in fiber is far superior to one that is not.

Fiber helps in the digestive process, is thought to lower cholesterol, help control blood glucose (sugar), protect against some cancers and reduce the risk of heart disease.

Types of Fiber

There are two types of fiber — soluble and insoluble.

Soluble fiber is found in fruits and vegetables, oat bran, barley and legumes. It dissolves in water and is thought to help lower blood fats and blood glucose (sugar).

Insoluble fiber, called cellulose, does not dissolve in water and does not have as many benefits as soluble fiber. It is found in whole grains and vegetables. As it passes through the intestines, it helps the body get rid of waste products. A major source of insoluble fiber is the bran layers of cereal grains, such as wheat bran.

Main Benefits of Fiber

Fiber and Your Intestinal Tract
Fiber prevents constipation as well as diarrhea; it also improves bowel transit time (the time it takes for food to pass through the intestines and be eliminated). A high fiber diet can decrease transit time by as much as 18 hours. This is an important step toward health since slow transit time allows toxins and excess hormones in the colon to be reabsorbed back into the blood.

Fiber, especially insoluble fiber such as cellulose (e.g., wheat bran) also helps keep the stool soft, bulky and moving easily through the intestines. It does this by functioning like a sponge, holding water and binding minerals and acidic materials. Softer, bulkier stools help to prevent constipation and hemorrhoids.

A high fiber diet also promotes a stable population of beneficial bacteria in the intestines while discouraging pathological organisms.

Fiber and Digestion
Fiber improves and modulates digestion by slowing the emptying of food from the stomach into the small intestine. The gradual rate of transfer prevents blood sugar fluctuations and improves pancreatic enzyme secretion and activity.

Fiber and Cholesterol

Fiber binds cholesterol in the stool, preventing it from being circulated in the blood, where it clogs arteries and contributes to heart disease.

Fiber and Cancer Protection

Fiber sustains bacteria in the intestines that produce beneficial short-chain fatty acids. Two of these fatty acids, propionate and acetate, are used as energy sources in the body. Butyrate, the third fatty acid, has anti-cancer activity in the bowel.

Fiber and Your Weight

Whole foods with a high fiber contents help you lose weight in a number of ways:
- Low calorie density, so you can eat a large volume of food containing less total calories.
- Provides a sense of fullness and satiety.
- Reduces glycemic and insulin responses to a meal. Helps to reduce insulin resistance.
- Slows down the rate at which you can chew, swallow and process food in your intestine. This gives your hunger-regulation hormones enough time to give your brain feedback about whether to eat more food or not.

Fiber and Estrogen

Some women with PCOS may have levels of estrogen that are too high.

A precise balance between estrogen and progesterone is essential for normal fertility. While normal estrogen levels are usually increased during the first half of your cycle, a failure to ovulate stops progesterone from reaching normal levels during the second half of the cycle, which is required for the proper balance between estrogen and progesterone. If estrogen levels continue cycle after cycle to be unopposed by progesterone, "estrogen dominance" can be the result, meaning that you have too much estrogen in relation to progesterone.

Results from various studies indicate that a generous intake of dietary fiber helps to reduce excessive levels of estrogen, thus helping to bring your body into better hormonal balance.[117]

The liver filters estrogens out of the blood and sends them down the bile duct into the intestinal tract. Fiber in the intestinal tract attaches to the estrogen, and the excess estrogen is excreted in the stool.

Fiber and Insulin Resistance

Many women with polycystic ovary syndrome or infertility have insulin resistance and excessively high levels of insulin. Many studies show that a high-fiber diet as opposed to a low-fiber diet reduces insulin resistance and peak insulin levels.[118] [119] Fiber also normalizes blood glucose levels.

Increased Fiber Curbs Appetite in Women

A recent study at the University of California (Davis) indicates that increased fiber content in a meal boosts feelings of fullness in women and increases levels of a certain hormone associated with satiety (feeling full and satisfied).[120]

The hormone CCK (cholecystokinin) is released from the small intestine when a fat-containing food is eaten. This hormone may be the chemical messenger that acts in response to fat to notify the brain that the body is getting full.

Now it appears that fiber can trigger the same signaling mechanism as fat.

The researchers fed a test group of men and women three different types of breakfast meals: low-fiber, low-fat; high-fiber, low-fat; or low-fiber, high-fat.

They found that both the high-fat and high-fiber meals resulted in greater feelings of satiety and significantly higher levels of CCK, than did the low-fat, low-fiber meals.

The inclusion of fiber in a meal increases your feeling of being full, due not only to fiber creating a greater volume of food in your gastrointestinal tract, but also to fiber promoting the release of CCK. The high-fiber foods in the healthy PCOS diet are a good way for you to help control your appetite.

High-Fiber Diet Helps Spare Your Gallbladder

A diet high in fiber has been shown to reduce the risk of gallstones. A lower risk of gallstones reduces the probability that you will need gallbladder surgery.

A recent study analyzed food consumption data from approximately 70,000 women starting in 1984.[121] The women were apparently free from gallbladder disease when the study began. By 2000, nearly 6,000 of the women had their gallbladders taken out (an astounding 9% of the total!).

Study results showed that women who consumed the highest amounts of fiber were 13% less likely to undergo gallbladder removal than those who consumed the lowest amounts.

Some Possible Consequences of Low Fiber Intake

Low fiber intake has been linked to a host of health problems, including: appendicitis, autoimmune disorders, colon cancer, constipation, deep vein thrombosis, skin conditions, diabetes, diverticulosis, gall bladder disease, gout, hemorrhoids, hypertension, irritable bowel syndrome, kidney stones, multiple sclerosis, obesity, pernicious anemia, pulmonary embolism, thyrotoxicosis, tooth cavities and varicose veins.

Sources of Fiber

Whole food sources of fiber are: vegetables, fruits, seeds, nuts, legumes and grains.

Fiber can be obtained in the PCOS diet through fresh vegetables, fruits, nuts and seeds. If you have been eating a low fiber diet, you could initially experience some gas when you increase fiber intake, so ease into it gradually and drink plenty of water (aim for a minimum of 2 quarts daily) to keep everything moving smoothly through your digestive system.

Caution with Supplemental Fiber

When obtained through whole foods, fiber is completely safe and beneficial.

However, occasionally some people who use supplemental fiber such as guar, psyllium, pectin, or carrageenan may experience difficulties when they use them in excessive amounts. For example, more than 2 cups of psyllium daily could disturb the walls of your GI tract, and excessive carrageenan could cause gastrointestinal damage.

4.6 Plant Foods

Plant foods are a lot more than "just another carbohydrate."

There are many hundreds (if not thousands) of compounds that affect human physiology in complex ways. Ancient medical traditions such as Ayurvedic and Tradition Chinese Medicine have used plants as healing medicines for centuries. Every year, new plant compounds are being discovered. The design of the majority of modern pharmaceutical drugs is based on the chemistry of plant compounds.

To a great extent, you are what you eat. It really is true. We know that ancient man has eaten plant material for hundreds of thousands of years. All of it was unprocessed and very high in fiber.

Today, Westernized cultures eat highly processed foods that do not contain the complete plant material. As a consequence, we do not get the benefit of plant compounds and fiber in the same combinations that our ancestors did. The vast bulk of our processed plant-based foods are very low in fiber and have many of their inherent nutrients removed in the refinement process. Moreover, poor agricultural practices have left our soils depleted so that, even though the plant looks the same, the level of nutrients in the plant is lower than in the same plant 100 years ago. We are left with foods that are calorie-dense but devoid of the plant compounds we need for good health.

In other words, refined foods cause us to be overfed and undernourished. A perfect example is the most widely consumed "vegetable" in America, the French-fried potato. No serious health practitioner or medical researcher would claim that eating more French-fried potatoes than any other vegetable is good for you. Yet that is what we are doing.

Consumption of more plant material in its natural state will help you to be adequately fed and optimally nourished. The beneficial effect of plant foods on human health is unmistakable.[122] Time and time again, studies have found foods of plant origin to reduce the risk of most major chronic illnesses suffered by the human population.[123] [124]

Natural plant foods include vegetation (leaves, stems, and roots), whole fruits, and raw nuts and seeds.

Plant Foods and PCOS

In addition to providing energy and essential nutrients, plant foods contain a wide array of "signaling" substances that influence what your cells do. This fact is especially important for women with PCOS. You have PCOS because your hormonal and other cell signaling systems are not working optimally. Eating fresh, whole plants foods will improve the ability of your body to function as it should.

Whole plant foods may have these beneficial effects:
- Reduction of hyperinsulinism and insulin resistance
- Increase in sex hormone binding globulin
- Reduction in free testosterone levels (reduction of hirsutism and acne)
- More effective metabolism and elimination of hormones
- Weight loss
- Lower risk of diabetes and cardiovascular disease
- Healthier ovarian function

Sex Hormone Binding Globulin (SHBG)

SHBG binds to hormones and thus makes them "inactive." High insulin levels cause the liver to produce less SHBG. Less SHBG means you have more "active" or bioavailable testosterone floating around. This is the testosterone that disturbs ovarian function, and causes hirsutism (excess body and facial hair and scalp hair thinning) and acne.

Women who eat a lot of high-fiber vegetables and fruits have higher SHBG levels.[125] So, for a variety of reasons, plant foods play an important role in controlling symptoms of PCOS.

Plant Pigments and Ovarian Function

Many plant foods are high in red, yellow and orange pigments called carotenoids. They are especially abundant in yellow-orange fruits and vegetables and dark green, leafy vegetables. Of the more than 700 naturally occurring carotenoids identified thus far, as many as 50 may be absorbed and metabolized by the human body.

Carotenoids provide antioxidant protection, improve cell-to-cell communication and support the immune system, in addition to other functions. We'll just mention two of the carotenoids here.

- **Beta-carotene:** The corpus luteum that appears on the ovary at ovulation contains the highest level of beta carotene in the body.

- **Lutein:** It appears to play a role in ovarian function. Originally lutein was isolated from the corpus luteum, hence the name "lutein." The corpus luteum of the ovaries contains high concentrations of lutein as well as other carotenoids.

The role of carotenoids in the ovaries is not entirely clear, although it may have to do with protection against free radicals. One study has noted that women with more consistent levels of carotenoids were more likely to become pregnant with in-vitro fertilization (IVF) than women who had more varying levels of carotenoids.[126]

A couple of studies have suggested that a free radical activity may interfere with the corpus luteum's ability to produce steroid hormones such as progesterone.[127] [128] Conceivably, carotenoids may help to control some of this free radical activity since they are well known as antioxidants.

It's also possible that increased intake of carotenoids may help to increase progesterone production. In a study of dogs at Washington State University, administration of supplemental beta-carotene increased their progesterone levels.[129]

Carotenoids may also be helpful for controlling insulin levels and reducing risk of diabetes. A study by the Centers for Disease Control has shown that people who had the highest levels of carotenoids were the least likely to develop diabetes or impaired glucose tolerance.[130]

We suspect that optimal levels of carotenoid intake via whole pigmented plant foods will contribute to ovarian health.

Plant Sterols and PCOS

Sterols are fats present in all plants, including fruits and vegetables. They affect your physiology and have anti-inflammatory, blood sugar control and hormone-influencing properties.

For example, some sterols help to prevent your blood sugar from going too high, apparently by stimulating your pancreas to produce insulin.[131] Another example is beta-sitosterol, which inhibits the conversion of testosterone into the more powerful dihydrotestosterone (DHT), which can cause hair growth and acne.[132]

4.7 Guidelines for Eating Carbohydrates

The best way to get the carbohydrates you need is in whole foods, not processed or refined foods. Consider the apple as an example. Which is better for you — a fresh apple, applesauce or apple juice?

Apple juice is totally unsuitable, since it is 65% fructose (way too much sugar) and is devoid of the fiber as well as most of the essential nutrients you need to regain your health. Drinking apple juice is a sure-fire way to worsen your PCOS problems. Applesauce is slightly better than apple juice since it does contain a modicum of fiber. Of course, applesauce loses some of it nutrients from processing. A fresh apple is a vastly superior source of carbohydrates and essential nutrients as compared to apple juice. And it is much better than applesauce.

Apply the same principle to any food you eat: choose the whole food, rather than a processed version of it. Most whole foods contain some carbohydrates, so you'll have little trouble getting enough for good health. On the other hand, whole foods, for the most part, do not contain excessive amounts of carbohydrates. Unlike most processed foods, whole natural foods give you a moderate amount of carbohydrates — not too much, and not too little.

Where Will My Carbohydrates Come From?

On the healthy PCOS diet, the bulk of your carbs will come from vegetables. The remainder will come from fruit, nuts and seeds. Grains and legumes are severely restricted, so you won't be getting much from these sources.

If you follow the principle of eating carbohydrates found only in whole foods, you'll be on a "natural," moderately low-carb diet without having to consciously worry about how many carb calories you are consuming.

How Much Carbohydrate Should I Eat?

If you're trying to lose weight, we suggest you consume about 40 to 60 grams of carbohydrate from the foods in the Recommended Level of our diet.

That doesn't sound like very much carbohydrate! 40 grams is only 1.4 ounces, and 60 grams is only 2.1 ounces. You might think that you are hardly allowed to eat any carbohydrate at all and that most of your food will have to be protein and fat. This is not the case.

Even if you are overweight, you can eat a very adequate amount of food that is nutritionally balanced. Your first task is to find out how much carbohydrate is in the food you want to eat.

Most processed packaged foods indicate the grams of carbohydrate on the label, so it's very easy to calculate the 40-60 grams of total carbohydrate you can eat. For example, Orowheat "Light" 9-Grain bread contains 7 grams of carbohydrate in each slice, and Honey Maid graham crackers have 3 grams of carbohydrate in each cracker. In this example, you would reach your 60-gram daily limit with 5 slices of bread and 8 graham crackers.

However, packaged and processed foods are not part of our recommended diet. So your carbohydrate calculations won't be as easy. For example, there's no label on a head of broccoli that tells you how much carbohydrate it contains.

Most of the carbohydrates in our diet come in vegetables and fruits. Fortunately, you can quickly find out the carbohydrate content of any vegetable or fruit by accessing the U.S. Department of Agriculture website:

www.nal.usda.gov/fnic/foodcomp/search

Using the data from the Department of Agriculture website, you can imagine what you could eat instead of 5 slices of bread and 8 graham crackers.

Here's an example of items from our recommended fresh foods list, consisting of a total of 60.5 grams of carbohydrate:
- 2 medium zucchini squashes (6.6 grams)
- 1 medium apple (13.8 grams)
- 1 cup broccoli flowerets (3.7 grams)
- 1 cup diced eggplant (4.7 grams)
- 1 cup shredded romaine lettuce (1.5 grams)
- 1 cup string beans (7.8 grams)
- 20 pecan halves (3.9 grams)
- 1 large kiwi fruit (13.3 grams)
- 1 cup asparagus (5.2 grams)

Which do you think would be more filling and more nutritious? 5 slices of "healthy" 9-grain bread and 8 graham crackers, or the above list of vegetables, fruit and nuts? The foods from our recommended diet are vastly more nutritious and more filling than is the bread and crackers. An added bonus is that if you are trying to lose weight, you can eat all the above food and still be within the recommended 40-60 grams of carbohydrate limit that will help you to burn off fat.

If you don't need to lose weight, you can consume considerably more carbohydrate that shown in this example.

Section 5

Protein

5.1 What's a Protein?

A protein is a complex biological molecule composed of a chain of units called amino acids. Proteins are required for the structure, function, and regulation of the body's cells, tissues and organs. Each protein has a unique function. Proteins may function as:

- Enzymes
- Hormones
- Hemoglobin
- Antibodies
- Genetic material
- A source of energy

Proteins are major constituents of every cell and body fluid except urine and bile. They act to maintain normal acid-base balance in the blood and to regulate salt and fluid balance in different body tissues. Proteins are required for the growth, repair and normal function of every part of bodies.

Proteins account for more than 50% of the dry weight of most cells and are involved in most cell processes. The amino acids of proteins are the building blocks of the cells. The cells need proteins to grow, to mend themselves and to create the product that is that cell's contribution to our physical system.

Protein is abundant in many foods such as meat, fish, poultry and eggs. Protein is also found in lower concentrations in legumes, nuts, seeds, grains, vegetables and fruit.

Optimally, proteins are broken down into amino acids in the gastrointestinal tract. However, it is not uncommon for some whole proteins to leak through into the bloodstream and cause inflammatory or allergic responses. Properly digested amino acids are stored until needed in the liver and individual cells.

Amino Acids

An amino acid is a chain of carbon and oxygen atoms with ammonia and hydrogen atoms attached. There are approximately 25 different amino acids.

A protein is a linkage of hundreds or even thousands of amino acids in varying combinations and patterns. There are many thousands — perhaps hundreds of thousands — of unique chains of amino acids in your body, each performing a specific function.

Amino acids can be used for energy just like fats and carbohydrates.

The body can change one amino acid into another, and to some extent, even create new amino acids. There are eight amino acids that cannot be made by our bodies and therefore must be obtained from the diet. These are called "essential amino acids."

The essential amino acids are: histidine, isoleucine, leucine, lysine, methionine, phenylalanine, threonine, tryptophan, and valine. Methionine, in particular, seems to be lacking in the typical American diet.

There are two "semi-essential" amino acids: arginine and carnitine. They aren't manufactured in sufficient amounts to guarantee optimal health and small amounts are required from the diet.

Recycling of amino acids is not 100% efficient; some are lost, requiring a constant re-supply from the diet.

We are particularly interested in those amino acids that are known to affect how we metabolize fat, as well as our moods and our appetite for certain foods.

The recently identified, poorly understood, and often therapeutic functions of individual amino acids were not considered when the Recommended Daily Allowances (RDAs) for individual amino acids were developed. The RDAs are based on the proper ratio of amino acids to maintain "nitrogen balance," i.e., nitrogen intake compared to nitrogen excretion, which is an estimate only of basic protein requirements. However, research shows pharmacological doses of individual amino acids, doses several times the RDA requirements, do affect fundamental physiological processes.[133]

What Amino Acids Can Do for You

- Increase lean muscle and energy output
- Accelerate muscle repair for fast recuperation from exercise
- Stimulate the production of growth hormone
- Reduce body fat
- Enhance oxygen and fatty acid utilization
- Increase mental concentration
- Stabilize blood sugar
- Accelerate ammonia removal to delay onset of fatigue
- Produce antibodies, enzymes and hormones
- Increase hair and nail strength
- Improve tissue and cartilage elasticity and regeneration

Minimum Requirement for Protein

About 30 grams of protein is used up each day just to keep the body going, although your need may vary according to body size, physical activity and other factors.

One formula to help you estimate the amount of protein you need:

Your weight / 2.2 x .87 = grams of protein per day.

What Happens When You Eat Too Little Protein?

What happens when you don't eat enough protein to keep your body running properly? Your body will rob protein from "lower priority" areas of your body such as your muscle tissue.

Very low calorie diets or fasting are not advisable unless you are under a physician's supervision. As soon as 12 hours after starting such a diet or fasting, stores of blood sugar (glucose) may be used up and your body is likely to start consuming a mix of protein and fat from the body for energy.

What Happens When You Eat Too Much Protein?

When there are amino acids (proteins) in excess of the body's requirements, they're sent to the liver, where they are converted into fat.

The conversion process produces ammonia as a byproduct, which is toxic. The ammonia is in turn converted into urea, which is somewhat less toxic. In order to excrete urea without damage to the kidneys, it must be highly diluted in water.

So to get rid of it, you need to drink large amounts of water. You may drink a lot of water, but inevitably it won't be enough. So your body will have to take water from its own tissues to dilute the urea. You lose weight quickly as a result of excreting lots of water. You may lose up to 12 lbs. of water weight on a high protein, low carbohydrate diet, regardless of how much water you drink.

If you have impaired kidney function, you should not embark on a high-protein diet unless under a physician's supervision.

Amino Acid Balance

The body will synthesize protein up to the point at which it runs out of adequate supplies of any essential amino acid. Any remaining unusable amino acids will be burned as energy or converted to fat.

You may have heard the term "biological value" or "net protein utilization" (NPU) of foods. The biological value of foods is the degree to which the amino acid distribution in a food matches the body's qualitative and quantitative requirements.

The net protein utilization (NPU) is the measure of biological value and protein digestibility of specific foods. Although there is no "perfect" protein source, eggs most nearly approximate the mix of amino acids required by humans. Thus, the egg is the standard by which other protein sources are measured.

The foods with highest NPU are, in descending order: eggs, fish, cheese, brown rice, red meat and poultry. Some protein powders made from fragments of milk proteins may have a NPU higher than eggs.

If you tend to avoid animal protein, or are a vegetarian, it may be a challenge for you to obtain all of the essential amino acids you need.

For example, let's take leucine, one of the "essential" amino acids, which you must get from your diet. A study at the University of Illinois has suggested that the amino acid leucine is a key to the positive outcomes of using a higher protein diet for fat because of its unique roles in regulation of muscle protein synthesis, insulin signaling and glucose re-cycling via alanine (another amino acid).[134] The investigators said that people wanting to lose weight may need to consume more leucine than is currently recommended by current dietary guidelines and dietary practices in the U.S.

Plant Proteins and "Complementary" Amino Acids

Animal protein foods such as eggs or meat contain all the essential amino acids. Therefore they are referred to as "complete" proteins. A problem is that they may also be high in fat and environmental toxins. It is essential to buy and consume organically raised and wild foods as much as you possibly can to avoid the chemical residues found in non-organically raised food products.

Plant foods have a kind of protein also, made up of the same amino acids, but in significantly different and incomplete combinations. It is possible that you can get some of your protein needs met from plant foods such as legumes, nuts, seeds or grains, even though they have some of the essential amino acids missing. However, because the protein content of plant foods is small and the carbohydrate content relatively much higher, you will eat too much carbohydrate if you try to satisfy protein needs with the amino acids found in plant foods.

If you're already at or near your ideal weight and don't need to shed fat pounds, you don't have to eat a perfect, complete protein such as eggs, meat, poultry or fish at every single meal. You can also have meals consisting of incomplete, plant-based proteins. However, the carbohydrates in plant-based foods will slow down the process of liberating stored fat for energy. Eating to lose fat and eating when we are at our ideal weight are two different processes. Food choices should be made according to your unique needs.

Protein and Appetite

A growing body of evidence shows that eating adequate protein at each meal is very helpful in controlling and even reducing your appetite.[135]

Researchers at the Harvard School of Public Health conducted a review of medical investigations on the effects of high protein diets on thermogenesis (metabolic rate), satiety, body weight and fat loss.[136]

Their conclusion: "There is convincing evidence that a higher protein intake increases thermogenesis and satiety compared to diets of lower protein content. The weight of evidence also suggests that high protein meals lead to a reduced subsequent energy intake. Some evidence suggests that diets higher in protein result in an increased weight loss and fat loss as compared to diets lower in protein, but findings have not been consistent…It may be beneficial to partially replace refined carbohydrate with protein sources that are low in saturated fat."

What's interesting in this survey of the medical literature is that increasing protein helps to reduce your appetite so that you will eat fewer calories without feeling hungry and deprived.

Protein and Blood Sugar

Some women with PCOS have blood sugar levels that are too high, or fluctuate to high levels. The increased blood sugar causes an unwanted increase in insulin. If the insulin increase is sustained over time, insulin resistance can result.

A number of studies have demonstrated that a relatively high level of protein in the diet will lower blood sugar levels. For example, the Minneapolis VA Medical Center recently completed a study of diabetics in which dietary protein was increased from 15% to 30% of total calories.[137] The carbohydrate content was decreased from 55% to 40%, i.e., the dietary protein replaced part of the carbohydrate.

The protein increase resulted in a decrease in glucose and glycohemoglobin, with a modest increase in insulin. The glycohemoglobin blood test result is significant because it reveals the average glucose levels over a 90-day period — it means that blood sugar remained lower over a period of time.

The study also showed that kidney function was not impaired by increasing the protein to 30% of total calories.

Protein and Body Composition

Inclusion of adequate protein in your diet may promote loss of fat weight. In a study of 24 overweight women at the University of Illinois, one group was given a high carb diet and the other group was given a high protein diet. The fat content was the same. Although both groups lost about the same amount of total weight, the high protein diet women lost about 60% more fat weight than the high-carb women. It's the fat that you want to lose, not muscle. So adequate protein is important.[138]

In summary, dietary protein is very important in the treatment of PCOS. The amount of protein you need relative to carbohydrate will depend on your health status and medical history.

5.2 The Problem with Milk

Thanks to the advent of refrigeration, the widespread consumption of dairy products was made possible. Today, cow's milk and products made from cow's milk make up a major portion of the standard diet in non-Asian countries. This phenomenon is unprecedented in human history. Is the pervasive consumption of dairy products a good thing or a bad thing? It appears the jury is still out on this issue. We view dairy products with a great deal of caution and think that heavy use of dairy products is unwarranted.

A Brief History of Milk

The earliest record suggesting man's use of animals' milk as food was unearthed in a temple in the Euphrates Valley near Babylon. The information was contained a mosaic frieze that was estimated to be about 5,000 years old.

In the 13th century, Marco Polo reported that Tartar armies drank a fermented form of mare's milk. Cows were first brought to the North American continent in the 15th century. Since then, there has been a phenomenal growth in North America of dairy cattle and consumption of their milk.

In 1909, Americans annually consumed a total of 34 gallons of fluid milk per person. 56% of that milk was consumed on the farms where it was produced. Less than 5 pounds of cheese were consumed and a tiny amount of ice cream was eaten. It's worth noting that most of this milk was consumed fresh from the cow and was not pasteurized or homogenized.

Today Americans consume about 23 gallons of fluid milk per person per year. However, they also eat 30 pounds of cheese plus 23 pounds of ice cream. These statistics do not include the huge volume of milk ingredients that are included in hundreds of processed food products.

Other parts of the world do not consume nearly as much dairy. For example, per capita consumption of dairy products in China is about 2 pounds per year.

Reasons to Be Concerned about Dairy?

We are concerned about dairy products for a number of fundamental reasons.

1. Milk Composition. Milk is designed to nourish and help baby mammals to grow. At some point, the baby animal is weaned and finds proper nourishment elsewhere.

The only exception to this rule is the human species. We are the only species of animal that consumes milk from the day we are born until the day we die. Is this a good idea? You should be aware that the composition of cow's milk is vastly different from the milk of primates.

Composition of Milk (per 100 g fresh milk)

Animal	Protein (g)	Fat (g)	Carbohydrate (g)	Energy (kcal)
Cow	3.2	3.7	4.6	66
Human	1.1	4.2	7.0	72
Monkey, rhesus	1.6	4.0	7.0	73

As you can see, the composition of cow's milk does not approximate human or primate milk. What are the consequences of consuming milk that is not meant to be a food for human adults?

2. Milk-Disease Link? We are the only animal species that consumes milk of other species, primarily from domesticated cows. Cow's milk contains growth factors to help baby cows grow rapidly. Have you ever seen a calf grow? They gain significant size and weight in a relatively short period of time, drinking only milk. Stop and think. Does it make sense for you to consume something that is optimized for making baby cows grow?

There is no conclusive evidence to establish that long-term consumption of cow's milk is healthier for you than not consuming it. In fact, studies of milk consumption in different countries suggest that milk may not be the health panacea you think it is.

- A study of seven countries with a high consumption of dairy products found that heart disease mortality rose as milk supply rose.[139]

- A study comparing heart disease death rates with food intake found that the highest correlation was with milk. "Changes in milk-protein consumption, up or down, accurately predicted changes in coronary deaths four to seven years later." The researchers noted that their analysis "strongly supports" previous conclusions that milk is the principal dietary culprit in hardened, narrowed arteries and that the problematic portion of milk is its protein, not its fat.[140]

- A study comparing coronary death rates with food intakes in 21 countries found that the food most highly correlated with coronary deaths was milk.[141]

It appears that casein, one of the milk proteins, may be responsible for these findings. There is some evidence to suggest that casein proteins may contribute to cardiovascular disease and possibly type 1 diabetes. [142] [143]

3. Milk and Genes. No adult humans ever consumed milk of any species until domesticated livestock were introduced about 5-10,000 years ago. It's an open question whether your genetic makeup has managed to adapt itself to dairy products.

4. Loss of Nutrients. Pasteurization destroys enzymes, diminishes vitamin content and damages milk proteins. Pasteurization does not kill viruses nor does it kill some resistant pathogenic bacteria. Anecdotal reports suggest that animals fed pasteurized milk do not thrive.

5. Herds Unhealthy? The health of commercial dairy herds is questionable.[144] Many herds have viral infections.[145] [146] Secondly, some dairy herds are fed hormones, growth promoters and antibiotics in order to increase milk production.[147] These substances end up in the milk or dairy product that you consume.[148] The container trucks that deliver milk from farm to factory are disinfected with chemicals, the residue of which is found in the milk supply as well.

6. Milk Allergies. A large number of people are allergic to cow's milk, especially to casein, which is a protein component of milk. Casein is a "gluey" kind of a protein that is difficult to digest. In fact, casein has many industrial uses, such as adhesives, binders and protective coatings.

As with many food allergies, a milk allergy can be hard to detect. Milk or milk components can be found in hundreds of processed of food products.

Any unidentified allergy creates an inflammatory condition and can only worsen PCOS symptoms.

7. Lactose Intolerance. Over 50 million Americans have difficulty digesting lactose (milk sugar) or other sugars. Most lactose intolerant individuals do not link their symptoms to lactose consumption. So you may be intolerant and not know it. This intolerance is an inherited metabolic inability to digest this sugar due to the absence of an enzyme in the digestive system. About 75% of the world's population does not tolerate lactose well. Asians, Native Americans and African Americans tend to have this milk intolerance. Caucasians may tolerate it in adulthood, but many do not. Many people seem to tolerate small amounts, but will have gastrointestinal symptoms such as constipation, cramping and bloat when larger amounts of milk products are consumed. Most people, as they get older, have diminished digestive power, leading to an increase in symptoms related to dairy consumption in later life.

8. Viruses in Milk. Are there viruses in dairy products, and should you care? Some dairy cows are infected with BLV (bovine leukemia virus), BIV (bovine immunodeficiency-like virus), BPV (bovine papilloma virus) or other viruses. Some of these viruses can infect other species such as sheep. Antibodies to these viruses have been found in humans. The health effects of these viruses in humans are not well understood. The evidence, scanty as it is, is not reassuring. Introduction of viruses of another species into your body is not good health building technique.

Does pasteurization kill viruses? Pasteurization is the process of heating milk in order to kill bacteria causing tuberculosis and undulant fever. It also extends shelf life of milk. However, it has not been proven that pasteurization kills all viruses. But even if a virus is inactivated by pasteurization, viral genetic particles can be absorbed into the body with unknown consequences. For example, BPV viral proteins can transform rat cells into cancerous cells.[149]

9. Ovarian cancer. Women who consume high amounts of milk and dairy products appear to have an increased risk of ovarian cancer.[150] [151]

Dairy Products and PCOS

We haven't yet come across any studies that discuss the consumption of dairy products in relation to PCOS, although there are some studies dealing with insulin and fertility. Here is a brief sampling of those studies.

Milk and Insulin
Researchers have found that even though milk and fermented milk products don't drastically raise blood sugar levels, they do cause significant insulin secretion.[152] In fact, milk and fermented milk products stimulate as much insulin secretion as whole wheat does. And some cheeses stimulate more insulin secretion than pasta or "all-bran" cereal, and almost as much as brown rice and popcorn.

Another study showed that adding milk to a low-glycemic meal increased insulin as much as a high-glycemic meal.[153]

In other words, dairy products have a low-glycemic value, meaning that they do not dramatically increase blood glucose. Since they do not rapidly increase blood glucose, presumably there is no need for increased insulin production. This is true for many foods, but it now appears this may not be true for milk, because even when the glycemic load of a meal is low, milk stimulates an increase in insulin.

In effect, consuming milk products with a meal increases your insulin levels, even if you are avoiding high-glycemic foods. Thus, the benefit of eating foods that are low on the glycemic index is defeated to some extent.

Milk and Infertility
In a study at Harvard University, researchers sought to determine whether there was a link between infertility and milk consumption by analyzing milk consumption in different countries.[154] They found that women who are able to digest milk sugar and who drank the most milk were the most infertile.

When milk sugar (lactose) is digested, it is broken down into glucose (blood sugar) and another sugar called galactose. Women who are able to digest milk sugar and who drink lots of milk thus have a greater exposure to galactose. There is some clinical and experimental evidence to suggest that galactose may be toxic to ovarian egg cells and lead to premature ovarian failure. Women who were lactose intolerant (not able to digest milk sugar) or who drank less milk had less exposure to galactose and had fewer fertility problems.

Another factor is that some women have impaired liver function, or have a deficiency of the enzyme required to metabolize galactose, which could lead to higher than normal galactose levels.

The possible role of milk in infertility has not been well studied. However, based on what little is known so far, we cannot recommend consumption of milk and dairy products.

Hormones, Growth Factors, Pesticides and Antibiotics in Dairy Products

Consider this startling statistic:

Year	Cows in U.S.	Milk Produced	Milk Produced Per Cow
1930	22.2 million	100.2 billion pounds	4,514 pounds
1998	9.3 million	156.6 billion pounds	16,838 pounds

How did US dairy producers manage to quadruple per-cow production within 68 years? Better breed of cow? Yes. Better milk extraction technology? Yes. More rapid culling of low producers? Yes. But these factors alone cannot account for such an enormous increase in milk production out of an animal.

Pesticides in the Cow's Diet?

It appears that dairy cows are not eating what they used to. As you know, dairy cows no longer graze in a pasture. They are confined in feedlots where there is nothing to eat except what is provided to them by the dairy operator. The operator will feed cows those particular feeds that are the cheapest while providing the maximum amount of milk. While some of the feed components appear to be healthy, others are nutritionally unbalanced or may be laden with pesticides that accumulate in the cow and its milk. For example, a common feed is cottonseeds or cottonseed hulls. Cotton is heavily sprayed with pesticides to stop boll weevils and other insects. However, the pesticides in the cottonseed are passed on to the cow. Some of the accumulated pesticides are then passed on into the milk.

By the way, the cottonseed hulls come from processing of cottonseeds, where the oil is extracted from the seed. The leftover byproduct is the cottonseed hull, which is sold to dairy operators. But what happens to the oil? It is sold to food processors, who put cottonseed oil into processed food products that you eat. So, you get the pesticides in cottonseeds, either directly by consuming the oil or indirectly from cow's milk. Check the label of every processed product you eat. Make sure it does not contain cottonseed oil.

Other sources of food for cows are routinely treated with pesticides, fungicides and fumigants. These chemicals are poisons, pure and simple. There is no "safe" amount you should be consuming.

Hormones

If you consume dairy products there's no way you can avoid consuming some amount of hormones.

Some of the hormones found in cow's milk are: estradiol, estriol, progesterone, testosterone, 17-ketosteroids, corticosterone, insulin-like growth factor (IGF-1), growth hormone (GH), prolactin, oxytocin and others. In addition, since the majority of cows are pregnant or recently pregnant, they may have elevated levels of some hormones.

We also have the issue of exogenous hormones (introduced from the outside). The main concern is with an injected hormone called rBGH (recombinant bovine growth hormone), also called BST. BST is a synthetic hormone that is injected into cows in order to stimulate milk production. Perhaps 30% of the U.S. dairy herd is injected with this hormone.

Cows injected with BST have 2-10 times as much IGF-1 in their milk as compared to untreated cows. What are the potential consequences of high levels if IGF-1 in cow's milk?

What is IGF-1?

IGF-1 stands for insulin growth factor-1. A growth factor is a small protein that is essential for a growth process to occur. There are many growth factors in the body, some of which are still being discovered.

The insulin-like growth factors (IGFs) have a structure similar to insulin. They can trigger the same cellular responses as insulin, including cell division. IGF-1 is one of the insulin-like growth factors.

Almost every cell in the human body is affected by IGF-1. In addition to the insulin-like effects, IGF-1 can also regulate cell growth and development. IGF-1 stimulates the growth of both normal and cancerous cells. Excessive levels of IGF-1 have been implicated in a variety of cancers.

All mammals produce IGF-1 molecules that are very similar. Human and cow IGF-1 are identical. Therefore, if BST (the growth hormone injected into some cows) stimulates higher levels of IGF-1, and if you drink that milk, it's logical to think that IGF-1 levels in your body would increase.

IGF-1 is not destroyed by pasteurization nor is there any assurance your digestive juices will destroy it in your stomach. Moreover, it's been known for decades that undigested or partially digested proteins will cross from the gut into the bloodstream.

Unfortunately, few human studies have been performed to verify how much of a cow's IGF-1 will get absorbed into your bloodstream. However, there was one study that analyzed two groups, one of which maintained their normal dairy intake while the other group maintained their normal dairy intake, but they added an extra three 8-oz. glasses of milk per day.[155] The group drinking the extra milk had their IGF-1 levels increase about 10% whereas the IFG-1 levels in the control group remained unchanged.

So, if this study is any indication of what actually happens when you consume a high level of dairy products, you should take heed. Too much IGF-1 is bad for you. On the other hand, too little IGF-1 is bad for you. You need a balance. But what happens when you get extra IGF-1 from your dairy products? We're not sure, although one study has suggested that ovarian cells of PCOS women have an exaggerated potential for IGF-1 stimulated cell division as compared to ovarian cells of normal women.[156] In other words, you may be more responsive to IGF-1 than other women.

It's hard to imagine that getting extra IGF-1 and other hormones from your food is a good idea. How can you know whether the dairy products you're eating contain IGF-1 or other hormones? You can't. There is no labeling law that requires a food product to say how much of any hormone, growth factor, pesticide or virus the product may contain.

Milk and Calcium

Dairy industry marketers have drummed into your head that you must drink milk in order to get your dietary calcium.

But consider this. The vast bulk of the world's population does not consume dairy products from cows. Therefore, you would think that multiple billions of people must be suffering from a calcium deficiency. The fact is that most of them are no more calcium deficient than you are. They simply get their dietary calcium from other sources. You can do the same.

You can get considerable calcium from vegetables, nuts, seeds, and some animal foods besides dairy.

In summary, dairy products are a very mixed bag. Until the health benefits of dairy products for PCOS and fertility have been convincingly demonstrated, we cannot recommend them as part of the healthy PCOS diet.

5.3 Guidelines for Eating Animal Protein

Here are some important points to keep in mind about protein in your diet.

Have Some Protein at each Meal

Some protein at each meal helps to ensure that you are getting enough protein for your needs. Protein at each meal is also important for regulating your hormones and preventing spikes in insulin production.

You might be concerned that the PCOS diet is asking you to eat too much protein. Remember that you'll be eating a substantial amount of vegetables and fruits. Also, your body will tell you in the unlikely event you're eating too much protein. If your liver and kidneys cannot process the amount of protein you're eating, you will get uncomfortable symptoms such as nausea, weakness or diarrhea.

We recommend that you visit your healthcare provider to be sure you do not have high blood sugar, or liver or kidney disease, before using the POCS or any other diet plan that emphasizes protein intake. You will avoid the above side effects and protect your liver and kidney by drinking enough water (a minimum of 2.5 to 3 liters daily) and consuming at least 40 to 60 grams of nutrient-dense carbohydrates daily.

Go Lean

As far as red meats are concerned, the leaner, the better. Trim off any visible fat before eating. However, some meats are "marbled," meaning the fat is mixed in with the muscle and can't be trimmed. You're advised to avoid any meat that is marbled with fat. But if you find yourself wanting to have meat with marbled fat, then at least let it cook long enough so some of the fat will be melted away.

The saturated fat from commercially raised cattle has been linked to health problems such as cardiovascular disease. The saturated fat in these animals is also high in a fatty acid called "arachidonic acid," which is pro-inflammatory if consumed to excess.

Go Range-fed

Most commercially fed animals are fed grains or agricultural byproducts in order to fatten them up.

One problem with these feeds is that they may contain petrochemicals, fumigants, fungicides, or pesticides such as DDT, PCBs and dioxins. They may also contain toxic metals such as cadmium or mercury. When livestock consume these pollutants, they accumulate in the flesh that you end up eating.

In addition, some of these livestock feeds are high in omega 6 fats and low in omega 3 fats, which cause the animals to have a higher level of omega 6 fats. Americans already consume far too many omega 6 fats and not enough omega 3. In excess, omega 6 fats are pro-inflammatory and contribute to disturbed cell function and a number of chronic disorders.

And finally, animals and poultry raised in large commercial facilities or feedlots typically are fed hormones and antibiotics. They are given hormones in order to make they grow or fatten up more quickly. They are given antibiotics because they are overcrowded and contagious diseases are always a threat.

In contrast, range-fed animals don't have any of these problems.

Go Wild

Wild game is quite low in fat, and what fat they have is of the highest quality. Wild game meat contains 15%-20% fat whereas a lean cut of commercially fed beef trimmed of visible fat contains 35%-40% fat, and some fatty cuts may have 65%-80% fat.

Cooking

Although more stable than other types of fat, animal fat will oxidize if heated to a high temperature. Oxidization creates unstable free radical molecules in the fat. When these free radicals get into your body, they create extensive damage and inflammation.

Cooking red meats at high temperatures produces charring and high levels of heterocyclic amines, which are cancerous.

Don't eat animal protein that is cooked with extremely high heat.

Section 6

Fats and Oils

6.1 What's a Fat?

There's hardly a dietary topic that is more confusing than fat. Many Americans have a mindset that fat is simply unhealthy and should be minimized. Saturated fats in particular have been singled out as unhealthy. We have been told to cut down on saturated fats in meats and consume products containing vegetable oil instead. Unfortunately, as food science has advanced some of this advice has been proven to be ill-founded.

We'll explore the issue of which fats are good for you and which are bad for you. But first, let's review what a fat is.

Fats are an essential food. You can't live for very long without fats. Fats can be either solid or liquid. They consist of one molecule of glycerol (just like the glycerin in a bar of soap) and 3 fatty acid molecules. These fats are commonly known as triglycerides.

Fatty acids are chains of carbon and hydrogen molecules of varying length and shape. They are the building blocks of fats, just like amino acids are the building blocks for protein. Different fatty acid molecules have different shapes, and that's why there are so many different types and forms of fats. The unique shape of each fatty acid determines the effect it will have in your body.

It's the fatty acid molecules that play such a crucial role in your health, including your success in dealing with PCOS. Fatty acid molecules are versatile because one end of the molecule is fat-soluble and the other end is water-soluble. They are an essential part of cell walls. They help to hold membrane proteins in place and play a role in the transport of nutrients and messages going in and out of the cell. Fatty acids perform a variety of vital functions in every cell of your body.

Some fats are absolutely required for health while others will cause serious damage. Whether a fat helps you or harms you depends on a number of factors:
- What kind of fat is it, and where did it come from?
- How has it been processed?
- Has it been exposed to light, oxygen, or heat?
- How old is it?
- How was it used in food preparation?
- How much was eaten?
- How frequently and for how long has it been eaten?
- What is the nutrient quality of the rest of your diet?

The fats and oils you eat will have a profound influence on your outcome with PCOS, including infertility, weight, insulin resistance and risk of diabetes and heart disease.

Fats provide critically important benefits to the body. They are:
- A crucial energy source
- Major components of cell membranes, and of the membranes of organelles inside the cells
- Required for your cells to function and to communicate

Important Note: The remainder of this chapter is pretty technical in places — but it provides helpful background information in case you're reading an article about fats or oils, or talking with your doctor about dietary fats, triglycerides or your cholesterol level. Since this is not a book about fats, we've provided rather skimpy explanations of an extensive and complex topic. If you don't understand something, just skim over it. If you want to really dig into the details about fats and oils, we recommend that you read *Fats That Heal, Fats That Kill*, by Udo Erasmus.

How Fats Are Categorized

Natural foods contain a combination of different types and proportions of fat. When scientists study fats, they tend to break them down into categories:
- Saturated or unsaturated
- Short chain or long chain
- Number of bonds

Saturated Fats

If you imagine the molecular structure of fatty acids as shaped like caterpillars, a saturated fatty acid would be a caterpillar with a relatively short, straight body. Their shortness makes them easy to digest and easy to burn in your metabolic engine. Butter and other animal fats are examples of saturated fats.

The term "saturated" means the fat is saturated with hydrogen atoms, which make it a more rigid, stronger structure. Therefore, they don't easily break down and become rancid.

Saturated fats are used for:
- Energy production
- Construction of cell membranes (providing rigidity)
- Source for conversion to certain unsaturated fatty acids
- Storage of fat energy for future use

Unsaturated Fats

Unsaturated fatty acids are like caterpillars with longer bodies that are bent. They contain a lower concentration of hydrogen atoms and are not as structurally strong as saturated fats. Unsaturated fats are much less stable than saturated fats, meaning that their structure can easily be altered.

Unsaturated fatty acids are used for:
- Construction of cell membranes (providing flexibility and fluidity)
- Generating electrical currents
- Attracting oxygen
- Conversion into hormone-like substances called eicosanoids
- Energy production (if not needed for other work)

Your body can manufacture some (but not all) unsaturated fatty acids as needed in order to perform necessary biological functions.

Common examples of unsaturated fats in the food supply are vegetable and seed oils, olive oil and fish oil.

Long Chain and Short Chain Fats

A long chain fat contains a longer string of atoms than does a short chain fat. The length of the chain of the fat will determine how it functions in your body. As needed, your body can make short-chain fats into longer ones.

Short chain fats are easy to digest and easy to metabolize. They are smaller and simpler than longer chain fats. Examples of short chain fats are butter, coconut oil and palm kernel oil. These fats tend to be used right away for energy.

Number of Bonds

Fats contain atoms that are "bonded" together by sharing electrons. (Electrons are tiny particles that circle around the atoms, just like the moon circles around the earth.) You can think of certain fat atoms as "holding hands" and thus forming a bond.

Some of the atoms in saturated fats have single bonds (holding hands with one hand). Unsaturated fats have double bonds (like holding hands with two hands).

Plants and animals can take a saturated fat and change it into an unsaturated fat by creating double bonds. The number and location of the double bonds will cause the fatty acid to have different biological effects. In the following chapter, we'll describe how this process works.

An unsaturated fat with two or more double bonds is a *polyunsaturated fat*. You see examples of these fats in the vegetable oil section of your grocery store.

A *monounsaturated fat*, such as olive oil, has one double bond.

Contrary to what you might think, a double bond is weaker than a single bond. And, the more double bonds there are, the weaker is the structure of the fat.

Cis- and Trans-Fats

"Cis" refers to the natural configuration of the double bonds in a natural fat. The "cis" configuration results in a fat molecule that has a bent shape. This bent shape allows unsaturated fats to do many things that saturated fats can't do.

In contrast, "trans-fat" refers to an unsaturated fat that has been "straightened out" by a special process called "hydrogenation." What you end up with is an unsaturated fat that behaves like a saturated fat, because it is straight just like a saturated fat is. We'll talk more about trans-fats in a bit.

Essential Fatty Acids (EFAs)

Certain types of unsaturated fatty acids are called "essential fatty acids" or "EFAs." These are essential for life and must be obtained from the diet; they cannot be manufactured by your body. EFAs are transformed by the body into eicosanoids, cellular hormone messengers that regulate many functions in all tissues.

If you have an inadequate intake of EFAs, or you cannot convert them into eicosanoids, it is impossible for you to be optimally healthy. That's why it's vitally important to know which dietary fats are good for you and which are not.

We'll complete the discussion of EFAs in the *Essential Fats and Eicosanoids* chapter.

Triglycerides

You may have heard about triglycerides, especially if you have a blood test and your doctor said your triglycerides were too high.

Most fats in our bodies are in the form of triglycerides. A triglyceride looks like 3 truck trailers backed up to a loading dock. The middle position prefers to hold an essential fatty acid. The two outside positions prefer to hold saturated fatty acids. However, if you eat a triglyceride from beef, the middle position will have a monounsaturated fat instead of an essential fatty acid. If you eat a completely hydrogenated fat, all 3 positions on the triglyceride will be saturated fatty acids.

Most triglycerides in your body come from eating fat in your diet. However, some are also created from excess blood sugar that cannot be stored into the cells. When there is no place left to store blood sugar, the liver will convert the excess into triglycerides, which are then stored as fat.

High levels of triglycerides in the blood encourage red blood cells to clump together, which decreases the ability of blood cells to deliver oxygen to your tissues.

Cholesterol

Not a fat, cholesterol is a hard, waxy, fat-like substance. It provides structural rigidity to cell membranes. It is also a precursor to the creation of steroid hormones (including your reproductive and adrenal hormones) and bile. There is some evidence that cholesterol may act as an antioxidant. Most cholesterol is created and broken down by the liver. Cholesterol is so important to life that nearly every cell in the body can produce it on demand; this is the cell's way to maintain stability of its membrane at all times.

When fatty acids and carbohydrates are broken down for energy, "acetate" is a byproduct. Since essential fatty acids are preferentially used for more important purposes than energy production, a high fat diet that is low in essential fatty acids will yield an especially high level of acetate.

This matters to you because acetate is the building block for cholesterol. So the higher the acetate level, the more pressure there is for the body to produce cholesterol. This often results in people who are on a "no cholesterol" diet, frustrated because they cannot get their cholesterol to come down. So they end up using medications like statin drugs.

By the way, as a side note, dietary cholesterol per se is not the cause of cardiovascular disease. Dietary cholesterol is not dangerous until you expose it to high temperatures. When you cook animal foods with high heat, the cholesterol in the food is oxidized. The oxidized cholesterol, which contains unstable free radical molecules, can cause damage to your cells. It's the overheating of cholesterol, not the cholesterol itself that creates a health problem. For this reason, we recommend you cook animal foods with a lower heat.

Hydrogenated Fats

Hydrogenation is the process of converting an unsaturated fat into a saturated or semi-saturated fat. This is accomplished by subjecting oil to high temperatures (248°-410°F) under pressure with hydrogen gas in the presence of a metal catalyst, usually nickel, for a period of 6-8 hours. The purpose of this process is to produce a "hard" fat from liquid oil by injecting hydrogen atoms and rearranging the molecular structure.

Complete hydrogenation. This is the creation of a totally saturated fat. Oil is saturated with hydrogen atoms so it will become stable and hard. This fat can be heated to higher temperatures before it begins to degrade. Usually made from coconut or palm kernel oils (which are 90% saturated to begin with), completely hydrogenated oils are used for specialty purposes, such as making chocolate. ("It melts in you mouth, not in your hand")

Partial hydrogenation. Here, the process of hydrogenation is not brought to completion. In other words, the "hardening" of the fat can be stopped at any point, depending on ultimate use of the product. Partial hydrogenation can produce a semi-liquid, plastic, or solid fat with unique properties of spreadability, "mouth feel" or texture, and shelf life.

Because hydrogenation is interrupted, there will be an unpredictable quantity of partially transformed fatty acids and other unidentified byproducts that may be detrimental to your health.

Transformed Fats - "Trans-Fats"

One of the partially transformed fatty acids resulting from hydrogenation is called a "trans-fatty acid." A trans-fat is similar to the original fat, only now an arm of the molecule has been twisted around and is facing in a different direction.

The problem is that trans-fats take up places in the body that were reserved for the original unprocessed fat. Trans-fats fit into the body's enzyme and membrane structures, but cannot complete the functions that the original fats are designed to do. This results in poorly functioning trans-fats blocking out the good fats that are essential for life; they take up space but do nothing helpful.

To make matters worse, trans-fats have a much higher melting point, which means they remain solid at body temperature and thus have a clogging, sticking effect in the body. This encourages fatty deposits in the arteries, liver and other vital organs. Trans-fats also make blood platelets stickier, forming small clots that float around in the blood. These clots can block circulation and slow down blood flow or even stop it altogether, causing a stroke or a heart attack.

Trans-fats alter the permeability of cell membranes, allowing undesirable materials to get in and letting molecules that would ordinarily stay inside the cell to leak out. This diminishes cell function and health.

Trans-fats do not have the same electrical properties that EFAs do. Therefore, trans-fats cannot participate in energy and electron exchange reactions that move your body chemistry along.

Trans-fats interfere with the conversion of EFAs into the highly unsaturated fatty acids found in the brain, sense organs and adrenal glands. Also, desirable hormone-like eicosanoids are not created, including those that improve arterial muscle tone, decrease blood pressure and prevent blood clots.

Are Trans-Fats a Threat to Your Health?

All of the available evidence suggests that trans-fats interfere with your ability to be healthy. They contribute to a host of metabolic problems. For example, a long-term study of 84,204 women conducted by the Harvard School of Public Health showed that consumption of trans-fats increased the risk of becoming diabetic.[157] The researchers said that simply replacing trans-fats with polyunsaturated fats would reduce diabetes risk by 40%.

In a companion study of 78,788 women, the Harvard researchers discovered that trans-fat consumption was associated with a higher risk of cardiovascular disease, especially among younger women.[158]

A third study of 823 women by the Harvard Medical School showed that consuming trans-fats was linked to increased systemic inflammation.[159]

Please bear in mind that women with PCOS have a higher risk for both diabetes and heart disease, as well as systemic inflammation. When you sum it all up, if you want to be healthy and get a handle on PCOS, trans-fats such as margarine are to be avoided like the plague. However, trans-fats are not always in obvious places such as margarine. In a study of pregnant women conducted by the University of British Columbia, 33% of the trans-fats consumed were in bakery foods, 12% in fast foods, 10% in bread, 10% in snacks, and only 8% in margarines or shortenings.[160] Nearly all of the unhealthy trans-fats were "hidden" in foods that we eat every day.

At present, there is no way for you to find out how much trans-fat is in processed foods or in foods that you eat at restaurants.

However, many food companies are reformulating their processed products in order to comply with future FDA regulations that will require trans-fat content be on the package label. Meanwhile, you can check the label for the terms "hydrogenated" or "partially hydrogenated." If you see those terms on a label, we recommend that you not consume that product.

Trans-fats may "naturally" be present in low levels in animal products.[161] They are the final metabolic products of livestock intestinal bacteria. This apparently results from overfeeding and the consequent passage of bacteria containing trans-fats into the small intestine. The bacteria are digested and the released trans-fats are deposited into the tissues and milk of the animal. In addition, livestock and poultry may be given commercial feeds that contain trans-fats. However, these natural trans-fats are a relatively minor health concern compared to the man-made trans-fats found in processed foods. Minimizing processed foods in your diet will minimize your intake of trans-fats.

How to Find Trans-Fats in Processed Food Products

Here's how to estimate the amount of trans-fats in a food product. First, read the label. If the product ingredients list contains the term "partially hydrogenated," then you know the product contains trans-fats.

Next, note the amount of total fat. Add up the grams listed next to each individual fat. You'll notice that the total of the individual fats is less than the grams of total fat. The missing grams are mostly trans-fat.

When only saturated fat amounts are listed and partially hydrogenated oil is the main fat in the product, the trans-fat amount is often equal to or more than the saturated fat amount.

Oxidized Oils

Unsaturated fats, usually found in the form of oils, have a much weaker structure than saturated fats. Unsaturated oils exposed to heat, light and oxygen will easily break down to form a host of toxic or "free radical" byproducts including ozonides and peroxides, hydroperoxides, polymers, hydroperoxyaldehydes, or cyclic monomers. The exposed oil is now "rancid" or "oxidized." It will have an "off" or stale smell to it unless it has been deodorized.

The amount of oxidized oils in your food supply is impossible to gauge with any accuracy. But you can rest assured that any food that contains unsaturated oils and is processed with heat, light and oxygen will contain some toxic residues. Of course, almost any oil that is extracted from seeds will have been exposed to heat, light and oxygen. That processed and oxidized oil is then exposed to further processing when a fabricated food is created.

For example, soybean oil is extracted from soybeans, using high pressure, which causes a great deal of heat in the presence of oxygen. The oil is now damaged. Your local baker adds the soybean oil to his dough. The dough is then baked under high heat for a considerable time, thus further degrading the oil. When you eat a donut or a few slices of bread, you don't really know the level of toxic byproducts you are ingesting.

Fats can also be oxidized inside your body. Remember that your body is warm and you are breathing in oxygen all the time. The oils in your body are exposed to this heat and oxygen and could become oxidized (turn rancid). It's OK for fats to be oxidized as part of the process of burning fat for energy. However, you do not want fats in the membranes of your cells to be damaged by oxidation. To keep oxygen in check, you have an antioxidant defense system that maintains a balance between too much oxidation and not enough. This antioxidant system depends on antioxidant nutrients that are derived from your diet. A few common examples of antioxidants are vitamins C and E, and the mineral selenium.

How Much Fat Should You Eat?

The amount and type of fat you need depends on many factors unique to you.
- Age
- Genetic tendencies
- Physical activity
- Physical environment
- Health status
- Your present fatty acid profile (deficiency vs. excess)

It's impossible to say exactly what percentage of your total dietary calories should be composed of fat. Popular diet experts have proposed percentages ranging from 5% to 30%. As a general guideline, we think it's OK to have 20% - 35% of total calories as fat — *if* they are **healthy** fats.

However, in North America and Europe, fats and oils make up over 40% of the 2,500 calories that an average human being consumes daily. This is 1,000 calories (110 grams) of fat every day! This is too much fat for most people. If you were building a log cabin in Alaska by hand, you would definitely need those fat calories. But if you're a sedentary office worker, you do not.

You should be especially careful with fats if you have insulin resistance or chronically high insulin levels. The University of Colorado recently completed a 14-year study of women with insulin resistance.[162] They found that a high-fat diet was a better predictor of weight gain than the amount of total calories consumed. If you are already overweight, and if you think you have insulin resistance, then a high fat diet may not be for you.

Keep in mind that if you're on a "low-carb" diet to lose weight, it's quite easy to replace the carbs with fat. We've noticed that some low-carb diets allow you to eat very substantial amounts of fats, including saturated fats. We do not recommend these diets for that reason.

Fat Grams vs. Fat Calories

Counting fat grams on product labels is good, but doesn't go far enough. A serving may consist of only a few grams of fat but when you look at the total calories of that serving, you may discover that the ratio of fat calories to total calories is quite high, making the food a high-fat, unhealthy food.

Remember, food manufacturers would prefer to put fat grams rather than fat calories on the label. Why? Because you would be shocked if you knew how many calories of fat you are actually getting.

For example, suppose you were to have one 28 gram serving of Que Pasa Tortilla Chips, containing 6 grams of fat, 19 grams of carbohydrate, and 3 grams of protein. You may think that this serving has a pretty low amount of fat — after all, there are only 6 grams of fat in the 28-gram serving. Based on grams alone, you would think the serving is only 21% fat.

But consider this: there are 9 calories in a gram of fat, but only 4 calories in a gram of carbohydrate or protein. So, our serving of tortilla chips is actually 38% fat, in terms of calories. Grams don't count — calories do!

When you eat processed foods, you often get a lot more fat calories than you think. This is one reason why the PCOS diet excludes most processed foods.

Is Fat to Blame for Obesity, Diabetes and Heart Disease?

A look into human history will help to answer this question. Quite a number of native or primitive cultures in the 20th century or earlier consumed a diet high in saturated fat. Yet they had very little heart disease, diabetes or obesity.

Moreover, heart attacks in Americans were almost unheard of at the beginning of the 20th century, but by the 1960s, heart attack was common — in spite of the fact that total fat consumption remained virtually the same during this period. How do we make sense of that? Has focusing on reducing fat and cholesterol in the American diet produced a healthier population? Clearly, it has not. Ongoing nutrition research is revealing the complexity of our situation, in which we have a highly manipulated food supply with a great deal of synthetic additives and chemical alteration of foods. These altered foods are not ideally suited to our internal chemistry. Chronic health problems are the result.

The American diet during the 20th century has undergone an astounding increase in the consumption of highly processed foods and beverages, many of which are laden with refined carbohydrates (sugars and starches) and refined vegetable oils. The processing has stripped away fiber and essential nutrients. It has degraded the proteins and fats naturally found in foods. Modern food technology has created "fabricated" food molecules that don't even exist in nature. Foods are contaminated with man-made chemicals and some chemicals are intentionally added for marketing reasons.

If you are focusing your entire attention on reducing fat in your diet, we believe you are misplacing your priorities. We think that fats *per se* are not dangerous to your health. However, if you consume the wrong type of fat, a processed fat, a man-made fat, a low-quality fat, then your health is *definitely at risk*. Of course, if your diet is overloaded with fat, even if it's "good" fat, your health may suffer.

Guidelines for healthy fat consumption:
- Eat fats that contain "essential fatty acids."
- Eat fats as they are naturally found — in the food itself.
- Avoid all processed fats, i.e., fats found in processed foods.
- Be moderate in your total fat consumption.
- Eat a variety of foods so you get a variety of fats.

We'll explore the reasons for these guidelines in the following chapters.

6.2 Essential Fats and Eicosanoids

There are two categories of unsaturated fats that are called "essential fatty acids" (EFAs). They are called "essential" because they must be obtained from your diet; you cannot manufacture them in your body. If you do not obtain these fats in your diet, you will become ill. Death from starvation is in part the result of a lack of sufficient essential fatty acids.

EFAs are transformed by the body into hormone messengers called eicosanoids, which regulate many functions in all tissues. If you have an inadequate intake of EFAs, or you cannot convert them into eicosanoids, fundamental biological processes necessary for health and well-being will not function. If you have an imbalance in the types of EFAs you consume, you will have a corresponding imbalance in eicosanoids. The inevitable result will be chronic disorders and disease.

To deal effectively with PCOS and infertility, and regain your overall health, you must pay attention to the types of fats in your diet.

Essential Fatty Acids (EFAs) and Your Cells

Essential fatty acids (EFAs) perform a variety of vital functions:

1. EFAs are involved in the creating life energy from food and they move that energy throughout your system.

2. EFAs attract oxygen. EFAs appear to facilitate the transfer of oxygen from your lungs to your red blood cells, which transport the oxygen to all parts of your body. EFAs then help move the oxygen from your capillaries, across the cell membrane and into special "furnaces" inside the cell where the oxygen is burned to create energy.

   They also appear to hold oxygen in the cell membrane, thus discouraging viruses, bacteria and other organisms from damaging a cell.

3. One of the EFAs helps to produce hemoglobin in your red blood cells which increases their capacity to carry oxygen.

4. EFAs are components of cell membranes and of membranes of sub-units inside your cells. They help maintain the structure of your cells by using their electrostatic attraction to hold proteins in place in your cell membranes.

   EFAs also increase cell "membrane fluidity." Because EFAs carry a negative charge, they repel each other and tend to separate. When you spill a tablespoon of vegetable oil (unsaturated fat) on the table, it will spread out. If you put a pat of butter (saturated fat) on the table, it will not spread out. The reason for oil spreading is that the molecules are repelling each other. This "spreading out" action in your cell membranes is what allows special channels, pumps and other biochemical mechanisms to function. Nutrients and messages can be easily and quickly moved in and out of the cell and the components within the cell.

5.   EFAs help you recover from fatigue. They facilitate the conversion of lactic acid into water and carbon dioxide. If you are on metformin (Glucophage) therapy, one of the possible side effects is a buildup of lactic acid. So if you're on metformin therapy, make sure you're getting your EFAs.

6.   EFAs have a universal effect on your health, including what happens with PCOS and all of its symptoms and future problems. A good way to appreciate the value of EFAs is to review the health problems that may develop if you don't get enough EFAs in your diet:

- Behavioral disturbances
- Edema
- Glandular atrophy (shrinking)
- Hair loss
- High blood pressure
- High triglycerides
- Impaired immunity
- Joint and tissue inflammation
- Kidney problems
- Liver degeneration
- Lower metabolic rate
- Mental deterioration
- Miscarriage
- Poor wound healing
- Neurological problems
- Skin disorders; dry skin
- Sterility in males
- Blood clot tendency
- Vision impairment
- Weakness

7.   EFAs are precursors to eicosanoids, as discussed below.

Eicosanoids

Eicosanoids are hormone-like substances that are made, and function, inside your body's cells. Unlike the hormones you've heard about (estrogen, insulin, cortisol, etc.), eicosanoids don't travel about in the bloodstream. They are created in the cell, go out the outer boundary of the cell, find out what is going on in the immediate vicinity, and then report back and tell the cell what to do. When their job is done, they self-destruct in seconds.

Eicosanoids have metabolic effects on your health that are every bit as powerful and important as the hormones you're more familiar with. You may not have heard about eicosanoids because everything we know about them has been learned under complex research conditions. There is no simple blood test through your doctor's office that can measure your eicosanoid status. However, medical research has established that eicosanoids have tremendous implications for your health.

Eicosanoids are divided into eight sub-groups. The most well known group is "prostaglandins." You or your doctor may have heard of them.

Eicosanoids and prostaglandins are commonly put into a "bad" (pro-inflammatory) or "good" (anti-inflammatory) category. What you want is a ***balance*** between the good and the bad eicosanoids, just like you want a balance between "good" (HDL) cholesterol and "bad" (LDL) cholesterol. (For example, "bad" LDL cholesterol is required to transport one of the EFAs in your blood, so without some LDL cholesterol, you would be in trouble). However, a chronic excess of bad eicosanoids over good ones will lead to degenerative disorders such as cancer, heart disease, diabetes, arthritis and depression.

"Good" eicosanoids have these actions:
- Inhibit platelet aggregation (blood clots)
- Promote vasodilation (expanding blood vessels for better circulation)
- Inhibit cell proliferation (cancer)
- Stimulate immune system
- Anti-inflammatory
- Decrease pain transmission

"Bad" eicosanoids have these actions:
- Promote platelet aggregation (blood clots)
- Promote vasoconstriction (constrict blood vessels for worse circulation)
- Promote cell proliferation (cancer)
- Depress immune system
- Pro-inflammatory
- Increase pain transmission

Dietary fats are the only source of essential EFAs that are needed to increase your "good" eicosanoids and keep the "bad" eicosanoids in check.

The Two Main Types of EFAs

The essential fatty acids (EFAs) we are concerned with are:
- Omega 6 fatty acids (linoleic acid)
- Omega 3 fatty acids (alpha linolenic acid)

The diet of nearly all Americans is way too high in omega 6 fats and seriously deficient in omega 3 fats. This imbalance occurs because of our over-reliance on refined, processed foods, especially altered fats and oils.

Each type of EFA has a complex metabolic pathway that results in very important health consequences. We'll briefly outline the metabolic pathways for the omega 6 and omega 3 fats below.

Omega 6 EFA (Linoleic Acid) Metabolic Pathway

Linoleic acid is found in fats throughout the food supply. However, it is most commonly found in vegetable oils derived from corn, soy, sunflower and safflower. Not only are these oils available in bottled form but they are used in the creation of hundreds of processed foods.

Anyone consuming the typical American diet will be exposed to very high levels of linoleic acid.

Here's what happens to linoleic acid in your body:

Step 1. Linoleic acid is converted into another fat called "gamma linolenic acid" or GLA. This conversion is caused by an enzyme called "delta-6-desaturase" or D6D. You can also get GLA directly by supplementing your diet with black currant seed, borage or evening primrose oils. This supplementation often temporarily relieves symptoms. Eventually however, supplementation interferes with the complex web of interactions involved with enzyme activity and the manufacture of GLA from the raw material of linoleic acid, so symptoms return.

Step 2. The GLA is then converted by another enzyme into dihomo-gamma-linolenic acid (DGLA). This conversion may be aided by calcium.

Step 3. We now encounter a fork in the metabolic road. DGLA is converted by enzymes into another fat called "arachidonic acid" (AA), or into anti-inflammatory "good" eicosanoid called PGE1.

This conversion process is handled by an enzyme called "delta-5-desaturase" or D5D. (D5D is not the same as D6D in Step 1). D5D is like a boulder in a stream that causes some of the water to go to the right, and some to go to the left. D5D diverts some of the DGLA down the "good" eicosanoid pathway, eventually resulting in the favorable PGE1 and similar eicosanoids. By the way, PGE1 improves production of hormones from the thyroid, adrenals and pituitary glands. It also inhibits the release of insulin from the pancreas. In other words, PGE1 would help dampen down any over-response of insulin to a meal.

D5D also diverts some DGLA down the "bad" pathway. DGLA is converted into arachidonic acid (AA). AA is then converted into pro-inflammatory "bad" eicosanoids such as PGE2, thromboxane A2 and leukotrienes. These unfavorable eicosanoids cause a great deal of trouble for the body.

For example, a small study conducted at Catholic University Medical School in Rome, Italy showed that ovarian tissue from PCOS women produced a higher level of pro-inflammatory eicosanoids (PGE2) than the ovaries of non-PCOS women.[163]

It is thought that you do not create most of the AA that is in your body. Some researchers think most of the AA in your body comes from eating flesh foods that contain AA. Examples are fatty red meats, egg yolks, and organ meats.

However, we should point out that arachidonic acid (AA) is not 100% "bad." It is one of the major fats in your body. You must have some AA. On the other hand, you can easily have too much AA in relation to the other fats, which tilts your body in the direction of inflammation and dysfunction.

As you can see, the D6D and D5D enzymes are critical for optimal fat metabolism.

Let's discuss these enzymes in more detail so that you can better understand why they are important to your health and managing PCOS.

The D6D Enzyme

The above metabolic steps are crucial to your health. Your cells simply cannot function properly without the creation of eicosanoids.

But there is a big problem in the metabolic pathway we just described.

Going back to step 1, you'll notice the D6D enzyme is required in order to proceed to the next step. However, D6D is a bottleneck in the metabolic pipeline. It will produce only a limited amount of GLA from the original linoleic acid. Therefore, you want to do everything you can to protect and promote the D6D enzyme. If you don't, you will have an eicosanoid imbalance and nothing can work right in your cells.

The D6D enzyme appears to be inhibited or blocked by these factors:
- Aging (the ability to make eicosanoids at age 65 is 1/3 what it was at age 25 - decline begins after age 30)
- Alcohol
- Caffeine
- Cancer
- Elevated cholesterol
- Environmental chemicals and carcinogens
- Genetic predisposition

- Hormonal abnormalities (insulin, catecholamines, cortisol, glucagon, thyroid)
- Hyperinsulinism (high levels of insulin - diabetes, high refined carbohydrate diet)
- Liver disorder
- Overabundance of alpha linolenic acid (ALA)
- Protein deficiency
- Radiation
- Saturated fat
- Smoking
- Stress hormones (elevated adrenaline, cortisol)
- Trans fats (hydrogenated vegetable oils such as margarine)
- Viral infection
- Vitamin and mineral deficiencies

As you scan down the above list, you'll notice that you probably have some of the factors that inhibit D6D. For example, many PCOS and infertile women have high levels of insulin and cortisol, an underactive thyroid, and high cholesterol. If you're on a low carb diet such as Atkins, you may also be consuming large amounts of saturated animal fats. So you may have several factors at play that are inhibiting your D6D enzyme.

Besides the above inhibiting factors, the D6D enzyme and other conversion enzymes need these co-factors if it is to function properly:
- Iron
- Magnesium
- Melatonin
- Vitamin B3
- Vitamin B6
- Vitamin C
- Zinc

Many women with hormonal and metabolic disorders have been found to be low in magnesium, zinc and vitamin B6. Women who have low levels of these vitamins or minerals will have impaired D6D enzyme function. This is one reason why a high-quality multi-vitamin/mineral supplement is often a good idea.

When you consider all of the factors above, you may realize that your health is impaired because you cannot create the GLA needed to create favorable eicosanoids.

There is very little GLA available in your diet. So you must have an effective D6D enzyme system in order to convert linoleic acid (which is plentiful in the diet) into GLA and thus create favorable eicosanoids. If the D6D enzyme system is impaired, it is likely you will develop a deficiency in PGE1, one of the good eicosanoids.

The D5D Enzyme

In Step 3 of the omega-6 metabolic pathway, the D5D enzyme plays a very important role. It will cause the production of either "bad" or "good" eicosanoids. The more active the D5D enzyme is, the more AA it produces, which is then converted into bad eicosanoids.

What causes the D5D enzyme to be more or less active? Insulin increases D5D activity, thus leading to more bad eicosanoids. Glucagon is a hormone that acts counter to the effects of insulin, including raising your blood sugar. Glucagon suppresses D5D. One of the omega-3 fats, EPA (eicosapentaenoic acid) will also inhibit D5D.

The PCOS diet is designed to help you reduce your insulin if it is excessive, and it provides good sources of the omega-3 fats. Thus the diet will help you to better control D5D and consequently reduce production of bad eicosanoids.

However, D5D is a rather "slow" enzyme, as is D6D. Therefore, the primary source of AA and bad eicosanoids may not be because of D5D activity. It is possible that much of the problem with eicosanoid imbalance comes from the over-consumption of commercially raised, grain fed red meats, which contain a lot of AA. This is one reason why we recommend that families eat meats from grass-fed animals or game meats as often as possible.

Omega 3 EFA Metabolic Pathway

Alpha linolenic acid (ALA) is a short chain omega-3 essential fat that is found in flax, hemp and pumpkin seeds, walnut, rapeseed (Canola), soybeans, dark green leafy vegetables and in some wild greens such as purslane.

Step 1. Alpha-linolenic acid (ALA) is converted, in a series of metabolic steps, into the long chain omega-3 eicosapentaenoic acid (EPA). Both the delta-6-desaturase (D6D) and delta-5-desaturase (D5D) enzymes are required for these steps to occur and for EPA to be created.

Please note that you cannot take the metabolic steps to create EPA unless your D6D enzyme system is working optimally.

EPA is the omega-3 fat that you have probably heard about — it is found in fatty fish and in fish oil. The nice thing about fish or fish oil is that you consume your EPA directly, allowing you skip Step 1 above and go directly to Step 2.

Step 2. EPA encounters a metabolic fork in the road — both forks are good. EPA can be converted into a series of favorable eicosanoids called PGE3. EPA can also ultimately be converted into docosahexaenoic acid (DHA).

You may have also heard about DHA, which is also found in fatty fish and fish oil. DHA is essential for the growth and functional development of the central nervous system (CNS) and brain in fetuses and infants, and is required for maintenance of normal CNS and brain function in adults.

DHA also inhibits the production of fat for storage and stimulates the burning of fat, which leads to lower triglycerides in the blood. Low levels of DHA are associated with increases in body weight.

The Relationship Between Omega-6 and Omega-3 EFAs

The omega-6 EFAs ultimately lead to both favorable eicosanoids (PGE1) and unfavorable eicosanoids via arachidonic acid (AA). The omega-3 EFAs lead to the favorable eicosanoid PGE3.

But the story does not end here. The two EFAs have a very complex interrelationship. For one thing, both the omega-6 and omega-3 EFAs compete with each other for the same enzymes, meaning that excessive consumption of one EFA will reduce the metabolism of the other EFA.

Moreover, a complex — but easily disrupted — series of metabolic events must take place for the dietary EFAs (omega-6 linolenic acid and omega-3 alpha-linoleic acid) to be transformed into eicosanoids. Their metabolic pathways have bottlenecks that reduce the amount and production rate of eicosanoids from EFAs. For example, just consuming more dietary omega-6 linolenic acid does not result in a corresponding increase in eicosanoid PGE1.

EPA inhibits the D5D enzyme. The higher the concentration of EPA in the diet, the more the D5D enzyme is inhibited and the less pro-inflammatory AA is produced. You'll recall that you can get EPA directly from your diet by eating fish or taking a fish oil supplement. Some EPA is also manufactured in your body from the omega-3 EFA, alpha-linoleic acid (ALA).

However, omega-3 ALA is an inhibitor of the D6D enzyme. This inhibition makes the formation of EPA from ALA more difficult. Therefore, if you want to get the greatest benefit from EPA, it will have to come from fish as opposed to vegetable sources rich in ALA such as flax. In other words, by eating fish, you are bypassing a metabolic bottleneck.

The second point is that you may have an impaired D6D enzyme system. In this case, consider eating more fish or taking fish oil so that you can bypass the omega-3 D6D metabolic step.

This is not all there is to know about metabolism of EFAs. If your head is already spinning from this much detail about EFAs, don't worry. The main point is that you need a dietary balance of omega-6 and omega-3 EFAs from a well-diversified diet of whole foods.

Why EFAs Are Important for PCOS

PCOS is characterized by an excess or a deficiency in one or more of these hormones: insulin, testosterone, cortisol, estrogen, progesterone, prolactin, follicle stimulating hormone (FSH), luteinizing hormone (LH), thyroid stimulating hormone and the thyroid hormones T3 and T4. In a serious case of PCOS, most of these hormones can be out of balance at the same time.

Essential fatty acids (EFAs) help your hormones do their job more efficiently. Here's how they do it. Once a hormone arrives at the cell's surface, it must find a "receptor" on the cell membrane that will accept the hormone. This is a like a lock and key system, where the key must fit properly into the lock in order for the lock to open. We said earlier that EFAs make your cell membranes more fluid. The increase in fluidity causes hormone receptors in your cells to change their behavior.

You might think of EFAs as "oil" you put into your lock to make it easier for the proper key to be inserted. Therefore, EFAs are important because they allow a smaller amount of hormone to get the job done. In other words, the proper amount and balance of EFAs should help you to reduce the excessively high levels of some hormones and to achieve an overall balance of your hormones.

EFAs and Insulin Resistance

Insulin resistance is a primary cause of PCOS and infertility.

There is now a range of evidence demonstrating strong relationships between the fatty acid composition of cell membranes and insulin action.[164] Improved insulin action is associated with:
* Increased proportion of omega-3 fats
* Less saturated fat
* Low omega-6 to omeaga-3 ratio
* Increased monounsaturated fats

Each of these four factors can influence insulin resistance. In combination, they may be even more powerful in reducing insulin resistance.

EFAs and Depression

Depression is a common symptom of PCOS. Omega-3 fatty acid supplementation (with fish oil) appears to prevent or relieve depression in susceptible people.[165] If you are depressed, consider increasing your omega-3 fats by eating more fish and possibly some cod liver oil or fish oil.

EFA Co-Factors & Metabolic Inhibitors

EFAs are the precursors for both "good" and "bad" eicosanoids. Whether the EFAs end up becoming good or bad eicosanoids depends to a great extent on "co-factors" and metabolic inhibitors which we listed earlier in this chapter.

Your diet, lifestyle, health status, environment, stress and levels of specific nutrients combine to have a great influence on production of good vs. bad eicosanoids. Remember that too many bad eicosanoids will make it extremely difficult for you to effectively manage PCOS or improve your chances of having a healthy pregnancy.

What is the Best Ratio of Essential Omega-6 to Omega-3 Fats?

Researchers and clinicians do not completely agree on this point. Some recommend a 4:1 ratio while others recommend a 1:1 ratio. The present ratio of omega-6 to omega-3 fats in the typical American diet is thought to be in the neighborhood of 20:1, which means that most Americans are consuming way too many omega-6 fats and not enough omega-3 fats.

The PCOS diet restricts the amount of omega-6 fats that you eat. The PCOS diet also strives to provide you with approximately the same ratio of omega-6 to omega-3 fats that most humans have been eating for thousands of years.

6.3 Other Fatty Information

This chapter covers a mix of topics and issues about fat in your diet.

Are Saturated Fats Bad?

Health authorities have told us that saturated fat contributes to cardiovascular disease and that we should eat much less of it. If this is true, how can it be that some French people consume more saturated fat than we do but have less heart disease?

The idea that saturated fat in animal meats is associated with cardiovascular disease, diabetes and other chronic problems, is supported by a lot of evidence; but interestingly, there are contradictory studies as well. For example, a number of native aboriginal cultures consume a traditional diet high in saturated fat, yet researchers find very little heart disease, diabetes or obesity in these communities (as compared to Americans).

We think that you cannot evaluate saturated fat in a vacuum. There are literally dozens of other factors besides saturated fat that contribute to heart disease, obesity, diabetes and other chronic conditions.

The flight of consumers from saturated fats into the arms of highly processed polyunsaturated vegetable fats has not resulted in a decline in cardiovascular disease, obesity, diabetes, cancer or any other health problem.

A recent study of 17 women with PCOS at the University of California at Davis illustrates this point.[166] After a 3-month habitual diet period, dietary fats were partly replaced with polyunsaturated oils for another 3 months. By the end of the study, their fasting blood sugar levels had risen from 76 to 95, and their glucose tolerance testing scores got significantly worse. However, their insulin and other hormones did not change, while other metabolic markers changed somewhat. Nevertheless, elevation of fasting blood sugar is by itself not a good thing.

This study shows that it's hard to generalize about fats. Later in this chapter, we'll discuss another study that draws a different conclusion.

Meanwhile, we should be cautious about "demonizing" saturated fats. Saturated fats provide a number of possible benefits:
- They are a source of energy
- They provide stiffness and integrity to cell membranes
- They protect the liver from alcohol and toxins
- They enhance the immune system
- They are needed to retain and protect unsaturated fats in cell membranes
- Some saturated fats are preferred reserve fuel for the heart
- They have anti-microbial properties

Butter vs. Margarine

Margarine is a Frankenstein-like product. The cheapest oils, already rancid, are mixed with a nickel oxide catalyst and then subjected to hydrogen gas under extremely high pressure and temperature. This process is called "hydrogenation," which is how an unsaturated liquid oil is turned into a saturated, solid mass. Hydrogenation yields a smelly, unpalatable gray substance that has emulsifiers and starch injected into it to give it a better consistency. This mess is then steam cleaned and bleached. Next, dyes and flavors are added to make you think you are eating something that is similar to butter.

The margarine hydrogenation process is somewhat uncontrolled, resulting in unpredictable and unknown fatty breakdown byproducts. Different batches of the same brand can have different contents. The fatty acids in margarine, because of their unusual structure, fit into receptor sites that were meant for EFAs (essential fatty acids). This interferes with critical enzyme systems and cellular membrane function. Margarine is a contributor to chronic degenerative disease including cardiovascular disease and cancer. There is nothing whatsoever in margarine that is healthy for you. Never use it for anything.

Butter is a mostly a saturated fat but it also has a lot more desirable monounsaturated fat. It has short chain fatty acids useful for energy production. But butter is high in cholesterol. Because it is a saturated fat, it can be used in cooking. Of course, butter tastes a lot better than margarine.

Butter is far superior to margarine. If you are deciding between margarine and butter, always choose butter, in moderate amounts appropriate for your activity level. Never choose margarine.

In some situations, you can use olive oil instead of butter for cooking.

Medium Chain Triglycerides

Medium-chain triglycerides (MCTs) are a class of fatty acids. They are found in coconut oil, palm kernel oil and butter. MCTs are also available as a supplement. They are more rapidly absorbed and burned as energy. In this respect, they resemble a carbohydrate more than fat.

MCTs increase calorie burning better than some other fats. However, a high level of MCTs may be required to make that happen. The evidence for using supplemental MCTs for weight loss or blood sugar control is not especially convincing.

Superunsaturated Omega-3 Fats

You can get the omega-3 essential fatty acids you need by consuming a mix of alpha-linolenic acid and fish or fish products.

Alpha-linolenic acid (ALA) is found in flax seeds, rape seed (Canola), hemp seed, soybeans, walnuts and dark-green leaves.

Eicosapentaenoic acid (EPA) and Docosahexaenoic acid (DHA) are essential fats that are found in cold water fish and marine animals. Salmon, sardines, mackerel and trout are common sources. Fish oil or oil derived from other marine animals will also provide EPA and DHA.

Polyunsaturated Omega-6 Fats

You also need some omega-6 fats in your diet.

The main omega-6 fat in your diet will be linoleic acid, found in most seeds and nuts. It's preferable that you get your linolenic acid from whole, raw seeds and nuts instead of from bottled oils.

The other omega-6 fat that we have already discussed is arachidonic acid (AA). AA is found in meats and other animal products. AA is the precursor to pro-inflammatory eicosanoids. There's no need to worry about getting enough AA. You will probably get plenty from your diet. Some individuals may need to restrict the amount dietary AA they have been consuming. Range-fed animal foods or wild game will be lower in AA.

Monounsaturated Omega-9 Fats

A monounsaturated fat is somewhere between a saturated fat (e.g., butter) and a polyunsaturated fat (e.g., vegetable oil). You can tell the difference when you put them into your refrigerator. Butter gets really hard. Vegetable oil stays as a liquid. Olive oil, high in monounsaturated fat, will be a viscous liquid, not quite hard but not quite free-flowing like vegetable oil.

The monounsaturated fat we are concerned with here is "oleic acid" (OA). OA is found mostly in olive, almond, avocado, peanut, pecan, cashew, filbert and macadamia nuts. Land animal fats and butter have some OA.

As with any particular fat, you can overdo it. Excessive amounts of OA may interfere with essential fatty acids.

Monounsaturated fats may be beneficial for reducing blood sugar and improving insulin metabolism, according to a study at the University of Kuopio, Finland.[167] After consuming a high-saturated-fat diet for 3 weeks, 31 individuals with blood sugar problems were assigned to either a high-monounsaturated diet, or a high-polyunsaturated diet for 8 weeks. At the end of the study, the monounsaturated group was significantly better able to process their blood sugar than the polyunsaturated fat diet group.

Another advantage of monounsaturated fats is that they may help you to burn fat. In a study at the Curtin University of Technology in Australia, twelve overweight postmenopausal women were given a meal that was either high in saturated fat (cream) or high in monounsaturated fat (extra virgin olive oil).[168]

Analysis five hours after the meal showed that the women who consumed olive oil instead of cream had a higher metabolic rate (thermogenesis) and were burning significantly more fat and less carbohydrate. A longer but similar study of men yielded similar results.

And finally, another study has shown that exercise has a different effect on monounsaturated fats vs. saturated fats.[169] This very interesting study of seven women (averaging 26 years of age) was conducted at the University of Wisconsin. The women were given different levels of exercise in the morning and then given a meal containing either a monounsaturated fat or a saturated fat. The women were monitored for the rest of the day.

The researchers found that women who had the monounsaturated fat meal and who exercised the most were the ones who burned off the most of the monounsaturated fat they had eaten. The women who exercised less or not at all burned less monounsaturated fat.

But what happened to the women who ate the saturated fat after exercising? Regardless of whether they exercised or not, the rate of burning saturated fat was the same.

This study suggests that if you eat more monounsaturated fat and less saturated fat, you can burn off more of the fat you eat rather than storing it in your fat cells. In addition, the amount of fat burned off increases as you increase your exercise.

The studies we've reviewed above suggest that you will benefit by including monounsaturated fats in your diet, including some olive oil and various nuts that contain monounsaturated fats.

Leptin and Canola Oil

In the *Evil Twins: Insulin Resistance and Leptin Resistance* chapter, we discuss leptin, a hormone produced by your fat cells that helps to control your appetite. We say that leptin needs to be kept in a normal range, not too low and not too high. Low levels can result in food cravings. Higher levels tend to suppress appetite but are also associated with tissues becoming less sensitive to leptin and thus contributing to craving and more weight gain.

An interesting study has shown that rapeseed oil (Canola) reduces leptin levels in women.[170]

A group of men and women were randomly assigned to one of three high-fat dietary treatments for four weeks: a diet high in olive oil (rich in monounsaturated fats), or rapeseed oil (rich in monounsaturated fats and alpha-linolenic acid), or sunflower oil (rich in omega-6 polyunsaturated fats).

On the rapeseed oil diet, the serum leptin concentrations of the women studied distinctly decreased. Both the olive oil and the sunflower oil diet did not affect serum leptin concentrations. The researchers suggested that the leptin levels were affected by the high amount of alpha-linolenic acid in rapeseed (Canola) oil. In contrast to the women, for unknown reasons, the serum leptin levels of the men studied increased slightly with rapeseed oil.

If you are insulin resistant and overweight, there's a good chance you're also leptin-resistant. In this case, foods containing monounsaturated fats and alpha-linoleic acid omega-3 fats (such as flax or Canola) may be helpful to you.

Fats and Blood Sugar

Some research has shown that the type of fat you consume will affect long-term blood sugar control.[171]

Long term blood sugar control is measured by the HbA1c (glycohemoglobin) blood test. It measures the amount of sugar that has attached itself to proteins in your red blood cells. This attachment of sugar to protein is called "glycation," and is an indicator of irreversible cell damage. People with blood sugar control problems have a high HbA1c. Chronically elevated blood sugar will result in excessively high insulin levels which contribute to insulin resistance.

HbA1c is higher in those people who consume high-fat diets. HgbA1c is also higher when a high ratio of saturated fat is consumed vs. polyunsaturated fats.

To better control your blood sugar, and reduce the need for insulin, intake of saturated fat should be kept at a modest level. Remember that saturated fat is not just found in meat. It is also found in processed foods that contain oils that have been converted into saturated fats by a chemical process.

Fats and Insulin Resistance

High-fat diets have been associated with insulin resistance, a risk factor for PCOS, infertility, diabetes and heart disease. The effect of dietary fat on glucose and insulin varies, depending on the type of fatty acid consumed. Saturated fatty acids have been consistently associated with insulin resistance. It appears that saturated, short-chain, and omega-6 fatty acids have the most undesirable effects on insulin action.

A number of studies show that saturated fat significantly worsens insulin-resistance, while monounsaturated and polyunsaturated fats improve it through modifications in the composition of cell membranes.[172] [173] [174]

A recent study has shown that shifting from a diet rich in saturated fatty acids to one rich in monounsaturated fat improves insulin sensitivity in healthy people. Replacement of saturated fat with unsaturated fat also reduces LDL "bad" cholesterol and triglycerides in insulin resistant individuals.[175]

Studies suggest that diets rich in monounsaturated fats (for example, olive oil) might be of benefit, especially for diabetics with insulin resistance.[176] A diet higher in monounsaturated fat appeared to provide an advantage over a fiber-rich, high-carbohydrate, low-fat diet on body fat distribution among diabetics. A high monounsaturated fat diet generates proportional body fat loss from both upper and lower body. In contrast, a fiber-rich, high-carbohydrate, low-fat diet resulted in disproportionate loss of lower body fat, worsening the ratio between upper and lower body fat distribution.

For purposes of reducing insulin resistance, replacement of saturated fats with monounsaturated fats is advisable. The most common monounsaturated fat you would be familiar with is olive oil.

Tropical Fats - Coconut and Palm

Tropical fats and oils include coconut, palm, palm kernel, cocoa and shea nut. These are traditional foods in some tropical cultures that have been consumed for centuries with no ill effects.

In this country, there has been a great deal of controversy as to whether tropical oils are good for you or bad for you. The argument has been that these oils are "saturated fats" and therefore contribute to cardiovascular disease. The idea that saturated fats in animal meats have been associated with cardiovascular disease, diabetes and other chronic problems is supported by much evidence, but not supported by other evidence. For example, a number of primitive cultures consume high levels of saturated animal fats but have low rates of cardiovascular disease compared to Americans.

As for coconut oil, it was used in the US prior to the advent of processing of vegetable oils, which are cheaper than coconut. There is a lack of convincing evidence to support the idea that coconut oil caused heart disease or any other disease, either in the U.S. or anywhere else.

Of course, any tropical fat will lose many of its health-giving properties when it is subjected to extensive processing. For example, palm oil is loaded with anti-cancer carotenoids. It also contains tocotrienols, a vitamin E-like substance that helps prevent cardiovascular problems and has myriad healthful benefits. However, these elements affect the appearance of these oils and are removed during processing in order to improve marketing appeal.

The unprocessed saturated fats in tropical plants do not appear to cause the same health problems that saturated fats in meats appear to cause. The reason may be because the molecular structure of tropical plant saturated fats is similar, but not identical to, the structure of animal saturated fats. Therefore, the biological effect may be different.

It is difficult to determine the quality of bottled tropical oils. However, fresh whole coconut is an excellent source of coconut oil.

What Fatty Acids Will You Find in Common Oils and Fats?

Most seed oils and animal fats have a combination of fatty acids. They are not just "polyunsaturated oils" or "saturated fats" only. For example, butter has about 500 different fatty acids. The table below lists the four basic fatty acids for common bottled oils and animal fats.

Oil	Saturated %	Mono Unsaturated %	Linoleic (Omega-6) %	Alpha Linoleic (Omega-3) %
Butter	66	30	2	2
Canola	7	61	21	11
Coconut	92	6	2	nil
Corn	14	25	60	1
Flax	9	19	14	58
Hemp seed	9	13	58	20
Lard	41	47	11	1
Olive	14	77	8	1
Peanut	18	48	34	nil
Safflower	9	13	78	trace
Soybean	15	24	54	7
Sunflower	11	20	69	nil

Of course, the relative percentages of fatty acids are only one factor in selecting a fat to include in your diet. Another extremely important factor is the quality of the fat, especially if it is a bottled oil.

6.4 Guidelines for Eating Fats

How much fat should you eat?

There is no "one size fits all" recommendation for the amount of fat you should consume. Every woman is biochemically unique. Health authorities, medical researchers and diet book authors do not agree on the amount of fat you should have.

Our impression is that most Americans consume too many calories in their diet and their diet is too high in fat. This means that most eat a large total amount of fat. However, we realize that many of you have already been dieting and may not be eating like the typical American.

As a starting point, we propose a fat intake of 20%-30% of total calories consumed. Since there are roughly twice as many calories in a gram of fat compared to a gram of protein or carbohydrate, the weight of fat in your diet would be about 10%-15% of the total weight of your food.

You might breakdown your fats this way:
- One third would be omega-6 and omega-3 essential fatty acids (EFAs)
- One third would be monounsaturated fats
- One third would be saturated fats

EFAs

As we said in the *Essential Fats and Eicosanoids* chapter, most people consume too many omega-6 EFAs and not enough omega-3 EFAs. However, our diet corrects much of this problem by removing some sources of omega-6 fats (such as most bottled oils and processed convenience foods) and recommending whole foods that contain omega-3 fats.

Even so, it's hard to say exactly how much omega-6 (linolenic acid) and omega-3 (alpha linoleic acid) fat you need. There is no "Recommended Daily Allowance" for these EFAs. The only way to know for sure is to get a fatty acid blood test. Meanwhile, focus on eating a variety of whole foods. Most of the foods in our diet contain some level of the EFAs.

We recommend you eat fish on a regular basis. If you don't like fish, consider taking cod liver oil or fish oil instead.

EFAs tend to stimulate metabolism. If you consume EFAs at the rate of 10%-15% of your total calories, you may increase the rate at which you burn fat and blood sugar. If you feel you have a sluggish metabolism, or need to lose fat weight, consider increasing your EFA consumption.

Monounsaturated Fats

You will find monounsaturated fats in our diet, including olive oil, olives, almonds, avocados, pecans, cashews, filberts and macadamia nuts. Animal foods will also have some monounsaturated fats.

Saturated Fats

Our diet emphasizes lean animal foods that are lower in saturated fat and cholesterol. For example, a serving of buffalo has 29.6 grams of protein and 5.4 grams of fat. In contrast, a comparable serving of beef sirloin (after the visible fat is trimmed off) is 30.1 grams of protein and 10 grams of fat.

We realize that buffalo may not be available in your local market — but you may be surprised if you live in the U.S. Grass-fed animals are known to be a better choice than a penned up animal fed with commercial livestock feed, and the consumer demand for these meats is growing. Bison is becoming a major market meat item in many areas. Ask you local grocery meat department to carry it for you.

Land animal fat contains longer-chain saturated fats that tend to cause your blood to be more "sticky" and thus not flow as well and more likely to form clots. In excess, they can interfere with the function of EFAs. So be very moderate in your consumption of land animal saturated fats.

In contrast, coconut, coconut oil and butter contain short-chain saturated fats that do not cause sticky blood, plus they burn more efficiently than longer chain saturated fats found in beef, lamb and pork.

Stay Close to the Source

The best way to get fats and oils in your diet is from the whole foods you eat. The worst way to get your fats is to eat highly processed convenience foods, fast foods, or to consume common vegetable oils found in your supermarket.

For example, eating walnuts is a better source of fats and EFAs than walnut oil or eating a Snicker's bar. The walnut also provides vitamins, minerals, protein, fiber and other important nutrients that aid EFA metabolism and improve your overall health.

In general, we advise you to stay as close to nature as possible when consuming fats and oils. Keep in mind that most fats are unstable when they are removed from their source food and exposed to light, heat and air. When a fat goes bad (rancid), it is very bad for you.

Minimize Bottled Oils

Most bottled oils are decidedly unhealthy and inappropriate for a person who wants to be healthy. You can understand why by knowing how the oil was created in the first place.

1. **Cleaning.** Oil seeds are mechanically cleaned.

2. **Cooking.** Seeds are cooked up to 2 hours at an average 120°C to destroy the cell walls that contain the oil.

3. **Extraction.** There are two ways:

   (3-a) Expeller Pressing. The seeds are squished in a continually rotating spiral-shaped auger (expeller press) similar to a kitchen meat grinder that pushes the seeds forward toward a metal press head. Under pressure of several tons per square inch, tremendous pressure and friction heat is produced, causing the oil to be forced out through holes in the side of the press head. The pressing process is completed in a few minutes under temperatures around 85° to 95°C. The higher the temperature and pressure, the better the yield of oil from the seed and the higher the profit.

   This oil is sold in health stores as "expeller pressed" or "cold pressed." Most processors do not exclude light and air, so the combination of light, air and high temperatures causes essential fatty acids to be destroyed.

   (3-b). Solvent Extraction. Oil is extracted from the seed by mixing and agitating seed meal with a solvent such as hexane at 55°-65°C. Once the oil-solvent mixture has been separated from the seed, the solvent is evaporated off and re-used. However, traces of solvent remain in the oil. Solvent extracted oil is sometimes mixed with expeller pressed oil and labeled as "unrefined" oil.

   Up to this point, the oil is still not acceptable to the supermarket consumer. The oil still has an odor, it is cloudy and it has a reddish or yellow color because it still has its original pigments.

4. **Degumming.** Valuable phospholipids such as lecithin are removed. Also removed are true gums, polysaccharides, and other valuable nutrients. The lecithin is packaged and sold separately to you in health food stores.

5. **Refining.** Caustic soda or other chemical compounds are used to remove free fatty acids, which indicate poor oil quality. Phospholipids, minerals and other nutrients are further removed. Refining occurs at 75°C.

6. **Bleaching.** Filters and activated clays are used to remove chlorophyll and beta-carotene pigments. This process produces toxic peroxides and essential fatty acids are further degraded.

7. **Deodorization.** The pressures, temperatures and chemicals of oil processing have by now produced altered oil that has odors and tastes that the original oil in the seed did not have. Therefore, the oil must be steam-distilled under pressure in a vacuum at extremely high temperatures ranging from 240° to 270°C (464° to 518°F) for up to an hour. The deodorization step removes the vitamin E, phytosterols and some toxins.

   The high temperatures in deodorization cause extensive rearrangements of the atoms in the molecules of the essential fatty acids to create fantastic, unnatural structures and shapes called "fatty acid breakdown products." Your body has absolutely no idea what to do with these misshapen molecules when they enter your body. Your body is looking for essential fatty acids that it must have — but gets instead something totally unusable, and must either try to get rid of it or store it someplace in your body.

   Finally, this oil can still be sold as "cold pressed" because no external heat was applied during the pressing of the oil. These highly refined, deodorized oils are found in the supermarket and some health food stores.

8. **Preservation.** Since the natural antioxidants beta carotene and vitamin E were removed, synthetic ones such as BHT, BHA, TBHQ, etc. are added to supermarket oils to extend shelf life and prevent rancidity. Defoamers are also added.

You now have a beautiful, shelf-stable product that is nearly devoid of nutrients and is loaded with toxic or unnatural processing byproducts. Wouldn't you rather just have some nuts or an avocado?

"High-Oleic" Bottled Oils

By now, you know that most of the bottled oils in the supermarket or in processed foods are not healthy. They typically include safflower, corn, sunflower, soybean and cottonseed oils.

But you may have heard about new "high oleic" oils that are supposed to be healthier. These are high oleic safflower and sunflower oils are higher in oleic acid, a monounsaturated fat that you also find in olive oil. These high-oleic oils come from hybrid plants. To the extent that these oils have more monounsaturated and less polyunsaturated fats, they are more stable and less likely to break down and become rancid.

However, as with any bottled oil, how do you know the oil is not damaged?

Acceptable Bottled Oils

Unrefined oils that still contain antioxidants and other valuable nutrients are hard to find.

The most widely available unrefined oil that is also not subject to tremendous heat during processing is "extra virgin" olive oil.

You may be able to find beneficial bottled oils in your health food store, including hemp oil or flax oil in opaque containers.

If a bottle of oil doesn't smell right, it's probably rancid and should be discarded.

The quality of bottled oils depends on the manufacturing techniques and quality control of the producer. It's difficult to judge the quality of an oil by its appearance, although if it is nearly colorless, that may suggest it is highly refined and therefore not a desirable oil.

After purchasing a bottle of any oil, break open 2-4 capsules of vitamin E and pour the vitamin E into the bottle. Vitamin E is a fat-soluble, powerful antioxidant that will help to prevent the oil from turning rancid.

Cottonseed Oil

Cottonseed oil contains small amounts of cyclopropene fatty acids, which have toxic effects on the liver and gallbladder, and at high levels, may interfere with female reproductive function. Cottonseed oil also contains high amounts of pesticide residues. Don't use cottonseed oil or consume any product that contains cottonseed oil.

Heated and Deep-Fried Oils

Heating of oils to high temperatures (320° F) creates toxic trans-fatty acids, cyclic fatty acid derivatives, cross-linked fatty acid chains, dimers, polymers of fatty acids, cross-linked triglycerides, bond-shifted molecules and molecular fragments.

Except for trans-fatty acids, there has been little research on the health effects of these fatty breakdown byproducts. However, you can rest assured that they do nothing to build your health. In fact, they may be as bad for you as trans-fatty acids, or even worse. These substances may cause fatty liver degeneration (discussed in our *Liver Health* chapter) or other liver problems, as well as cell damage anywhere in your body.

Frying with Fats

We're not fans of frying foods. But if you must fry some food, you can lubricate the pan with butter, lard or olive oil. Butter and lard can take more heat than olive oil without being damaged.

Part 2

The Healthy PCOS Diet

Section 7

Introduction to the Diet

7.1 PCOS Diet Levels

The PCOS Diet has two levels:
- Recommended level
- Maintenance level

You may choose the level that is most appropriate for you.

Recommended Level

The Recommended level diet is designed to help you:
- Balance your hormones
- Reduce PCOS symptoms such as insulin resistance
- Lose fat weight
- Improve your fertility
- Improve your basic health and vitality
- Increase your lifespan

To succeed with the healthy PCOS diet in this book, start at the Recommended level and stay at this level for at least one month. There is no maximum period of time you should stay at the Recommended level — you can stay at this level for several months, several years or the rest of your life.

The Recommended level foods are considerably more restricted than the Maintenance level foods.

At the Recommended level, you only eat foods on the "Best Foods" lists. However, if you unwilling or unable to restrict yourself to the "Best Foods," you can *occasionally* use foods from the "Good Foods" lists.

Maintenance Level

The Maintenance level is a more liberal diet that allows you a wider choice of foods but is still a healthy diet for most people. At the Maintenance level, you continue to eat foods mostly from the Best Foods lists, but you occasionally add foods from the Good Foods lists.

After you have completed at least one month at the Recommended level, you can decide whether to continue at the Recommended level or move to the Maintenance level. Every woman is biochemically and genetically unique. You may need to stay at the Recommended level for the rest of your life or you may be able to move on to the Maintenance level in a month or two.

If you switch to the Maintenance level and your symptoms or weight begin to return, go back to the Recommended level and remain there until you get the health results you're looking for before again attempting to move on to the Maintenance level.

Food Lists

Within each major food category outlined in this book, the healthy PCOS diet ranks foods according to: best, good and not good.

Best foods lists. Foods on these lists will provide you the best possible health results. While you are at the Recommended diet level, you will be eating foods on this list only.

Good foods lists. You can eat foods on the Good foods lists occasionally if you are at the Maintenance level of your diet. These foods are relatively healthy for the average person. However, some of them may cause you to regress. Every woman is unique, so we can't predict whether specific foods on the Good list will benefit you, have no effect, or cause you problems.

Try not to replace foods on the Best lists with foods from the Good lists. Foods on the Good list may be eaten on special occasions or once in a while. They do not form the daily core of your diet.

Unhealthy or possibly unhealthy foods lists. Some foods on these lists may not be appropriate for some women, while other foods on these lists should not to be eaten at all. If you are serious about dealing with PCOS, infertility, weight and your general health, view these foods with caution.

Each Woman Is Unique

There is substantial genetic variation among PCOS women. To get results, some will need to be at the Recommended level indefinitely. Others may be able to transition to the Maintenance level fairly quickly. Still others will be somewhere in between.

You will have to experiment to some extent to determine what Diet level or what mix of Diet levels works best for you.

Some women are slim. Some are obese. Some are in between. Slim individuals may benefit from the Recommended level of the diet. Other slim women may not need to be at the Recommended level at all.

Overweight women may have the biggest challenge. Some are "locked in" to fat-building mode because of insulin resistance. Others who are overweight have serious hormonal disorders that cause appetite dysregulation and binge eating. Overweight women will probably need to be at the Recommended level for a longer period of time. If they wander off into the Maintenance level or indulge in "bad" foods, they may get themselves into metabolic trouble.

Diversions from the Recommended level are OK but "your mileage may vary." For some, a diversion will have minor negative consequences. For others, if they have some cheese for example, they will feel like they have gained a pound.

The "Recommended level" is just that — recommended, not mandatory. If you are willing to settle for a more modest health result, you can include the Maintenance level foods and even occasionally indulge in the disallowed foods.

Diet Alone Is Not Enough - Exercise Is Essential

We should point out that diet alone may not be enough to effectively deal with your symptoms of PCOS. You will also need to exercise on a regular basis. Exercise is an essential part of your strategy to normalize your hormones and get rid of unwanted fat. Think of diet as your right leg and exercise as your left leg. You can't go very far or fast if you try to walk on just one leg. But if you use both legs, you can go much further and faster. Please see our *Exercise* chapter for additional information about exercise.

The Choice Is Yours

The PCOS Diet will ask much of you. You will be asked to completely revamp your diet and eating habits.

To a great extent, the outcome of your disease depends on what you do — or don't do. That includes what you eat. Your food is your medicine. Which "medicine" do you want to take? The one that is good for you, or the one that is not good for you?

There is no such thing as a totally convenient, totally easy health diet. You can't drop in at your local supermarket, restaurant or deli and pick up a completely healthy prepared meal that you can pop into the microwave or eat in your car.

A healthy diet takes commitment, determination and persistence. The path of least resistance is to eat packaged and prepared convenience foods or to mindlessly follow a simple "fad" diet. This path will inevitably lead you to heart disease, diabetes and a host of other chronic disorders that could end in a premature death.

The path of least resistance is not the path we recommend. We recommend a more challenging path where you create your own meals and diet plan — discarding unhealthy foods and replacing them with healthy ones.

The diet we recommend is neither easy nor hard. All it takes is focus and persistence. On a daily basis, make a steady progression toward a healthy diet.

Is this a "deprivation diet?" Depending on how you perceive life, it could be. For example, if you stopped smoking would you feel "deprived?" For a while, you might — until smoking is no longer something you think about and you don't miss it at all. In the end, you are glad you stopped smoking — you save money, your clothes and home smell better, you can breathe better, you have more energy and you've greatly reduced your risk of lung cancer.

We're asking you to do the same with your food. If you're like most Americans, you're habituated to eating unhealthy foods. On this diet you're going to stop eating them. At first, you may feel deprived because the new foods won't give you the taste pleasure or transitory lift you're accustomed to. But gradually you will get used to the new flavors and textures. Most importantly, you should begin to feel better, which will give you lots of positive reinforcement that you are on the right track.

Finally, please bear in mind that you have a serious disorder that is difficult to treat and cure. We are proposing that you use a healthier diet as a tool to take control of your PCOS symptoms, and reduce your risk for developing heart disease and diabetic problems. Your lifespan will also probably be lengthened . . . to say nothing of being able to get pregnant and have a family! So you have a lot at stake!

Our Promise to You

What is the definition of success or failure? The diet plan in this book is simply a way to eat that will "make good things possible." Our diet plan reflects the way we were genetically designed to eat, based on hundreds of thousands of years of human history.

This is not a "diet," as in "weight loss diet." It is a way of living — the way all of us lived until very recently. A wholesome diet and lots of physical activity is how we have lived since the dawn of human history. It is natural. It is what our bodies thrive on and are looking for. It is a diet that is harmonious with our being.

Our promise is to "make good things possible" if you follow the guidelines we've outlined in this book.

7.2 What to Eat

This book is not a weight-loss diet book where we tell you to eat "x" grams of protein, "y" grams of carbs, and "z" grams of fat. Nor do we tell you to limit yourself to "x" calories per day. Most of the popular diet books have a "one size fits all" approach. This approach does not work for PCOS.

Women who have PCOS are not a homogeneous population with a single problem. Some are extremely obese, some are very lean and many are somewhere in between. Some have insulin resistance while others do not. Some have serious multiple hormonal disorders but others have a less disordered profile.

Some can eat a lot of food and not gain weight while others gain a pound if they even look sideways at food. Some are binge eaters while others don't eat enough food.

Some will benefit from a very high-protein diet while others will not get any results. Some don't have the enzymes to digest milk sugar while others do. Some are on medications that alter dietary needs, but not all are. The types of metabolic problems will vary among PCOS women.

Moreover, your genetic pattern is specific to you. Other PCOS women will be slightly different. From the genetic perspective, a diet ideal for you is not ideal for the next woman.

PCOS women are located in every country of the world. The types of foods that are available vary greatly from country to country.

And some readers of this book are convinced they have PCOS but they actually don't. For example, some may have insulin resistance that generates some PCOS-like symptoms but don't meet all the diagnostic criteria for polycystic ovary syndrome. These individuals may have metabolic syndrome, "Syndrome X," or diabetes. (However, they can still benefit from the healthy PCOS diet).

As you can imagine, PCOS is an exceedingly complex collection of symptoms and disorders. It would be misleading to suggest that one specific diet or another would be the "right one" for all of you.

Guidelines - What to Eat

The diet presented in this book is a set of food selection guidelines, based on human history, volumes of medical research and years of clinical experience.

Within our guidelines, it's up to you to select the specific foods to eat and the specific amounts to eat.

Section 8 of the book, *Main Components of the Diet*, provides you with extensive lists of foods to eat. The most preferable foods will be found at the "Recommended Diet Level" in each major food category. Foods found at the "Maintenance Diet Level" may also be appropriate if your PCOS symptoms are not severe.

Above all, we want you to eat the healthiest possible foods. By healthy, we mean unprocessed and unaltered by human hands to the greatest extent possible. We can't emphasize this point enough. The evidence is overwhelming that a diet high in refined foods is bad for your health, which means it's especially unsuitable for a serious disorder such as PCOS.

Our guidelines do impose some rather severe restrictions. For example, at the Recommend Diet Level, we ask that you not consume any grains, dairy or beans. If you eliminate grains, dairy and beans, most processed products will automatically disappear from your diet.

You will replace the missing processed foods with vegetables, fish, poultry, meat, fruit, nuts and seeds. These foods provide all the dietary nutrition you need. Simply have a variety of these foods. Our 30-day Meal Plans and Recipes (see the *Meal Plans & Recipes* section) will give you some ideas for varieties and selection of food. If you are especially hungry at a particular meal, have extra vegetables.

Guidelines - How Much to Eat

Some women need to restrict their caloric intake more than others. Eat modest-sized meals. The foods in our diet are high in fiber, so you can eat a relatively large volume of food containing fewer calories as compared to an equal amount of processed food. Please do not eat less than 40 grams of carbohydrate daily. A range of 40 to 60 grams of recommended carbohydrate foods is an effective general guideline for most women using the diet plan in this book.

Use common sense. If you need to lose weight, don't eat a big handful of nuts just because they are on the diet. If you need to restrict your calories but have a big appetite, you may consume additional amounts of various vegetables from our Recommended list for vegetables.

7.3 What Not to Eat

Most of the foods you will find in a typical supermarket or food outlet will not improve your health. For the most part, they will actually impair your health. They should *not* be consumed.

"Convenience" Foods

Consumption of refined, processed foods is clearly detrimental to your health. These are also known as "convenience" or "junk" foods.

A convenience food is created when a whole food is refined, heated, extracted, extruded or otherwise processed and then combined with an unknown number and quantity of chemicals to alter the appearance, texture, shelf life, color and general appeal of the food. During the processing, most of the nutritional component of the food is destroyed.

Convenience foods are very easy to identify. They are almost always found in attractive containers such as cardboard boxes, plastic containers or plastic wrap. The food itself will have an attractive shape, color and texture. It may also contain ingredients to stimulate you to eat more.

Convenience foods may be purchased almost everywhere, in every market and in all fast food convenience outlets.

These foods generally have little or no nutrient value; they only provide "empty" calories. Your body must expend energy and stored nutrients in order to digest or eliminate these foods, thus resulting in a loss of body reserves.

Convenience foods present additional problems because they are likely to contain:
- Partially hydrogenated (altered) oils which disrupt cell membrane function
- Oxidized (rancid) oils which cause free radical damage to cells
- A variety of food additives that are unhealthy and which contribute to disease
- Refined carbohydrates that cause blood sugar fluctuations and hormone imbalances
- Toxic metals, pesticides, fungicides, petrochemicals, antibiotics, hormones
- Pathogenic microorganisms (bacteria, viruses, parasites)
- Excessive amounts of salt or sweeteners
- Genetically modified foods.

The presence of these items makes convenience foods something you don't want to put into your mouth.

The average American consumes about 9 lbs. of food chemicals and additives per year. This places a huge burden on your detoxification system. If you cannot detoxify these substances, they will take up permanent residence in your body and lead to degenerative disease.

Regular consumption of unhealthy convenience foods can lead to allergy problems, skin disorders, migraine headaches, gastrointestinal disorders, fatigue, nausea, depression, hyperactivity and a host of other disorders.

To better control PCOS and regain your health, stay completely away from refined, highly processed "convenience" foods.

Oily, Fatty Foods

Most of the foods we eat contain highly processed, heated, oxidized or chemically altered oils and fats that seriously interfere with cell function, contain unknown byproducts of processing, and directly damage cells, including their DNA. These toxic oils and fats are sold "as is" or may be hidden in a wide variety of food products.

For a more complete understanding of this complex but important subject, please read *Fats That Heal, Fats That Kill: The Complete Guide to Fats, Oils, Cholesterol and Human Health* by Udo Erasmus.

In addition to their toxic effects, oily or fatty foods affect your circulation. Recent scientific studies have shown that the heart has to work almost twice as hard during exercise after a high-fat meal as after a high starch meal. Fat not only interferes with utilization of oxygen, but also requires twice as much oxygen for its breakdown into energy as compared to protein or carbohydrate. Reducing dietary fat helps to increase the ability of our blood to carry oxygen to all of our tissues.

Sugary Foods

In addition to fats and oils, most of the foods we commonly eat are laden with sweeteners such as sugar or corn syrup. Incredibly, the average American consumes an estimated 150-170 lbs. of sweeteners per year, nearly 1/2 lb. per day! This is perhaps five times the amount of sweeteners consumed a century ago. Sweeteners and refined carbohydrates such as white bread and breakfast cereals cause blood sugar fluctuations that in turn create chronic hormonal imbalances.

Foods to Avoid Lists

In following chapters, we have lists of specific "unhealthy" foods in each of the major food categories. Please avoid these foods.

The unhealthy foods listed in these chapters are most likely part of your diet. In fact, the unhealthy foods on our lists may form the core of your diet. By asking you to stop eating these foods, we are turning your dietary habits upside down. Please consider that these foods are a major cause of your present health problems. To improve your health, you need to improve your diet first.

For example, wheat products such as bread, bagels, crackers, cookies and other baked wheat products are on our "do not eat" list. It's likely you eat some of these products on a daily basis. Baked wheat products have several problems because they:

1. Can quickly elevate your blood sugar beyond acceptable levels and trigger an unhealthy hormonal response because they have sugars and refined flour

2. Contain oils which have been subjected to oxygen and high temperatures, converting them into unstable free radicals which damage your cells

3. Contain gluten (gliadin) proteins to which you may be sensitive, thus causing damage in your GI tract and other health problems.

You may feel temporarily deprived because we are taking away refined grains as a staple of your diet. But we provide you with plenty of alternatives. Gradually you'll become accustomed to the new foods and not think about how much you miss a slice of bread or a fresh pastry.

We acknowledge that you are moving from the familiar to the unfamiliar. We're asking you to change lifelong habits. This can be challenging, but it won't be too long before you have established new, healthier dietary habits. Be patient. Be persistent. You will be successful!

Section 8

Main Components of the Diet

8.1 Meats

Best Meats for Recommended Diet Level

These are the meats on the Best Foods list.

Beef
- Any cut (except ribs), range fed only, all visible fat trimmed off
- Beef liver - free range fed only or organic only
- Ground beef - free range fed only, 90%-95% lean

Other Meats
- Buffalo - any cut
- Rabbit
- Goat

Game Meats
- Alligator
- Antelope
- Bear
- Caribou
- Deer
- Elk
- Frog legs
- Kangaroo
- Pig (wild)
- Reindeer
- Snake
- Any wild game

Good Meats for Maintenance Diet Level

You may occasionally eat the following meats from the Good Foods list if you are not on at the Recommended diet level.

Lean Beef, commercially fed, all visible fat trimmed off
- Chuck steak
- Filet mignon
- Hamburger (95% lean only)
- London broil (flank steak)
- Roast beef (top round or rump)
- Round steak
- Sirloin

- Tenderloin
- Veal
- Any other lean cut

Lean Pork (all visible fat trimmed off)
- Chops
- Ham, lean, boiled
- Loin
- Any other lean cut

Lean Lamb (all visible fat trimmed off)
- Chop
- Leg
- Roast

Organ Meats - (Free-range, organic only)
- Livers - beef, lamb, pork, chicken
- "Sweetbreads" (thymus gland or pancreas) - beef, pork, lamb

Unhealthy Meats - Avoid

- Bacon
- Bologna
- Corned beef
- Hamburger (less than 90% lean)
- Honey turkey
- Hot dogs (any kind)
- Jerky (unless free of salt and preservatives)
- Liverwurst
- Pastrami
- Pork sausage
- Ribs - pork or beef
- Salami
- Tongue, beef
- Veal
- Any lunch meats or processed meats
- Any meat containing substantial visible marbled fat

Notes

Bacon, Lunchmeats, Sausage, and other Cured Meats. Bacon and other cured meats provide the highest source of nitrites in the diet. Used as a food preservative, nitrites are converted into carcinogenic nitrosamines in the body. It is known to produce stomach cancer and possibly other cancers. Bacon and cured meats are mostly fat. Bacon and sausage are usually subjected to very high heat to get the desired result. High-heat cooking oxidizes the fats, thus creating free radicals that damage your cells. Some cured or processed meats have additional food additives that are harmful to your health.

Ground Beef. Buy the leanest ground beef you can find. However, be aware of what is meant by "lean." Although a steak or other cut of beef labeled "lean" must have no more than 10% fat by weight, and "extra lean" no more than 5% by weight, these standards do not apply to ground meat. Raw ground beef labeled 75% lean is 25% fat by weight. That's a lot of fat! Raw "lean" ground beef is, on average, 21% fat by weight. Raw "extra lean" ground beef is, on average, 17% fat by weight — still a lot of fat. Look for ground beef that says "95% lean," which suggests it is only 5% fat.

The surest way to get the leanest ground beef is to buy a cut of very lean beef and have your butcher trim off all fat and then grind it (or you can grind it at home with a meat grinder or food processor).

After cooking ground beef, blot it on paper towels (30 seconds on each side) to remove surface fat. If it is crumbled, you can rinse it in a strainer or colander to remove even more fat. While draining and rinsing beef can dramatically reduce the amount of fat it contains, the protein, iron, zinc and vitamin B-12 content is not significantly affected.

How Beef is Graded. Beef is graded by the U.S. Dept. of Agriculture (USDA) according to its "desirability." You will want the lowest and cheapest grade (which is the "Select" grade) because it is lowest in fat.
- Prime Beef: This is the most expensive and contains the most fat. Restaurants buy this and it is typically not available in grocery stores.
- Choice Beef: The second most expensive and contains the second highest levels of fat.
- Select Beef: This is the most economical and contains the least fat (compared to the same cut that is graded Choice or Prime).

Some markets do not have their meat graded by the USDA. However, they may indicate on the label which cuts are "lean" (not more than 10% fat) or "extra lean" (not more than 5% fat).

Grass-fed Beef. Pasture-fed cattle not only have a lower fat content, they also tend to have higher levels of conjugated linoleic acid, or CLA. CLA has been shown to have an anti-cancer action and there is some suggestion it is helpful for weight loss. Pasture-fed cattle may also be lower in pesticides or other pollutants.

8.2 Seafood

Seafood, especially fish, is an excellent source of protein. Fish are your best dietary source of highly beneficial omega 3 fats.

Best Fish and Seafood for Recommended Diet

- Barracuda
- Bass
- Bluefish
- Clams
- Clams (from unpolluted area)
- Cod
- Crab
- Crayfish
- Drum
- Eel
- Flounder
- Grouper
- Haddock
- Hake
- Halibut (higher in desirable omega 3 fats)
- Herring (higher in desirable omega 3 fats)
- Lobster
- Mackerel, Pacific (higher in desirable omega 3 fats)
- Mahi mahi
- Monkfish
- Mullet
- Mussels (from unpolluted area)
- Northern pike
- Octopus
- Orange roughy (higher in desirable omega 3 fats)
- Perch
- Pickerel
- Pollack
- Pompano
- Porgy
- Rockfish
- Salmon
- Sardines (higher in desirable omega 3 fats)
- Scallops
- Scrod

- Sea trout
- Shad
- Shark
- Shrimp
- Smelt
- Snapper
- Squid (calamari)
- Striped bass
- Sturgeon
- Sunfish
- Tilapia
- Trout
- Turbot
- Walleye
- Whitefish
- Whiting
- Yellowtail
- Any other fish

Good Fish and Seafood for Maintenance Diet

- Same as for Recommended Diet
- Tuna, in moderation

"Possibly" Unhealthy Fish and Seafood - Use Caution

- Catfish (domestic)
- Caviar (domestic, China)
- Croaker (may be high in pesticides in some areas)
- Mackerel, Atlantic (may be high in pesticides)
- Oysters (may be high in pesticides in some areas)
- Shark, except possibly Thresher shark (may be high in pesticides)
- Swordfish (may be high in mercury)
- Tilefish (may be high in pesticides in some areas)
- Trout (farm-raised; some areas of eastern US)
- Tuna (may be high in pesticides or mercury)

Notes

It's difficult to assess the risk of eating the fish and seafood listed above in the "possibly" unhealthy section. In general, we think you're better off with fish caught in unpolluted waters.

Large fish at the top of the food chain. Swordfish, and to some extent tuna and shark, may be high in mercury, pesticides or other pollutants. It has not been conclusively proven that mercury found in these fish is a major threat to your health. Tuna and shark are OK in moderation and if you are not pregnant. Although large fish are an excellent food, they are at the top of a polluted food chain and tend to accumulate more chemicals than smaller fish.

Fish and seafood from contaminated areas. Some parts of our coastline, and many lakes and rivers are badly polluted. Fish from these waters may not be safe to eat. Check with your local health authorities about which bodies of water near you are unsafe. Any fish or seafood harvested from such areas will have higher levels of unhealthy chemicals or toxic metals.

Farmed fish. Some commercial oyster beds or fish farms may be located in areas polluted with chemicals or toxic metals. Also, farmed fish may be exposed to feeds that contain pesticides or other chemicals. These harmful materials could end up in your farmed seafood. Farmed seafood includes salmon, catfish, tilapia, trout and some shrimp.

Raw fish. Avoid eating raw fish in order to reduce exposure to parasites.

Canned fish. Canned fish is OK, but not as good as fresh or frozen fish. Some canned fish, such as tuna, is cooked in the can at very high temperatures, sufficient to cause some oxidation of the cholesterol and fats in the fish. These oxidized free radical molecules cause cell damage in your body.

When buying canned fish, try to find it without salt, packed in water instead of oil. The added oil is high in omega 6 fats, which are undesirable. If the fish is canned with water and salt, you can rinse the salt off.

Shopping. When buying fish, the nose knows. If it smells fishy, it's not fresh. If buying a whole fish, look for clear, bright, bulging eyes; bright, shiny skin with tightly attached scales; and bright red gills and flesh that springs back slightly when pressed. Fillets should show no trace of browning or drying around the edges. When buying frozen fish, choose packages that feel solid.

8.3 Poultry

Poultry is a good source of protein.

Best Poultry for Recommended Diet Level

- Chicken breast
- Game birds: turkey, pheasant, goose, duck, pigeon, quail, partridge, grouse, etc.
- Ostrich
- Pheasant (available in some supermarkets)
- Turkey

Good Poultry for Maintenance Diet Level

- Chicken thighs
- Cornish game hen (remove skin before eating)
- Duck (remove skin before eating)
- Goose (remove skin before eating)

Unhealthy Poultry - Avoid

- Breaded chicken
- Chicken nuggets
- Chicken roll
- Chicken wings
- Deep fried chicken
- Fried chicken
- Honey turkey
- Turkey roll

Notes

Poultry Guidelines

1. Breast meat of poultry is preferable because it is lower in fat than thighs, legs and wings. Wings in particular have little meat and lots of fatty skin and should be avoided.

2. Always remove the skin before eating.

3. Don't have commercially raised goose or duck except for special occasions. These birds have a lot of fat.

4. Buy free-range, organic chicken, if available.

5. Avoid packaged, processed poultry meats.

6. Avoid deep fried chicken in restaurants, especially fast-food outlets.

7. You can bake, broil, grill, boil or stir-fry poultry — just don't fry or deep fry it.

8. After baking or broiling a whole bird, put it on some paper towels to let the excess fat drip off.

Cooking of Game Birds

Because it is so lean, game meat can become dry and leathery when cooked. Cook game birds slowly with relatively low heat in a covered container with some water in it to maintain moisture. Rub the birds with olive oil before cooking. While cooking, baste several times with oils or oil-based marinades or sauces. Cooking your game bird this way will make it more moist and tender.

8.4 Eggs

Eggs are an excellent source of protein and are more easily digested than muscle meats. Eggs also contain important nutrients besides protein.

Best Eggs for Recommended Diet Level

- "Omega 3" eggs - higher levels of beneficial omega 3 fats (available in some markets)
- Free range or organic eggs (available in some markets)

Good Eggs for Maintenance Diet Level

- Regular eggs if you cannot find Omega 3 or free range eggs

Unhealthy Eggs - Avoid

- Egg substitutes
- Omelets in restaurants - too much fat and oxidized cholesterol
- Scrambled eggs in commercial buffets or in restaurants, unless you can verify they are made from fresh eggs (many are made from cheap, unhealthy spray-dried eggs)

Notes

Egg Guidelines

1. Hard boil, soft boil, or poach most of your eggs.

2. Frying or scrambling of eggs is not recommended. But if you do fry or scramble, use the lowest heat possible, even if it takes longer.

3. Avoid omelets unless they are made without cheese. Use the lowest possible heat when cooking.

4. Eat eggs in moderation. Consider having less than 6 eggs a week. Before the advent of agriculture, man did not eat many eggs since they were only seasonally available.

Egg Quality Guidelines

1. You can minimize your exposure to antibiotics, hormones and viruses by finding stores that offer eggs from free-range chickens. Check the box to make sure the eggs are free range and organic.

2. Don't consume an egg if there is a crack in the shell. You can determine this by immersing the egg in a pan of cool water. If the egg emits a tiny stream of bubbles, there is a hole or crack.

3. If the egg white is watery instead of gel-like or the yolk is not upright and firm or easily bursts, the egg is not fresh and shouldn't be eaten.

4. Discard any eggs that have a smell.

Raw Eggs vs. Cooked Eggs

Cooked eggs have some distinct disadvantages: vital nutrients are destroyed if eggs are heated and the protein can be damaged and altered in a way that can cause an egg allergy.

Another big problem with cooked eggs is cholesterol. You probably have avoided eggs because you've been told they are very high in cholesterol and therefore may cause heart disease. However, you must draw a distinction between natural (uncooked) and oxidized cholesterol (cooked).

We are not aware of any studies that established a causal link between uncooked cholesterol and heart disease. It is cooked or "oxidized" cholesterol that has been linked to heart disease. When natural cholesterol is heated, its chemical composition is changed and it becomes a reactive agent that may cause free radical damage and other problems inside your body. The more you heat it, the worse it gets. (The same is true for any fat or oil.)

Therefore, if you are going to cook an egg, use the lowest possible heat and try not to expose too much of the egg yolk to the air. Frying or scrambling eggs exposes much of the egg's surface to both heat and air, thus oxidizing the cholesterol. In contrast, poaching or slowly boiling the egg with low heat keeps it intact and thus it has less exposure to both heat and air.

If you want to preserve the egg's nutrients, the best way to eat it is raw. However, we understand you may find eating a raw egg disagreeable. You may also be concerned about salmonella infection. Salmonella are pathogenic bacteria that can make you feel sick. The risk of salmonella infection appears to be quite low.[177] Less than 1% of the U.S. egg supply is infected. If you are going to eat a raw egg, dip the shell into a mild solution of Clorox and water before you crack the egg open. This will further reduce your possible exposure to salmonella.

Eggs and chicken from agricultural "factories" are more likely to have salmonella, as well as antibiotics or growth hormone.

The antibiotics are necessary because of rampant infection in U.S. flocks caused by the birds being raised in close quarters. However, while antibiotics stop bacteria, they do not stop viral infections. Much of the U.S. chicken flock is virally infected. Therefore, eggs from free-range chickens are preferred.

Nutritional Notes

Biotin
Eggs are exceptionally rich in biotin, one of the B-vitamins. Increased biotin helps PCOS women in two ways.

First, biotin is important for hair growth and health. If you're having a problem with hair loss, biotin can help.

Second, biotin appears useful if you're having trouble with glucose (blood sugar).[178] [179] Biotin causes improvements in disordered glucose metabolism by stimulating glucose-induced insulin secretion by the pancreas and by improving glucose handling by liver and pancreas. Animal studies suggest that a high biotin diet improves the metabolism and utilization of glucose without increasing insulin levels. A deficiency of biotin results in impaired glucose tolerance.

Lutein
Eggs provide the most bioavailable source of lutein,[180] a yellow pigment that belongs to the carotenoid family (beta carotene is another carotenoid you may be familiar with).

Not only is lutein critical for eye health, it also appears to play a role in ovarian function. Originally, lutein was isolated from the corpus luteum, hence the name "lutein." The corpus luteum of the ovaries contains high concentrations of lutein and other carotenoids. The role of carotenoids in the ovaries is not entirely clear, although they may be involved in protection against free radicals. One study has noted that women with more consistent levels of carotenoids were more likely to become pregnant with in-vitro fertilization (IVF) than women who had more varying levels of carotenoids.[181]

Dr. Peter D'Adamo[182] has this to say about lutein and the ovaries: "Lutein especially, has been shown to decrease the amount of cystic formation on the ovary by its antioxidant abilities. The female ovary is a very metabolically active organ, and the follicles must cut their way out when a woman ovulates, by secreting an enzyme to bore a hole to the exterior."

"Normally there is quite a bit of lutein in the ovarian tissue to snuff out the inflammation that results. If not, the tissue becomes cystic. It is interesting to note that lutein is the yellow pigment in plants (lutea is Latin for "yellow"). Many tissues which are metabolically unstable, such as the retina of the eye ("macula lutea") and the ovulatory product ("corpus luteum") are yellow from the deposition of lutein."

"Unhealthy ovaries tend to be whitish colored at autopsy because of an inability to deposit lutein or an inadequate amount in the diet."

Cholesterol in Egg Yolks

Some people are obsessed about avoiding egg yolks because they contain cholesterol. The concept is that if you eat cholesterol, your blood cholesterol will go up and you will get cardiovascular disease. Therefore, these people strictly avoid eggs. However, the evidence for this viewpoint is inconclusive.

The fact is that some people are "sensitive" to dietary cholesterol while others are not. In other words, some people can eat many eggs and their cholesterol does not go up. On the other hand, other people can eat a few eggs and experience an increase in their cholesterol level.

8.5 Dairy Products

Until the health benefits of dairy products for PCOS have been conclusively proven, we cannot recommend them as part of the PCOS diet. What dairy products should you eat?

Best Dairy for Recommended Diet Level

- No milk
- No dairy products of any kind
- No foods containing dairy products

Good Dairy for Maintenance Diet Level

We do not recommend dairy products for the reasons outlined in *The Problem With Milk* chapter.

However, we recognize that some individuals feel they cannot live unless they have some dairy in their diet. If you are one of these individuals, and if your PCOS and fertility symptoms are no longer a serious problem, you could consume the following the foods listed here and also listed in the Maintenance Level section.

These dairy products should be consumed in moderation and only occasionally. Consider them as condiments or accessories to your diet, not to be consumed every day.

- Butter (for cooking only)
- Feta cheese
- Kefir
- Lite Swiss cheese
- Low-fat yogurt (non-sweetened)
- No-fat cottage cheese
- No-fat ricotta cheese
- Parmesan cheese (1 tablespoon or less per serving)
- Whey protein powder

Unhealthy Dairy - Avoid

- Bavarian cream
- Butter (except for cooking)
- Butter sauces
- Buttermilk
- Cheese (most)
- Cocoa drinks and mixes
- Cream
- Evaporated/condensed milk
- Half & half
- Hydrolyzed protein (may contain milk proteins - read the label)
- Ice cream
- Malted milk
- Milk
- Milk chocolate
- Sour cream
- Whipped cream
- Yogurt, sweetened
- Skim milk.

A large number of foods also contain milk or milk proteins. Read food labels carefully, especially for the words "casein" or "caseinate," which are milk proteins commonly found in food products. If you're in a restaurant, ask your server if there are any dairy products in the food you are ordering.

Here is a list of foods that usually contain milk or milk proteins. Check the labels when possible. If these foods contain milk or milk proteins, add them to your "always avoid" list. Many of these foods are also unhealthy for other reasons besides containing milk.

- Au gratin foods
- Baked bread
- Bars - energy, nutritional
- Biscuits and biscuit mix
- Bisque
- Blanc mange
- Bologna
- Cake mix
- Cakes
- Candies
- Chicken broth
- Chowders
- Cookies
- Crackers
- Cream sauces

- Creamed foods
- Custards
- Desserts
- Diet drinks/shakes
- Donuts
- Fritters
- Frosting
- Frozen desserts
- Gravies
- Hamburger
- Hard sauces
- Hash
- Margarine
- Mashed potatoes
- Meat loaf
- Muffin mix
- Non-dairy creamers
- Omelets & scrambled eggs
- Pancakes & pancake mix
- Pie crust & pie crust mix
- Protein powder (casein)
- Rarebits
- Salad dressing
- Sausage
- Scalloped potatoes
- Sherbet
- Sorbet
- Soufflé
- Soups
- Spumoni
- Tofu desserts, frozen
- Waffles & waffle mix

Notes

Do not consume dairy products if you are allergic to milk proteins or have lactose intolerance.

8.6 Legumes

Legumes and products made from legumes are not part of the Recommended level of the healthy PCOS diet.

Best Legumes for Recommend Diet Level

No beans unless they are sprouted.

Good Legumes for Maintenance Diet Level

- Aduki beans
- Asparagus peas
- Bean sprouts - any bean
- Black beans
- Black-eyed peas
- Great Northern beans
- Lentils
- Miso
- Mung beans
- Navy beans
- Peas
- Pink beans
- Shoyu
- Soymilk*
- Tempeh*
- Tofu*
- White beans.

* We suggest you minimize or avoid these foods if you have hypothyroid problems.

Possibly Unhealthy Legumes (For You) - Avoid

Beans affect different people in different ways. The following beans or bean products may be troublesome for you.

- Chickpeas (Garbanzo beans) - (high in galactose)
- Hummus (contains Garbanzo beans)
- Kidney beans (a problem for some people)
- Lima beans (a problem for some people)
- Peanut butter

- Peanuts
- Pinto beans (a problem for some people)
- Refried beans
- Soybeans (a problem for some people)

Unhealthy Legumes - Avoid

- Texturized vegetable protein (TVP).

What Is TVP?

TVP (texturized vegetable protein) is a manufactured food made by treating soybeans with high heat and various alkaline washes to extract the bean's fat content or to neutralize their potent enzyme inhibitors. The soybean protein isolate is extruded under high temperature and high pressure. This processing damages the protein, rendering it harder to digest.

In addition, MSG, a neurotoxin that damages your hypothalamus gland, is frequently added to TVP to mask the "beany" taste and make it taste more like the various foods it imitates. The label on the final food product may not tell you that MSG was added to the TVP. Artificial flavorings besides MSG are often added to TVP.

TVPs are used extensively in school lunch programs, commercial baked goods, diet beverages and fast food products. TVP is in hundreds of different products. Be sure to read the label of any processed product you buy.

TVP is also known as "textured vegetable protein," "texturized vegetable protein," "hydrolyzed vegetable protein," or "vegetable protein." Usually, these are highly processed soy products that are found in a wide variety of foods.

Avoid TVP unless you are absolutely certain it is free of MSG and other food additives. You may be able to find TVP that is free of MSG and food additives in some health food stores.

Legume Guidelines

1. Sprouted legumes are OK - many of the "anti-nutrients" in legumes go away when sprouting occurs. See the *Sprouts* chapter for more information.

2. For more information on legumes and soy see these chapters: *Antinutrients in Grains and Legumes* and *To Soy or Not to Soy*.

3. Whether soy will improve or impair fertility and other PCOS symptoms depends on the unique health attributes and genetic pattern of each individual.

4. Peanuts and peanut butter (except organic) are not recommended because they may be high in pesticides and possibly aflatoxins (a toxic mold). Most of the U.S. peanut crop is free of aflatoxin but foreign peanuts are not.

5. Avoid soy or any other legume if you know you are allergic to it.

6. Minimize soy protein concentrate or soy protein isolate unless you are having it as part of a weight-control shake or as part of a dietary program prescribed by a doctor.

7. Restrict yourself to fermented soy products such as miso, shoyu or tempeh, or lightly processed soy products such as soy milk or tofu.

    A minor problem with fermented soy foods is that the fermentation process releases a sugar called galactose. There is some evidence that galactose may be detrimental to ovarian function. We don't know whether the galactose in fermented soy foods will cause you a problem. Most women do not need to worry about this.

Notes

Tofu is a curd made from soybeans that is pressed into large cubes. It is found in most supermarkets. It is a bland, versatile food that can be combined with almost any other food and can be prepared in many ways.

Soy sauce is traditionally made by a long process of fermentation. In Japan, this soy sauce is called "shoyu" or "tamari." In the U.S., soy sauce is not fermented and has wheat, salt, added chemicals and colorings. It is inferior in all respects to the traditional Japanese soy sauces. Do not consume U.S. soy sauce. Ethnic sections of supermarkets, ethnic markets or health food stores should have the traditional type of soy sauce. Use soy sauce or tamari sparingly. Make sure is it the "low sodium" variety.

Miso is a fermented soy paste that is used in cooking; it adds a unique flavor to soups and other foods.

Tempeh is a fermented soybean cake that can be eaten "as is," or added to salads, soups or other foods.

Soymilk is an increasingly popular beverage that is usually found in plain, vanilla or chocolate flavors. It is the liquid extracted from soybeans that have been soaked and pureed.

8.7 Grains

Grains and products made from grain are not part of the Recommended Level of the PCOS diet.

We are cautious about grains for four basic reasons:

1. Many grains contain gluten, which with gastrointestinal problems as well as some chronic disorders. Many individuals are also allergic to the gliadin molecule, which is in the gluten.

2. Many grains have a high glycemic index if they are refined and when they are cooked. Refining and cooking breaks down the starch in the grain. This causes it to be more easily and quickly assimilated into your bloodstream, thus raising its glycemic value and your blood sugar. Unnecessarily high increase in blood sugar will have unfavorable implications for your hormonal balance. Since most grains are refined and cooked, they are problematic for you.

3. Some grains have been sprayed with pesticides, fumigants or fungicides.

4. Some crops are genetically modified, with unknown health consequences.

Best Grains for Recommend Diet Level

- Wheatgrass
- Powdered barley or wheat sprouts

Good Grains for Maintenance Diet Level

The following foods are high in cooked starchy carbohydrates, which may cause problems for you unless you consume them only occasionally and in small quantities.
- Oatmeal (slow cooked, ***not*** instant) - in moderation
- Buckwheat - in moderation
- Quinoa - in moderation
- Amaranth - in moderation

Unhealthy Grains (For You) - Avoid

- All grains and grain products except those listed above, especially:
  - Wheat* (durum, semolina, kamut, spelt)
  - Rye
  - Barley
  - Triticale
- Corn and corn products

*Wheat or wheat gluten is truly ubiquitous in our food supply. Wheat materials are found in hundreds if not thousands of food products, far too numerous to list here.

Notes:

In the *Anti-Nutrients in Grains and Legumes* chapter, we recommended that you not consume gluten grains. So you may be surprised to see that we allow oatmeal as part of the Maintenance diet level. Oats — unlike wheat, barley and rye — do not contain gliadin, which is the molecule in gluten that is responsible for much of the trouble with these grains. However, these grains are all processed with the same machinery. Therefore, some gliadin from wheat, barley or rye gets mixed in with the oats that are being processed. This is why oats are prohibited in some health diets along with wheat, barley and rye. In spite of this mixing problem, the gliadin level of oats is quite low.

8.8 Vegetables

Vegetables are the mainstay of a healthy PCOS diet. The fiber, vitamins, minerals and other nutrients found in vegetation are essential for optimal cell and body function.[183]

A surprising and not well-known characteristic of fresh vegetables is that they are an excellent source of high quality EFAs (essential fatty acids), especially the highly desirable omega-3 fatty acids.

Best Vegetables for Recommended Diet Level

You may eat unlimited quantities of these vegetables, as often as you wish:
- Alfalfa sprouts
- Artichoke
- Artichoke, Jerusalem (sun choke)
- Arugula
- Asparagus
- Bamboo shoots
- Bean sprouts (see next chapter)
- Beet greens
- Bok choy*
- Broccoflower*
- Broccoli*
- Broccoli raab (rapini)
- Brussels sprouts*
- Cabbage - common, nappa, red, Savoy*
- Carrot
- Cauliflower*
- Celeriac
- Celery
- Celery root
- Chicory (curly endive)
- Chili peppers
- Chives*
- Cilantro
- Collard greens
- Cucumber
- Daikon radish
- Dandelion greens
- Eggplant
- Endive
- Escarole
- Fennel

- Fiddlehead fern
- Garlic
- Ginger root
- Horseradish
- Jicama
- Kale
- Kelp
- Kohlrabi (cabbage turnip)*
- Lamb's lettuce
- Leeks*
- Lettuce - Boston, green leaf, butter, red leaf, romaine
- Mushrooms
- Mustard greens
- Okra
- Onions - green, pearl, red, white, yellow*
- Parsley
- Pea pods - snow peas
- Peppers, bell - green, red, yellow
- Peppers, hot
- Pimento
- Prickly pear
- Purslane
- Radicchio (Italian chicory)
- Radish
- Radish sprouts
- Scallions
- Shallots
- Spinach
- Sprouts (see next chapter)
- String beans - green, yellow snap, wax
- Summer squash - zucchini, crookneck, pattypan
- Swiss chard
- Turnip greens
- Water chestnuts
- Watercress

* Indicates the vegetable may cause gas in some sensitive people. If they cause GI irritation, discontinue. Even though they may cause some gas, these vegetables are very healthy.

Possibly Permissible Vegetables for Maintenance Diet Level

- Beets
- Pumpkin
- Rutabaga
- Squash - acorn, banana, Hubbard, butternut, spaghetti
- Turnip

(See Notes below)

Possibly Inappropriate Vegetables (For You) - Minimize

If you have insulin resistance, you may need to restrict or avoid these vegetables (especially regular potatoes):
- Cassava (yucca)
- Parsnip
- Potatoes, any kind
- Taro
- Sweet potatoes
- Yams

Unhealthy Vegetables for Everyone - Avoid

Always avoid these foods:
- Deep fried vegetables
- French fries
- Hash browns
- Onion rings
- Rhubarb (because it is usually cooked with sugar)
- Tempura vegetables

Notes

1. Be moderate with most starchy root vegetables, except those in the onion family. Eat only occasionally. If you have an insulin resistance problem, minimize starchy root vegetables or avoid them entirely.

2. A preponderance of raw vegetables is generally preferable, if they agree with you. However, if raw vegetables cause you any digestive problems, switch to lightly cooked vegetables.

3. Eat a variety of vegetables. Don't get stuck in a groove where you repeatedly eat only two or three.

4. If you have arthritis, you may wish to avoid tomatoes, eggplant, white potatoes, green/red peppers, cayenne pepper or paprika. These plants belong to the "nightshade" family to which some arthritic people are sensitive.

5. Choose organic vegetables whenever possible. The majority of non-organic vegetables contain significant levels of pesticides. Organic vegetables also have a much higher nutrient value.

6. These vegetables may be waxed: cucumbers, eggplant, peppers, pumpkins, rutabagas, squashes and sweet potatoes. Plain water will not remove wax. Use a mild detergent for washing these vegetables.

7. Corn is not listed as a vegetable because it is a grain, not a vegetable. Corn is not a part of the PCOS diet. Peas are not listed as a vegetable because they are legumes. Legumes are not part of the Recommended Level of the PCOS diet. However, we consider pea pods a vegetable.

8.9 Sprouts

A "sprout" is a sprouted seed or legume.

Best Sprouts for Recommended Diet Level

There is no limit on the quantity and variety of sprouts you can eat. The more, the better!

- Adzuki beans
- Alfalfa
- Amaranth
- Arugula
- Barley (hull-less)
- Broccoli
- Broccoli raab
- Buckwheat
- Cabbage
- Canola
- Fenugreek
- Flax
- Garbanzo beans
- Oats (hull-less)
- Kamut.
- Lentils
- Millet
- Mung beans
- Mustard
- Peas
- Quinoa
- Radish
- Red clover
- Rye
- Soy beans
- Sunflower
- Triticale
- Watercress
- Wheat

Good Sprouts for Maintenance Diet Level

Same list as above.

Notes

You've undoubtedly seen "bean sprouts" in the grocery store, or had them in a restaurant. This common bean sprout comes from the mung bean. As you can see, there are many other kinds of sprouts beside the common bean sprout.

Sprouts have several advantages:
- Excellent source of quality nutrition — they are high in:
  - Protein
  - Fiber
  - Vitamins and minerals.
- Organic — pesticides and artificial fertilizers are not used in the growing of sprouts.
- Fresh — they are still alive and growing until you eat or cook them. This is a food that is at its energetic and nutritional peak when you eat it.
- Enzymes — since sprouts are alive, they still contain enzymes that ease digestion and improve health.
- More nutrient-dense than vegetables but they retain the advantages of a vegetable.

You can buy sprouts in the store or you can grow them yourself. You can ensure maximum quality and freshness if you grow them yourself.

They are an excellent addition to salads, can be added to vegetable dishes or used in a stir-fry. They can be eaten on their own, as a snack or as part of a meal.

How to Grow Sprouts

There is a wide variety of sprouting equipment available that can make your sprouting activities more productive and convenient. You can find this equipment online or in your local health food store. The simplest piece of equipment you will find is a Mason jar with a screen mesh lid. The most expensive sprouting equipment will be semi-automated operations with an electric water pump.

However, if you've never done sprouting before and just want to get your toe in the water, here's one way to get started:
- Put about 1/4 cup of your beans or seeds in a quart jar filled with water and soak them overnight.
- Drain the soaked beans or seeds the next day by pouring them into a strainer. Or, you can cover the jar with cheesecloth (secured with a rubber band) and then turn the jar upside down.
- Rinse the beans or seeds and drain them again.
- Turn the jar upside down and leave it in a darkish place that doesn't get too hot or cold (room temperature). Leave the strainer or cheesecloth in place so that the sprouts won't fall out.
- At the end of the day, rinse the sprouts again in order to keep them clean and moist.

- Repeat this rinsing process twice a day for at least three days, until the sprouts are as long as desired.
- On the last day or two, put the sprouts in a sunny spot so they will turn green.

When to Harvest Your Sprouts

Let your preferences dictate when to harvest your sprouts. Some people like them when they are small or young while others may prefer to let them grow until they have sprouted a few small leaves. For example, if you are sprouting mung beans, you could eat the sprout when it is mostly a juicy stem with hardly any leaves, or you could wait until it develops very small leaves. Some sprouts can eventually get a little "woody" or chewy. You can sample some of the sprouts in your jar every day. Harvest them when they taste "just right" to you.

Put your sprouts into a closed container in the refrigerator, where they can be stored for up to 8-10 days. You can even freeze sprouts, but they won't retain their crispness.

8.10 Fruits

Fruits are an important element of good nutrition. They contain vitamins, minerals, enzymes, fiber and a wide variety of beneficial "phytonutrients" such as bioflavonoids.

Best Fruits for Recommended Diet Level

You may have up to 1 - 3 modest servings of these whole fruits daily:
- Apple
- Apricot
- Avocado
- Berries - blackberry, blueberry, boysenberry, raspberry, gooseberry, linganberry, dewberry, elderberry, youngberry, loganberry
- Cantaloupe
- Cherry
- Cranberry
- Grapefruit
- Grape (in moderation)
- Guava
- Kiwi
- Lemon
- Lime
- Nectarine (organic only)
- Olives
- Orange
- Passion fruit
- Peach (organic only)
- Pear
- Plum
- Strawberries (organic only)
- Tangerine
- Tomato

Good Fruits for Maintenance Diet Level

- Asian pear
- Coconut (whole, fresh)
- Fig (fresh only)
- Kumquat
- Mango
- Melons - canary, Crenshaw, honeydew, casaba, musk, Persian
- Papaya

- Persimmon
- Pineapple (fresh only)
- Plantain
- Prickly pear
- Prunes
- Quince
- Star fruit
- Watermelon

Inappropriate Fruits (For Some of You) - Minimize or Avoid

- Banana
- Bitter melon (may cause problems with certain blood types)
- Breadfruit
- Dried fruit (most)
- Pomegranate (may cause problems with certain blood types)

Inappropriate or Unhealthy Fruits for Everyone - Avoid

- Candied or pickled fruit
- Canned fruit
- Fruit drink
- Fruit juice
- Fruit-flavored soda pop
- Jams
- Jellies
- Raisins (may have mold, pesticides; find organic source)

Fruit Guidelines

1. Whole, fresh fruits are best. Frozen is OK. No canned fruit.

2. Fruit juice is not recommended because the fiber and other nutrients have been removed and the concentration of fructose may be too high.

3. Avoid dried fruits because they have a high glycemic index and are fumigated. Organic dried fruit is OK in moderation if you soak it in water until it is fully reconstituted. In particular, avoid raisins because of their high pesticide content; organic raisins in small quantities are OK. Occasional dried fruits (1-2 pieces) are OK if you are at the Maintenance Level.

4. Minimize consumption of baked or cooked fruit since it is digested more quickly than raw fruit.

5. Eat a variety of fruit. You can have up to several modest servings a day.

6. Don't eat a large quantity of fruit at one sitting. A large amount of fructose (fruit sugar) is not helpful for your condition.

7. Choose fresh organic fruits whenever possible. The majority of non-organic fruits contain significant levels of pesticides. Organic fruit also has a higher nutrient value.

8. If you have a choice, select domestic or local fruit instead of imported fruit. Some imported fruit may be higher in pesticides.

9. These fruits may be waxed: apples, avocados, some melons, citrus, passion fruit, and peaches. Plain water will not remove wax. If you detect wax, either peel the fruit or wash with a mild detergent to remove the wax.

8.11 Nuts and Seeds

Nuts and seeds are an excellent complement to vegetables and fruits. They provide a much more calorie-dense source of nutrition than vegetables.

Best Nuts & Seeds for Recommended Diet Level

- Walnuts (preferred - high in omega 3 fats)
- Flax seeds (preferred - high in omega 3 fats)
- Macadamia nuts (preferred - high in omega 3 fats)
- Almonds
- Brazil nuts
- Cashews
- Chestnuts
- Hazelnuts (filberts)
- Pecans
- Pine nuts
- Pistachios
- Poppy seeds
- Pumpkin seeds
- Sesame seeds
- Almond butter (use sparingly!)
- Cashew butter (use sparingly!)
- Hazelnut butter (use sparingly!)

Good Nuts & Seeds for Maintenance Diet Level

- Nut flours, freshly ground
- Sesame tahini (sesame paste)
- Sunflower seeds

Inappropriate or Unhealthy Nuts & Seeds - Avoid

- Peanuts
- Peanut butter
- Nuts or seeds roasted in oil
- Salted nuts or seeds

Nuts & Seeds Guidelines

1. Nuts and seeds can be habit-forming. If you have a weight problem, restrict yourself to 2-3 ounces or less per day.

2. Eat raw nuts and seeds only. Never eat nuts or seeds that have been cooked in oil. Also avoid dry roasted. Heating nuts and seeds causes oxidation of the fats in them, thus converting them into free radicals that damage your cells and cause inflammation.

3. To make nuts and seeds more digestible, you could soak them overnight in pure water. Drain the water, rinse, pat dry and refrigerate. Soaking activates enzymes that cause the nut/seed to become "alive" and start the growing process.

4. Avoid nuts and seeds coated with salt, sweeteners, food colorings and additives. They are unhealthy or increase your appetite.

5. Avoid peanuts, which are legumes, not nuts. Most legumes are excluded from the Recommended Level of the PCOS diet. Peanuts are a common cause of food allergies and may contain pesticides.

6. The fats in nuts and seeds are easily oxidized when they are exposed to heat, light and air. Buy nuts in the shell, if possible. The shell insulates the meat of the nut or seed from air, light and heat. You can also buy shelled "whole" nuts and seeds in vacuum packed packages. Whole nuts are less likely to be oxidized (rancid) than nut pieces. Nuts and seeds should be refrigerated.

7. Organic nuts and seeds are your best choice, if you can find them.

8. If you have a coffee bean grinder, flax seeds can be ground up and sprinkled on your salad or breakfast cereal. Flax seeds are a good source of omega 3 fats that your body needs.

9. Some nuts may be rancid when you buy them. If you notice an "off" taste, or if the nuts look discolored, don't eat them.

10. Commercial nut butters such as almond butter are a refined food and should be used sparingly. Because they are processed, they have been subjected to heat, light, and air, which stimulates unhealthy oxidation (rancidity). To minimize further oxidation, keep nut or seed butters tightly sealed and refrigerated at all times. You can also minimize oxidation by adding the contents of 3-4 vitamin E capsules and mixing it into the nut butter.

11. Be very moderate with nut butters, especially if you have a weight problem. Some individuals are very fond of nut butters and may end up consuming too many calories.

Notes

If you're avoiding nuts and seeds because you think all they do is make you fat, consider the following information.

Nuts are an excellent source of:
- Healthy monounsaturated or polyunsaturated fats
- Fiber
- Arginine (an amino acid)
- Vitamin E
- Magnesium, potassium, copper and other essential nutrients

Consumption of nuts has been shown to reduce the incidence of both heart disease and diabetes, both of which are major concerns of women with PCOS.[184]

The arginine in nuts stimulates nitric oxide, a potent vasodilator (expansion of blood vessels). Human feeding trials using almonds and walnuts in place of traditional fats caused an 8-12% reduction in LDL "bad" cholesterol.[185] Most studies have shown that eating nuts frequently reduces the risk of coronary heart disease by 30-50%.

Possible mechanisms by which nuts may be cardioprotective include reductions in LDL cholesterol, the antioxidant action of vitamin E, and the effects on endothelial and platelet function due to higher levels of nitric oxide derived from arginine in nuts.

A 16-year study of 83,818 women revealed that those who consumed a 1-ounce serving of nuts more than five times a week had a 27% less chance of developing type 2 diabetes, compared with those who never ate nuts.[186] The high fat content of nuts did not cause them to gain weight.

Another study of postmenopausal women showed that frequent nut consumption provided modest protection against the risk of death from all causes as well as cardiovascular disease.[187]

Replacement of complex carbohydrates with nuts also helps you to lose weight, according to a study from the City of Hope National Medical Center in Duarte, California.[188]

8.12 Fats & Oils

We believe that the best dietary source of fats and oils is from eating the whole food that contains the oil. Fatty foods such as avocados, olives, nuts and seeds will provide you with all the fat you need.

In general, bottled oils are a much inferior source of getting the fats necessary for good health. They are inferior primarily because they are highly processed and the oil has been altered and degraded to some extent.

However, some individuals experience their food as unpalatable unless bottled oils are used. If you're one of these individuals, this chapter is for you.

The classification of oils below is somewhat arbitrary because there is no way for us to accurately assess the quality of bottled oil. For example, the fat in an avocado is quite healthy. But avocado oil undergoes a great deal of "purification" in order to give it an appearance and smell that the marketers think you will be comfortable with. We honestly don't know whether a particular avocado oil will be good for you or not. The same holds true for most other oils.

The only bottled oil we feel entirely comfortable with is "extra virgin" olive oil because of how it is processed.

Best Fats & Oils for Recommended Diet Level

Oils
- Flax oil
- Hemp oil
- Macadamia nut oil
- Olive oil
- Walnut oil

OK for Cooking
- Olive oil

Good Fats & Oils for Maintenance Diet Level

Oils
- Sesame oil
- Almond oil
- Canola oil
- Coconut oil
- High oleic safflower oil

OK for Cooking
- Butter
- Lard
- Palm kernel oil

Possibly Unhealthy Fats & Oils - Minimize

- Avocado oil
- Peanut oil

Unhealthy Fats & Oils - Avoid

- Most vegetable oils found in your supermarket
- Butter spreads (most of them)
- Butter substitutes
- Corn oil
- Cottonseed oil
- Cream
- Lard
- Margarine
- Safflower oil
- Shortening
- Soybean oil
- Sunflower oil

Notes

Oils are refined foods that are loaded with calories. Be quite moderate with oils, consuming 4 or less tablespoons a day, especially if you are prone to gain weight. Use good judgment — a little oil can go a long way.

To prevent oxidation of bottled oils, squeeze 1-2 capsules of vitamin E into the bottle after opening. Keep tightly sealed and refrigerated.

Medicinal Use of Oils

Cod liver oil and flax seed oil may be taken to increase omega-3 fatty acid intake. Consult with a qualified health professional as to the amount of these oils that you may need. As a general guide, one or two teaspoons a day of cod liver oil would be a good place to start. You may wish to gradually increase up to 3 tablespoons, unless it causes some bowel discomfort.

Section 9

Water and Beverages

9.1 Water

This morning you may have had milk on your cereal and then some coffee before going to work; then more coffee or a soft drink at work. Lunch may have included a large diet Pepsi or possibly a milk shake; then a sparkling fruit drink, a soft drink, or coffee with your afternoon break. After work you went to the gym and drank some water from the fountain or had Gatorade. Before dinner, you had a couple of beers. Then wine, a soft drink or milk with dinner. Amazingly, this approximates what a typical American consumes.

Many thousands of years of human evolution did not design the human body to consume an array of beverages and chlorinated tap water. Until a couple hundred years ago, people mostly drank plain water. Since then, we've concocted a bewildering array of beverages. At the same time, we've badly polluted our water supply. What we're drinking now is hurting our health.

You Are Water

If you have PCOS, you've probably given some thought to trying the Atkins diet or modifying your diet in some other way. You have thought about your exercise program. But how much thought have you given to what you're drinking?

Water is required for life and good health. Water is necessary for:
- Blood and lymphatic circulation
- Digestion and assimilation of nutrients
- Elimination of metabolic waste
- Temperature control of your body
- Lubrication inside your body (extra-cellular fluid)
- Energy production
- Other biochemical processes

It's also important to keep in mind that you are mostly water:
- Your body is over 70% water
- Your blood is 80% water
- Your brain is 75% water
- Your liver is 96% water

Therefore the quantity and quality of the water you drink is critical to your health and plays an important role in overcoming any illness or disorder.

Why Drinking Water Is Important for PCOS

Besides being critical for all life processes, water is especially important for women with PCOS.

1. Water is an anti-inflammatory.
As we noted in the first two chapters, PCOS has an inflammatory component. Water helps to reduce inflammation in a couple of ways.

- First of all, water is a solvent. As such, it dissolves many inflammatory toxins and waste products in the body and carries them out of your body in urine, feces and sweat.

- We also discussed earlier that a lot of inflammation is due to oxidant stress, which means there are too many unstable free radical molecules circulating in your body and causing cell damage. Most people don't realize that water is also an antioxidant that reduces oxidant stress. For instance, water "disarms" a type of free radical called "singlet oxygen" by absorbing its energy as heat. Because of water's high heat capacity and high intracellular concentration, it very likely constitutes your body's first antioxidant line of defense against singlet oxygen free radical attack

2. Water helps you regulate weight and metabolism.
If you have a weight challenge, drinking enough water helps you in several ways:

- Water is an appetite suppressant. When you are feeling hungry, have a glass of water 10 minutes before you begin eating. You may find your desire to eat a large portion has diminished.

- Your cells require water in order to produce energy (burning of glucose or fat).

- Although it sounds paradoxical, drinking more water may cause you to lose water weight. Dieters sometimes restrict their water intake because they fear that it will lead to water retention. The opposite appears to be the case. Some of the "fat" on overweight people is actually retained water. When your body doesn't get enough water, it will tend to hold on to what it has. When you drink enough water, your body can eliminate excess fluids.

- Drinking plenty of water accelerates removal of toxic substances, which is important when you're losing weight. As accumulated fat is released to be burned as fuel, the stored toxins in the fat are released into the bloodstream. Water helps these toxins get removed from your body.

- An optimally functioning liver is important for fat and sugar metabolism, detoxification and hormone balance. Since your liver is mostly water, it can become stressed and reduce its level of function if it is dehydrated. Dehydration also inhibits your kidneys from removing waste materials via your urine.

3. Water increases your energy.

Many women with PCOS report that they feel tired or fatigued. Your energy level is proportional to your water intake. A 5% drop in body fluids may cause a 25%-30% loss in energy. A 15% drop in fluids will probably result in death. It's estimated that 3/4 of the U.S. population may suffer some energy loss due to minor dehydration.[189]

4. Water reduces high blood pressure.

Although high blood pressure is not a primary characteristic of PCOS, it's a concern for some women.

A contributing factor to hypertension (high blood pressure) is your body's adjustment to blood volume loss. The most common cause of lower blood volume is dehydration. Since your blood is more than 80% water, its total volume is strongly influenced by the amount of water you drink.

When your body detects a loss of blood volume, it closes off less active capillary beds (tiny blood vessels) in order to maintain adequate blood flow to the more active or important areas. These vessel closings cause a rise in blood pressure. In addition, as you lose blood volume from lack of adequate water, your blood becomes "thicker" or more viscous. So it takes more pressure to make the blood circulate.

A lack of sufficient water also increases blood pressure because your blood system still has to pump water into each cell. If there is less water available in the blood to be pumped into the cells, pressure has to be increased to compensate for the lack of available water.

5. Dehydration may disturb hormone balance.

When you're dehydrated, the volume of your cells may diminish. Some functions of the cell are altered, including the action of insulin. It appears that disturbances in water balance (such as dehydration) may interfere with insulin function and lead to insulin resistance.[190] [191] There is also some evidence that estrogen function could be impaired.[192]

Cell hydration is an important element in the regulation of liver metabolism by hormones.[193] Changes in cell hydration also influence uptake of amino acids and may create oxidative stress (production of free radical molecules that damage cell function).[194] [195]

6. Water helps you metabolize hormones.

Unneeded hormones are metabolized by your liver and excreted in your stool and urine. The importance of water for producing urine is obvious.

But water is also necessary for creating a properly formed stool and avoiding constipation. Constipation slows down the excretion of unwanted hormones and causes them to be re-circulated into the body, thus contributing to a hormonal imbalance.

For example, about 20% of metabolized estrogen is excreted via your GI tract. When you're constipated, some of that estrogen sits in your lower intestine for a long time where some of it is reabsorbed from your lower intestines back into your "portal vein," which is the main blood vessel that connects your GI tract to your liver. So your liver receives back the same estrogen that it got rid of earlier. The effect is to build up estrogen levels in your liver and your body, leading to overall hormonal imbalance.

7. *Water helps you absorb vital nutrients.*
Water is needed to make it easier to transport nutrients in your food and vitamins from your GI tract into your bloodstream. If you're dehydrated, the simple sugars will still be assimilated but the more complex nutrients and your vitamins may not be. You end up absorbing what you don't want (sugars that unbalance your blood sugar level) and not absorbing what you do want (important nutrients and vitamins).

8. *Water reduces your risk of colon cancer.*
Water is a particular health benefit for women. Research conducted at the Fred Hutchinson Cancer Center in Seattle found that among women who drank more than five glasses of water a day, there were fewer cases of colon cancer.[196] Their risk was about half of what it was for women who drank less than two glasses a day.

9. *Water is the ultimate "low-cal" drink . . .*
because it doesn't have any calories at all! So if you have a weight challenge, don't bother with lo-cal soft drinks. Drink water instead.

How Much Water Should You Drink?

The amount of water you need depends on a number of factors:
- Your size
- Your health
- Your activity level
- The season and humidity
- The temperature and your exposure to heat

So it's tough to generalize; every person is unique. But as a general guideline, daily optimal water intake in ounces for the average person is estimated to be roughly 40% of your body weight. So if you weigh 160 lbs., you should drink at least 64 ounces of water (160 lbs. x 40% = 64 oz.). That's equal to eight 8-oz. glasses of water. If you are ill, undergoing a detoxification program, exercising vigorously, or have chronic inflammation, you'll need more water than the average person. For example, you can lose 3 quarts of water just by jogging for one hour on a warm summer day.

If you're like most Americans, you don't drink enough water. When you are chronically dehydrated, the thirst centers in your brain stop sending signals that you need water. So waiting to drink until you are thirsty is waiting too long and may lead to chronic dehydration. Once you start drinking enough water, it will take you about a month to re-establish the normal function of your thirst centers. In the beginning, you may have to force yourself to drink water until it becomes a normal, regular habit.

While you are sleeping, you will become slightly dehydrated from loss of water vapor through your lungs. It's wise to rehydrate yourself with 8 to 16 oz. of water within 30 minutes of waking.

You can also drink a glass of water about 30 minutes before a meal. This encourages stomach acid production and helps digestion.

"I Can't Drink All that Water!"

Even if you know you need to drink more water, you may discover you do not stick with it. That's understandable. During the first few days of drinking more water than your body is accustomed to, you may find yourself going to the bathroom every 20 minutes. This can be a little discouraging as well as interfering with your usual work routine. It seems as though for every glass you drink, you pee at least a glass and therefore all this drinking is a waste of time.

Be patient. Your body is rebalancing itself and good things are happening. It's flushing itself of the water it has been storing throughout all those years of "survival mode." As you continue to give your body all the water it wants, it gets rid of what it no longer needs. It may release water from your ankles, hips, thighs and belly. You are releasing much more than you realize. The flushing of old stored water will eventually cease and your runs to the bathroom will normalize.

If you just can't stand another glass of plain water, add a squeeze of lemon for flavor.

Do Beverages Count?

No, beverages don't count as substitutes for water. Nature didn't create Pepsi. Your cells are designed to work with water, not some artificial liquid. For women with PCOS, beverages are not an acceptable substitute for your water needs.

When thirsty, drink water, not a liquid containing food or chemicals. If you want to have a beverage, it should be in addition to your water intake not a substitute for it.

Ice & Ice Water

Avoid ice unless you feel secure about the purity of the water from which it was made. Remember that automatic ice makers use unfiltered tap water. Freezing kills most parasites but does not kill bacteria or viruses.

We also suggest that you avoid ice-cold drinks with your meals. Iced drinks cool your stomach lining to a temperature that is unnatural and not optimal for digestion. The stomach's reflexive reaction to cold causes blood vessels to constrict, which reduces circulation and delays the release of digestive enzymes. Delayed or incomplete digestion can lead to malabsorption and putrefaction. You don't want to lose any benefits of the fresh, wholesome foods you're eating just for the sake of an iced drink!

Have your cold drinks at least a half-hour before, or an hour after, a meal.

9.2 Purified Water

Tap water is not suitable for women with PCOS.

Chemicals in chlorinated tap water appear to alter ovarian function and the length of the menstrual cycle.[197] There is also some evidence to suggest that chlorinated tap water may contribute in some way to spontaneous abortions.[198]

Tap water is laden with all kinds of chemical pollutants and microorganisms. Chlorine is a poison that is used to make your water "safe." Chlorination and its byproducts contribute to atherosclerosis and other degenerative diseases. The addition of chlorine in water creates trihalomethanes, which are carcinogens that naturally form when chlorine reacts with organic compounds in water.

Organochlorines may be linked to breast cancer. They don't degrade very well. They accumulate in fatty tissue such as the breast. Organochlorines can be found in body fat, blood, mother's milk and semen. They may cause mutations, suppress immune function and interfere with the natural control of cell growth.

Chlorination kills most disease-causing bacteria and some viruses, but it does not kill the cyst forms of parasites like giardia or cryptosporidium.

There have been reports of estrogens in drinking water. The vast quantities of synthetic hormones administered to both humans and livestock over the past fifty years have not simply vanished into thin air. Rather, they have gradually reappeared in our water supply because water treatment plants cannot filter them out. The same is true of millions of pounds of synthetic chemicals in pesticides that are hormone mimics, i.e., they are not hormones but act like hormones when they get inside your body.

Because your hormones are already out of balance, you don't want to make that imbalance any worse by drinking tap water.

For all the above reasons and because drinking water has over 700 known contaminants, we recommend that you drink only purified water. If you can't afford to buy purified water or a water purifier, then you should at least find out what is in your local water supply.

You should be able to get local drinking water information at the Environmental Protection Agency (EPA) website (www.epa.gov/safewater/dwinfo.htm), or call the EPA Safe Drinking Water Hotline at 800-426-4791.

Water Purifiers

The mechanisms for purifying water have improved and proliferated over the past 20 years. Today, you have a bewildering array of choices.

The most common methods to purify your water are:
- Solid block or granulated carbon filters
- Reverse osmosis
- Distillation
- Ultraviolet light
- Special additives such as tricalcium phosphate or lead-sorbent matrix to trap heavy metals

Many water purifiers employ more than one of the above methods, because no one method by itself will remove 100% of all possible contaminants.

So which water filter unit would be best for you? We can't give you recommendations specific to your water supply, but we do suggest you go to do some research on the Internet.

You can also check out the National Sanitation Foundation at www.nsf.org. This is an independent non-profit organization that evaluates water purifiers and bottled water.

Bottled Water

The quality of bottled water is variable. It is probably not as desirable as water purified at home but is generally better than tap water.

Some bottled water comes from municipal water supplies. To discover the source of any bottled water, call the bottler and request documentation about the nature and purity of the source, or check out your brand of bottled water with the National Sanitation Foundation. For safety, bottled water that comes from municipal water supplies or lakes should be treated by your bottler with reverse osmosis filtration before being bottled.

9.3 Coffee

The coffee bean contains a large number of known and unknown substances. When the bean is roasted and then brewed, some of these substances end up in your coffee cup. The data about coffee is contradictory, so we can neither condemn it nor give it our blanket approval.

From the hydration (water) standpoint, caffeinated beverages such as coffee, tea and soft drinks are undesirable because caffeine acts as a diuretic, causing water loss unless you compensate by drinking more water.

In terms of dealing with PCOS, coffee is a mixed bag.

Regarding infertility, a few studies suggest that coffee consumption delays conception or otherwise increases infertility.[199] [200] Another study indicates that coffee consumption has no influence on fertility.[201] However, it appears that women who consume the most coffee seem to have a higher tendency for infertility.

Other research indicates that tannic acid may increase infertility. However, it's not clear whether the caffeine or the tannic acid in coffee might be responsible for the increased infertility and spontaneous abortions.

Caffeine is found in coffee, tea, some soft drinks, chocolate, cocoa and many over-the-counter medicines. Tannic acid is found in coffee, tea, cocoa and red wine.

Unfortunately, decaf coffee may not be a good option. In one study, consumption of 3 or more cups per day of decaffeinated coffee more than doubled the risk of spontaneous abortions.[202] Some coffee companies still remove caffeine from coffee beans with chemical solvents such as trichloroethylene, methylene chloride, or ethyl acetate. Some of these chemicals are suspected carcinogens. They may also have an effect on hormone receptors, thus adversely influencing your hormonal balance.

Aside from the fertility issue, coffee is not a good idea for women who are taking metformin (Glucophage). Metformin causes an increase in homocysteine, which is dangerous to your health if the level gets too high. A number of studies have shown that coffee consumption raises homocysteine.[203] However, caffeine alone does not appear to be the primary cause, although it does contribute to higher homocysteine.[204] Apparently, there is something else in the coffee, or the way it is prepared, that may be causing homocysteine to go up.

On the other hand, coffee may be of some benefit for women with a concern about diabetes. A very recent study at the University of Amsterdam showed that people who drank coffee reduced their risk of diabetes.[205] The more coffee they drank, the lower their risk. Individuals who drank seven or more cups daily were 50% less likely to develop diabetes.

Here's our take on coffee. In general, you're better off without it. We don't like the fact that some coffee beans have high pesticide levels. A roasted bean, seed or nut of any kind should not be your first food choice. When coffee beans are roasted, free radicals are created that contribute to oxidant stress. Roasting also creates acrylamide, a substance that is a suspected carcinogen.

Coffee disturbs your nervous system, indirectly leading to increased stress. One of your goals in your quest to control PCOS is to reduce stress, not increase it. And finally, if you're trying to get pregnant, we recommend that you avoid all coffee, tea (except herbal) and caffeinated beverages.

In general, we don't view coffee as a major health threat. If you're addicted to coffee because of the caffeine lift, we recommend you switch to green tea, which has much less caffeine, but still enough to give you a mild lift.

9.4 Tea

A growing body of research indicates that tea, especially green tea, is much better for you than coffee. Before we review green tea, let's mention the four basic categories of teas.

- **Black tea.** Black teas are produced by withering, cutting, rolling, fermenting and drying of tea leaves. The drink is red in color with an astringent taste. Black tea accounts for about 95% of the world market.

- **Oolong tea.** Oolongs are semi-green teas, produced by stopping the fermentation process just as the leaves start to turn brown. The leaves are then fired or dried. They make a yellowish tea with a malty flavor.

- **Green tea.** Green tea has been picked, steamed and rolled before firing. This stops the fermentation process, so that the leaf does not turn brown. The brewed tea is pale yellow or green in color, with a slightly bitter taste.

- **Herb tea.** There are literally hundreds of herbs from which a tea can be made. Herbal teas have been used for centuries to treat many medical conditions.

Green Tea

Green tea is thought to retain superior health benefits because it is less processed than black or oolong tea. A large body of evidence suggests that green tea offers these health benefits: anticancer, antibacterial, antiviral, antioxidant, lowers cholesterol and triglycerides. It also reduces inflammation, aids detoxification, reduces blood pressure, protects DNA reduces clotting (platelet aggregation) and improves digestion.

Green tea may help with PCOS in several ways:

1. Women with PCOS who are leaning toward diabetes are more likely to be under oxidant stress and thus have more inflammation and cell damage. Green tea is a strong antioxidant that slows down this process.[206]

2. Some women with PCOS also have "estrogen dominance," which contributes to infertility, increases the risk of cancer and creates other health problems. A recently released study from the University of Southern California shows that there is a relationship between tea consumption and estrogen levels. This study analyzed the estrogen levels of 130 post-menopausal women. The researchers discovered that those who drank the most tea had the lowest levels of estrogen.[207]

3. A troublesome aspect of PCOS is an excessive level of male hormones. The visible signs of this hormonal imbalance are acne, excessive facial hair and body hair distribution

similar to a male.

Studies from the University of Chicago and Mayo Graduate School indicate that ingredients in green tea reduce the effect of male hormones by two different mechanisms.[208] [209] [210] One mechanism is by inhibition of the male hormone receptors on your cells. The other is by inhibition of the 5-alpha-reductase enzyme that converts testosterone into the more potent dihydrotestosterone (DHT). DHT is found in your skin and is thought to be an important factor in hair growth and acne.

4. Ingredients in green tea may play a role in appetite control and weight management according to scanty evidence from rat studies.[211] [212]

Herbal Teas

Most herbal teas that you find in a health food store are acceptable, if consumed in moderation. Regarding special herbal tea formulas or teas consumed in large quantities, you're advised to first consult with your naturopathic physician or qualified herbalist. Herbs can have a strong effect on your body, depending on their amount, quality, combination and frequency of consumption.

Bottled Tea Drinks

Check the label of any bottled tea drink before you purchase it. Most of them contain sweeteners or other additives. These added substances either disturb your blood sugar control, or they are simply extraneous materials that you liver has to metabolize and dispose of. You'll probably want to avoid most bottled tea drinks.

9.5 Soft Drinks

We can only shake our heads in disbelief when it comes to soft drinks. The U.S. Dept. of Agriculture has reported that annual consumption of soft drinks is 53 gallons per person. In fact, it's been reported that we drink more soft drinks than water!

There is nothing whatsoever in the typical soft drink that is healthy. So why drink them? Even the trendy, "healthier" drinks with added vitamins or herbs should be viewed with caution.

There's such a proliferation of soft drinks and soft drink ingredients that we can't talk about them in detail. But here is a sampling of things you should know about soft drinks:

- Most soft drinks are high in phosphorous, which binds magnesium in your GI tract, thus preventing its absorption into your bloodstream. Colas are especially high in phosphorous. Magnesium insufficiency is one of the factors creating insulin resistance, which is a primary problem in PCOS.

- Phosphorous in soft drinks also increases urinary calcium excretion. Calcium plays an important role in weight management. Women consuming less calcium are more overweight than those who consume plenty of calcium.[213] Calcium also plays a role in egg maturation and follicular development. Excessive phosphorous increases the amount of parathyroid hormone, which causes calcium to leave the bones. Teen girls who drink carbonated beverages are at greater risk of bone fractures compared to other girls their age.[214]

- Soft drinks contain sweeteners, some of which can disturb your blood sugar balance and lead to insulin problems.

- Soft drinks contain "non-nutritive," empty calories. Your body has to expend metabolic effort to process the empty calories but gets nothing in return. Drinking lots of soft drinks actually reduces your stores of vitamins and minerals.

- Aspartame, an artificial sweetener found in some soft drinks, has been associated with a higher incidence of brain disorders in lab animals.[215] In addition, chronic aspartame ingestion may have cumulative negative effects, possibly because of formaldehyde formation.[216]

- Some soft drinks contain chloroform — a known cancer promoter. This may be hard to believe, so let us explain. Chloroform is a by-product of the chlorination of tap water, which is used in soft drinks. So if your soft drink bottler uses chlorinated tap water, you can expect some chloroform in your favorite beverage. Very few bottlers go to the expense of purifying the water they use for their beverages.

- Besides chloroform, soft drinks are a nasty brew of unidentified chemicals, colorants, stimulants and sweeteners that are totally devoid of nutritive value and only weaken your health. Some of these materials do nothing except make your liver and kidneys work overtime to detoxify them. Any amount of unnecessary liver or kidney stress is undesirable, particularly if you are on metformin or other medications.

- Mice given cola drinks instead of water for up to 8 weeks developed DNA damage.[217] Damage was not detected in mice given tap water or non-cola beverages. Although there's not a lot of research in this area, it's possible that flavoring agents in cola drinks could contribute to cell damage and abnormal cell behavior.

- Brominated oils are used in bottled fruit drinks to provide a cloudy stability to drink ingredients and to prevent ring formation in the neck of the bottle. With bottled natural fruit juices stored over time, some material settles to the bottom, while some dries out and forms a ring in the neck of the bottle. From the marketing perspective, rings and settling are undesirable, so brominated oils are added to reduce this tendency. However, studies of lab animals indicate that brominated oils may have a deleterious effect on the heart, thyroid, liver (fatty liver) and kidneys.[218] Consumption of brominated oils by rats resulted in impaired reproduction and behavioral abnormalities.[219] There is one report of a person drinking large amounts of cola and developing "bromism," characterized by headache, fatigue, ataxia and memory loss.[220]

There is no conceivable reason why you should consume soft drinks. We strongly recommend that you never consume them.

9.6 Alcoholic and Other Beverages

We've discussed coffee, tea and soft drinks. But what about other beverages?

Alcoholic Beverages

Is it OK to drink alcohol? Mounting evidence suggests that modest alcoholic beverage consumption is mildly beneficial.

A recent study of the dietary habits of Americans has showed that those who consumed 20 drinks or more per month had a 66% reduction in risk for "metabolic syndrome."[221] The researchers noted improvement in symptoms, especially increased HDL ("good") cholesterol, lowered triglycerides, reduced waist circumference and reduced insulin levels. Metabolic syndrome symptoms are also common PCOS symptoms. The benefits were achieved by drinking beer or wine but not hard liquor.

Light to moderate alcohol consumption appears to be associated with improved insulin sensitivity and reduced risk for cardiovascular disease.[222] [223]

One interesting study, recently completed at the University of Cambridge, reported that women who drank any kind of alcoholic beverage had a lower level of HbA1c (glycohemoglobin) than women who did not drink any alcohol.[224] (The median level of alcohol consumption was 3 drinks per week). HbA1c is blood test marker that indicates your average blood sugar level for the past 3 months. The lower your HbA1c, the lower your average blood sugar level has been. A high HbA1c indicates you are possibly diabetic or pre-diabetic and that you have generalized cell damage.

However, drinking a lot of alcohol is counterproductive. Not only does a large amount of alcohol cause blood sugar fluctuations, it also impairs liver function. Chronic high levels of alcohol intake are obviously very unhealthy and could lead to addiction. We also recommend that you drink only with meals, in moderate amounts.

We suggest you use your own good judgment. If you do drink, we think wine and beer is preferable to other alcoholic beverages, because they contain antioxidants and plant materials that are beneficial to your health. Choose organic, low-sulfite wines when possible to avoid ingesting unnecessary chemicals that can place further stress on your liver or trigger allergic reactions.

Cocoa, Kool Aid, Tang, Etc.

There are abundant varieties of artificial drinks that are not carbonated soft drinks.

Common examples include cocoa and coffee mixes, Kool Aid and Tang.

The unhealthy aspects of these drinks fall into three basic categories:

- Too much sugar. Most of them are so loaded with sugar or other sweeteners that your blood sugar balance will be thrown off and you will have an unwanted increase in insulin.

- Unhealthy oils. Some drink mixes contain unhealthy vegetable oils. Look for "partially hydrogenated" oil on the label. We explained earlier how these oils contain trans-fatty acids that disturb the function of every cell in your body.

- Artificial additives. Artificial colorings, flavorings and other agents provide no nutrition whatever, plus they may stimulate your immune system into action. At the very least, they are additional work for your liver and kidneys as your body tries to get rid of these materials.

We strongly recommend you avoid all artificial drinks so long as you have PCOS.

Milk

Should you drink milk? The jury's still out on that. However, our basic viewpoint is that cow's milk is ideally designed for baby cows, not for humans. There's not much evidence to show that people who drink milk are healthier or have better calcium status than those who do not drink milk. For more information, refer to *The Problem with Milk* chapter.

Milk is not included in the healthy PCOS diet. If you continue to consume milk or dairy products, it would be wise to get a milk allergy test and a lactose intolerance test to determine to what extent dairy is compromising your health.

Fruit Drinks & Fruit Juices

Women with PCOS should avoid fruit drinks and minimize fruit juices because they cause blood sugar fluctuations and may contribute to elevated triglycerides (blood fats) and insulin resistance.

A fruit "drink" is a concoction of fruit juice, water, natural or artificial sweeteners, other flavorings and additives. Most fruit drinks are extremely high in refined sugars and should not be consumed. Look carefully at the label of any bottled or frozen fruit beverage. If it says it's a "drink," don't buy it.

Fruit "juice" can be either "100% juice," or something less than 100%. In either case, because of the high content of fructose (fruit sugar), we recommend you not drink it. A small amount may be OK on special occasions with a meal, but don't drink fruit juice without food. In animal studies and some human studies, a high intake of fructose or sucrose may worsen insulin sensitivity.[225]

It's estimated that in 1910, the annual per capita consumption of fructose from all food sources was around 15 lbs. Today, due to the pervasiveness of high fructose corn syrup in foods and beverages, consumption of fructose from all sources is estimated at *70 lbs. per person per year.*

What happens to all this fructose? It is preferentially converted by the liver into triglycerides, a fat that is carried in the blood and deposited into fat cells.

To complicate matters, the metabolic work required for handling fructose in the liver creates lactic acid, an undesirable byproduct. You'll recall that metformin, a drug used to improve insulin sensitivity, also increases lactic acid production, leading in a few cases to a dangerous condition called lactic acidosis. It has also been suggested that fructose can cause an increase in uric acid (associated with gout).

We recommend that you avoid all sweetened beverages and drinks. Although fruit juices have more nutritional value than soft drinks or fruit drinks, they have a concentration of sugars that is too high for many women with PCOS. If you have a craving for orange juice, have an orange instead. By eating the whole fruit instead of its juice, your greatly diminish the "sugar shock" to your body, plus you get needed fiber and other essential plant nutrients that build your health.

Sparkling Water

Sparkling water is a better choice than fruit juices, fruit drinks, or any artificial or soft drink. Unflavored sparkling water on ice is pleasant and enjoyable. You can also find sparkling water that is mildly flavored with various fruit flavors. If you buy flavored sparkling water, check the label to see what is in it.

Section 10

Other Elements Of Your Diet

10.1 Herbs, Spices, Seasonings and Condiments

If healthy food does not taste good to you, you won't eat it. How a food tastes is the primary reason we eat a food — or avoid it. The purveyors of processed foods know this and have concocted hundreds of products that have a very enticing flavor, texture and "mouth feel."

For the most part, you will no longer be eating those foods. Instead, you will be eating more "whole," natural foods. You can make them more palatable and enjoyable if you add seasonings to enhance their natural flavors.

Here is a list of condiments, seasonings and herbs you can add to your food for better flavor. Be a little wild. Try different things, in different combinations. With a little experimentation, you can make any dish or meal delicious!

Salt and Insulin Resistance

Should you salt your food, or is salt to be avoided because it is bad for you? This is a question to which there is no definitive answer.

Many Americans consume way too much salt, much more than they need. Excessive sodium intake may contribute to high blood pressure, water retention and other health problems.

Others completely avoid salt, often at the advice of their doctors. Salt restriction appears to reduce high blood pressure in some — but not all — individuals.

However, sodium, which is a component of salt, is a necessary nutrient that must derived from food, or from salt, or both. The issue is complicated because the sodium needs of individuals differ with their level of physical activity, body size and other factors.

Our concern here is the relation between salt consumption and insulin resistance. Insulin resistance is a primary causal factor in PCOS.

Either too much salt, or too little, appears to contribute to insulin resistance.[226] [227]   One study has suggested that even moderate salt restriction may worsen insulin resistance.[228]

We honestly don't know what the "right" amount of salt is for you. We can only recommend that you not heavily salt your food. Nor do you want to completely eliminate salt unless required to do so by your physician. You'll want to find a very moderate level of consumption that works for you.

If you do salt your food, we recommend that you also consume liberal amounts of leafy greens and modest amounts of nuts, all of which contain potassium and magnesium. To operate properly, your cells must have the right balance of sodium, potassium and magnesium. The healthy PCOS diet provides good quantities of potassium and magnesium.

The recipes in this book are designed to be tasty and complete without the need to add a lot of salt. If you're accustomed to heavily salting your food, try instead some of the herbs, spices, seasonings and condiments listed in this chapter. You do not have to rely only on salt to flavor your food.

Seasonings and Condiments

Salt-free all-purpose seasoning: A homemade blend (recipe included) of herbs, spices and dried vegetables that is free of salt, yeast, gluten and sugar. Recommended for use with meat, fish, poultry and vegetables.

Braggs Liquid Aminos: Braggs is a liquid protein concentrate, derived from non-GMO soybeans. It's not fermented or heated and is an excellent replacement for tamari. Great on salads and dressings, in soups, on veggies and for use in stir-frys.

Mrs. Dash: A commercial salt-free, gluten-free blend of various vegetables, herbs, seeds, dried fruits and vegetables; available at most grocery stores in the spice section. Comes in 12 varieties.

Fines Herbs: A seasoning mixture comprised of equal parts of tarragon, chervil, chives and parsley. Delicious seasoning for all meats, vegetables, salads and salad dressings.

Herbs de Provence: Distinctly French and used in French cuisine, this seasoning mixture is made up of marjoram, thyme, summer savory, basil, rosemary, sage, fennel seeds and lavender. Can be purchased commercially or you can make the mixture yourself.

Tamari: Tamari is a dark sauce made from soybeans. It has a distinctively mellow flavor and doesn't contain as much salt as commercial soy sauce. Try to get a "low sodium" and "wheat-free" version of tamari if you can. Examples of wheat-free tamari are Eden Organic tamari and San-J Wheat-Free Organic tamari. Wheat-free tamari is available in some health food stores.

We have included minimal amounts of tamari in some of the recipes for this diet. Treat tamari as an "optional extra;" if your taste allows you to get by without it and to substitute one of the many other options in this chapter, feel free to do so. Tamari can be quite helpful in making food taste better.

Spike: A blend of 39 granulated or powdered herbs, vegetables and spices from the kitchen of gourmet nutritionist, Gaylord Hauser. It comes in salt or salt-free versions. Spike contains: toasted onion, nutritional yeast, garlic, celery root, dill, horseradish, mustard, lemon peel, orange, parsley, red bell peppers, green bell peppers, white pepper, rose hips, summer savory, mushroom, safflower, white onion, spinach, tomato, sweet paprika, celery seed, cayenne pepper, turmeric, cumin, ginger, coriander, fenugreek, cloves, cinnamon, oregano, tarragon, sweet basil, marjoram, rosemary and thyme. There is 24 mg. potassium in the salt-free version per 1/4 serving. It can be purchased in most grocery stores.

Dijon mustard: Most commercial brands of Dijon mustard contain some combination of white wine, onion, garlic, dry mustard, a little honey, oil, salt and Tabasco sauce. We have included a honey-free recipe in this book.

Morton Salt Substitute: Regular table salt is sodium chloride. This product is potassium chloride and may be a better choice than regular salt if your doctor has told you to reduce sodium intake.

Dulse and other seaweeds (nori, kombu, kelp): High in minerals and micronutrients, specifically iodine (which supports thyroid function) and calcium, dried seaweeds add an interesting flavor to foods, particularly soups and salads. They can be purchased in powdered or flake form. Use moderately because of its high sodium content, but go ahead and experiment a little. They'll add some variety to your culinary experience. They can be found at most health food stores or purchased online.

Dark chocolate chips: In some health food stores or other retail outlets you can find dark chocolate chips that do not contain milk. If you're yearning for a bit of a treat, you can occasionally use a small amount of chocolate chips to liven up your meal or snack. For example, if having raw nuts as a snack is too boring, add a few chocolate chips. It doesn't take many chips to render a pleasant chocolate flavor to a snack or meal.

Herbs and Spices

Herbs are healthful and delicious additions to any diet, and certain combinations give certain ethnic foods their own unique personality. For example:
- **Oregano, Marjoram, Rosemary** - used a lot in Greek and Italian dishes.
- **Thyme, Savory (Winter or Summer) and Tarragon** - provide a mild herbal flavor
- Basil - delivers a strong, delicious herbal flavor.
- **Cayenne, Chili Pepper, Cumin** - for people who like spicy food; used widely in Mexican dishes.
- **Cardamom, Curry, Ginger, Turmeric** - exotic combinations used in Asian and East Indian cuisines.
- **Cinnamon, Nutmeg, Allspice, Anise, Cloves, Ginger** - deliver sweet, pungent and distinct flavors.

So here are some favorite herbs and spices that can add all kinds of delight to your menus.

Mix, match and experiment. Learn what tastes best to you…and enjoy!

Allspice: Tastes like a combination of nutmeg, cloves and cinnamon. Used in both savory and sweet dishes. A welcome addition to fruit salads.

Anise: Use both seeds and fresh leaves. Has a sweet licorice flavor.

Basil: Pungent flavor reminiscent of cloves and licorice, but distinctly herbal. Used in Mediterranean and Thai cooking. Most basil has green leaves, but opal basil is a beautiful purple color. Also, try lemon basil and cinnamon basil for some interesting and delicious flavors. Great in vegetable dishes and salads.

Bay Leaves: Used to flavor stews, soups, vegetables and meats but too much can make the dish bitter. Remove before serving.

Cardamom: Has a pungent aroma and a spicy, sweet flavor. It's widely used in Scandinavian and East Indian cooking.

Caraway: Aromatic seeds that have a nutty, delicate anise flavor and are widely used in German, Austrian and Hungarian cuisine. Use to flavor stews, meats and vegetables.

Cayenne: Made from the dried pods of chili peppers. Cayenne has little aroma but it is *extremely hot* to the taste. Adds zing to any dish…but be careful.

Chili Powder: A powdered mixture of dried chili peppers, oregano, garlic, cumin, coriander and cloves. Combines well with lime and is used in South American and Mexican dishes. Great sprinkled on eggs.

Cilantro: Cilantro is the green leaves of the coriander plant (and the ground seeds are used in curries and other East Indian dishes). Cilantro is also called Chinese parsley and it has a pungent fragrance. Use just the leaves since too many stems make a dish taste "soapy." Used in Asian, Caribbean and Latin American cooking. Its distinct flavor lends itself to spicy dishes.

Cinnamon: Widely used in sweet dishes, but also makes an intriguing addition to savory dishes such as stews and curries. Sprinkle sparingly on fruit for a taste of the exotic; particularly good with apples. Studies suggest it helps regulate blood sugar.

Cloves: Gives a sweet, spicy flavor to food; very intense; a little goes a long way.

Coriander Seed: Available in seed form or ground. Use in curry dishes and soups.

Cumin: Cumin is aromatic, nutty and peppery all at once. It is available in seed and ground forms.

Curry Powder: Curry powder is a blend of up to 20 spices, herbs and seeds. Among those most commonly used are chilies, cardamom, cinnamon, coriander, cumin, nutmeg, cloves, fennel seed, fenugreek, mace, red and black pepper, poppy and sesame seeds, saffron, tamarind and turmeric. Used in East Indian and Asian cooking mostly, but a dash of curry can liven up an egg salad like you wouldn't believe. Also delicious in chicken soup.

Dill: Fresh dill weed is far superior to dried; however it quickly loses its fragrance during heating, so don't add it until toward the end of the cooking time. Dill weed is used to flavor salads, vegetables, meats and sauces. If neither fresh nor dried leaves are available, you can use dill seed, which, when heated, is stronger and more potent than the leaves.

Dry Mustard: Dry mustard is just ground mustard seed. Use to spice up sauces and main dishes and as an ingredient in salad dressings.

Fennel: Fennel bulbs and stems are used as a vegetable, but the leaves and seeds are used as herbs, for garnish as well as flavor. It has a delicate, sweetness that complements both sweet and savory foods. Promotes good digestion.

Garlic: Garlic is a cousin to leeks, chives, onions and shallots. Mincing, crushing, pureeing or pressing garlic releases its essential oils and provides a stronger flavor than slicing it or leaving it whole. Garlic has a number health-building qualities and is highly recommended.

Ginger Root: Pungent, slightly sweet and spicy, ginger root is primary to Asian and Indian cooking but finds its way into almost all cuisine around the globe. Grate, grind or sliver it. Good with fruits as well as savory dishes. Promotes good digestion and has anti-inflammatory properties.

Marjoram: Delicate flavor somewhat like a mild oregano. Marjoram is used to flavor many foods, particularly meats and vegetables. Best added toward the end of cooking time so its flavor doesn't completely disappear.

Nutmeg: Spicy and sweet, nutmeg is sold ground or whole. Whole, grated nutmeg zest is superior to what you buy in the store, pre-ground and dried. Nutmeg is excellent when used on fruits and vegetables.

Oregano: Belongs to the mint family; is similar to both marjoram and thyme, although not as delicate as marjoram. It's pungent so use with caution. Dried is more potent than fresh.

Parsley: Used as a flavoring and garnish.

Pepper: Pepper enhances the flavor of both savory and sweet dishes; stimulates gastric juices and therefore supports good digestion when used in moderate amounts. Peppercorns come in three basic types: black, white and green. The most common is black; it's slightly sweet and hot and the strongest flavored of the three.

Peppermint: Peppermint is a pungent herb and great digestive aid. Use chopped as part of a recipe or use as garnish for fruits and vegetables.

Rosemary: Highly aromatic, with the resinous flavor of pine and a hint of lemon. Rosemary is used in a variety of dishes including fruit salads, vegetables, soups, vegetables, meat, fish and egg dishes, salads and salad dressings.

Saffron: Pungent and aromatic; primarily used to flavor and tint food, but is essential to many dishes such as bouillabaisse (fish soup).

Sage: Slightly bitter and strongly pungent, sage is a good herb to use with poultry. Pineapple sage is a possible addition to fruit salads when used in small amounts.

Savory: There are two types of savory, winter and summer. Both have a strong fragrance and flavor that hints of both mint and thyme.

Tarragon: Aromatic herb known for its distinctive flavor which is a bit like anise but more herb-like. Tarragon gives a class French flair to food and is delicious with chicken, fish and vegetables.

Thyme: Garden thyme has a slightly minty/lemony flavor; lemon thyme is more lemony. Thyme is widely used in cooking, adding flavor to vegetables and soups, as well as meat, poultry and fish dishes.

Turmeric: Turmeric has a pungent, bitter flavor and yellow-orange color. It is used in East Indian cooking and is almost always used in curry preparations. It's also a primary ingredient in making mustard, giving commercially prepared mustard its color. Has anti-inflammatory and other important health properties.

Vanilla: Fruit of the orchid, vanilla adds a sweet, full, creamy flavor to fruits and smoothies.

10.2 Sweeteners

In general, added sweeteners are not recommended. If you find you must have an added sweetener, use stevia.

Best Sweeteners for Recommended Diet Level

- Stevia
- Whole fruits from Recommended Level list

Good Sweeteners for Maintenance Diet Level

- Stevia
- Whole fruits from Recommended or Maintenance Level lists
- Maltitol (use sparingly)

Unhealthy Sweeteners - Avoid

- All food products and beverages containing fructose (except whole fruit)
- All food products and beverages containing corn syrup or high fructose corn syrup
- Amasake
- Apple juice
- Aspartame - possible adverse long-term health effects - use at your own risk
- Brown rice syrup
- Concentrated fruit sweetener
- Corn syrup
- Corn syrup solids
- Dairy products containing corn syrup or high fructose corn syrup
- Date sugar
- Fructose (also known as levulose or fruit sugar)
- Fruit juice concentrate
- Fruit juice sweetener
- Fruit Source (granulated sweetener made from grape juice concentrate and rice syrup
- Glucose
- High fructose corn syrup
- Honey
- Invert sugar
- Lactose (if you are lactose intolerant)
- Maltose
- Maple syrup

- Molasses
- Saccharin
- Sucanet (made from evaporated sugar cane juice)
- Sucralose (Splenda)
- Sucrose (table sugar)

Notes

Below is some additional information about various sweeteners. Except for stevia, we're not recommending these sweeteners; we're just informing you about them.

Amasake
Amasake is a traditional Japanese product made by fermenting sweet brown rice into a thick liquid. It is a creamy, quickly digested beverage used by athletes after a workout or as a sweetener in cooking or baking.

Aspartame
Aspartame, an artificial sweetener found in some soft drinks, has been associated with a higher incidence of brain disorders in lab animals. In addition, chronic aspartame ingestion may have cumulative negative effects, possibly because of formaldehyde formation. A great deal of controversy swirls around the possible adverse health effects of aspartame. Until the actual long-term safety of aspartame has been proven, we strongly recommend you stay away from it.

Barley malt
Barley malt is a thick, dark, slow-digesting sweetener made from sprouted barley. It has a malt-like flavor and is most widely known for its use in brewing beer. Malted barley has a high complement of enzymes for converting its starches into simple sugars. Pure malt extract, which is relatively expensive, is sometimes adulterated with corn syrup, which is cheap. Barley malt extract (available in powder and liquid forms) is also used medicinally as a bulking agent to promote bowel regularity.

Brown rice syrup
Brown rice syrup is a naturally processed sweetener, made from sprouted brown rice. It is thick and mild-flavored.

Date sugar
Date sugar is a powder made from dried, ground dates.

Fruit juice concentrates
Fruit juice concentrates are made by cooking down peach, pineapple, grape and pear juices to produce a sweeter, more concentrated product. The product is then frozen to increase shelf life.

FruitSource®

FruitSource is the brand name of a granulated sweetener made from grape juice concentrate and rice syrup.

Honey

Honey is a sweet substance made from plant nectar (sucrose) by the honeybee. About 40% of the sugar in honey is fructose. Honey is available raw or pasteurized. Commercial honey is heated to 150 to 160°F (65.5 to 71°C) to prevent crystallization and yeast formation whereas "organic" or "raw" honey has not been heat-treated.

Although honey many contain clostridium botulinum spores (the bacterium that causes botulism), the high sugar content of the honey prevents the spores from germinating in the gastrointestinal tracts of normal adults. However, this is not true in infants under one year of age.

Maple syrup

Maple syrup is made from the boiled sap of sugar maple trees. The taste and color vary depending on the temperature at which the sap was boiled and how long the sap was cooked.

Sucanat®

Sucanat is a branded ingredient made from evaporated sugar cane juice. It resembles raw sugar in appearance and taste, though it is slightly less sweet. It is considered to be less refined than raw sugar.

Stevia

Stevia is derived from a South American shrub *(Stevia rebaudiana)*. A good quality leaf is estimated to be 300 times sweeter than cane sugar, or sucrose. Also known as "honey leaf" and "yerba dulce," stevia is not absorbed through the digestive tract and is therefore non-caloric.

Although stevia adds sweetness to foods, it cannot be sold as a sweetener because the FDA considers it an unapproved food additive. However, under the provisions of the Dietary Supplement Health and Education Act (DSHEA) passed in 1994, stevia can be sold as a dietary supplement. Stevia also appears to have medicinal properties. Preliminary evidence suggests that it may lower blood pressure, prevent and reverse diabetes, and possess anti-viral properties.

We recommend stevia as a substitute for aspartame and sucralose. You can find stevia in some health food stores or online.

Sucralose (Splenda)

Sucralose is manufactured by chlorinating sugar (substituting chlorine atoms for hydroxyls) and is much sweeter than sucrose (table sugar).

The FDA has pronounced sucralose as "safe." However, there are no long-term studies to establish that there are no adverse health effects from chronic consumption of sucralose. We simply don't know. Experimental administration of sucralose to lab animals is not reassuring.

It could be argued that sucralose is less problematic than aspartame. Nevertheless, we recommend you not use sucralose (Splenda).

10.3 Snacks

If you're at the office, traveling, or just between meals at home, you may want to have a snack. Here are some possibilities:

1. **Fresh fruit** such as berries, apple or grapes. Have a few nuts with your fruit for added protein and fat to help stabilize your blood sugar.

2. **Raw vegetables** are portable and handy. Eat alone or with a guacamole/salsa dip.
   - Broccoli
   - Carrots
   - Cauliflower
   - Celery
   - Cherry tomatoes
   - Cucumbers
   - Jicama slices
   - Mushrooms
   - Radishes
   - Tomato & avocado slices

3. **Dehydrated vegetables**
   - Any home-dehydrated vegetable

4. **Raw nuts or seeds** — anything you like except peanuts

5. **Animal protein snacks**
   - Broiled chicken breast slices (cold, skinless)
   - Homemade beef jerky (no salt)
   - Hard-boiled egg or deviled egg
   - Lean beef, cold slices
   - Homemade meat jerky

6. **Seafood**
   - Homemade dehydrated salmon strips
   - Sardines, small tin
   - Shrimp, cold, cooked — peel and eat

7. **Sprouts**
   - Crunchy sprout mixes
   - Bean sprouts
   - Radish sprouts

8. **Soups**
   - Hot soup in a thermos
   - Soup heated anyplace where there is a microwave

9. **Miscellaneous**
   - Olives, green

10.4 Meal Replacement Shakes

Meal replacement shakes, protein powders and beverages for weight loss are intensely marketed by the weight loss industry. But do they work?

They can be effective for weight loss *if* they are part of an overall healthy diet, and *if* the meal replacement product is of the highest quality.

Meal replacement products are not part of the health PCOS diet. We recommend that meal replacement shakes not be a regular part of your diet unless you are under a doctor's supervision, or you are using them as an occasional snack or meal substitute when a normal meal is not available.

Types of Meal Replacement Products

Meal replacement products generally fall under these main categories:
- **Very low carb.** Almost all protein, very few carbs, not a balanced meal replacement
- **High protein.** Generally high protein mix with low amounts of fat and carbs
- **"Balanced."** Roughly 40% protein, 30% fat, 30% carb - similar to Zone diet
- **Weight gainers.** High calorie drink mixes for those who need to gain weight
- **Carbohydrate drinks.** For "quick energy"

You'll want to avoid the weight gainers and carbohydrate drinks. You'll want to carefully evaluate the low carb and "balanced" meal replacement products.

Quality of Meal Replacement Products

Price competition is fierce among meal replacement products. Therefore, there is constant pressure to use the cheapest ingredients and consequently the product quality varies widely. The cheapest product may not be the best product. When you read the product label, you may encounter a lot of "smoke and mirrors." For example, one popular "low carb" meal replacement powder contains "beef protein." That appears to be a nice way of saying "gelatin." Gelatin is not high quality protein.

They Are a Processed Food

Keep in mind that all meal replacement products and protein powders are highly processed foods. Therefore they may be lacking in food components that you need.

One prominent example is fiber. Dietary fiber is necessary for gastrointestinal health and helps to regulate absorption of nutrients into the bloodstream. Yet most meal replacement products are low in fiber. In fact, some have no fiber whatsoever.

Another problem, especially with the "low-carb" products is that processed protein is very bitter. This bitterness must be masked by sweeteners. But to keep the carb calories down, they don't use sucrose (table sugar) or fructose (high fructose corn syrup). Instead, they resort to artificial, non-caloric sweeteners such as sucralose (Splenda), aspartame or acesulfame potassium. The health consequences of habitual consumption of artificial sweeteners are unknown. All we can say is that these sweeteners do not help you build good health.

Some of the "balanced" meal replacement products use fructose. A little fructose is OK, but some products have excessive amounts. In addition, the fructose is absorbed quickly since it is refined product, separated form the plant from which it came. A lot of fructose entering your system all at once is not desirable.

Some products contain inexpensive vegetable oils. The quality of these processed oils is unknown. They may also give you plenty of unwanted omega-6 fatty acids but none or not enough of the more desirable omega-3 essential fatty acids. Some of the products use "high-oleic" oils that are relatively low in omega-6 fatty acids and relatively high in monounsaturated fats, which is better.

The proteins in the products may be allergenic. Allergies to soy, milk and egg are fairly common. Most proteins in the products come from these sources.

And finally, the processed protein in meal replacement products is denatured and damaged to some extent during the refining process. The damaged protein is not as good for you as the undamaged protein found in whole foods.

When to Use Meal Replacement Products

Meal replacement shakes or products can be used occasionally if you are not able to eat a normal meal. A high-quality meal replacement shake is far superior to munching on processed snacks or convenience foods because you are hungry.

If you intend to use meal replacement shakes instead of eating meals as a way to lose a lot of weight, we strongly recommend that you do so only under a doctor's supervision. Licensed naturopathic physicians, for example, are familiar with the use of quality meal replacement products as part of a carefully controlled dietary program to get healthier and lose weight. These programs utilize very specific meal plans to ensure nutritional adequacy. You progress is carefully monitored to ensure you do not get into trouble.

How to Make a Meal Replacement Shake

By themselves, many meal replacement products don't taste very good. To make them taste better, put some water into a blender and then add your meal replacement powder. Add some fresh or frozen berries (any kind). You can use other fruit, although berries are your best option.

If you like your shakes thick and cold, add some ice or frozen fruit. Then blend and drink. (However, it's preferable to not use ice since the cold can impair digestion).

If you are using a product that contains little or no fat, consider adding some flax seed oil or ground up flax seeds. You might also add some macadamia nut oil, which adds a nutty flavor and is mostly unsaturated fat.

Personally, we like to add cod liver oil or fish oil to a shake, in order to get some beneficial omega-3 fatty acids. Cod liver oil also has some vitamin D, which may be helpful to PCOS women. Lemon-flavored fish oil is available so that you can mask the fishy taste.

A final option is to add some powdered fiber. There are quite a number of powdered fiber products to choose from.

"Medical Foods"

Some companies produce protein or meal replacement powders that are marketed primarily to health professionals, who then in turn prescribe them to their patients. These protein powders are generally of the highest quality and have added nutrients to help the patient achieve certain health goals. They are typically fortified with vitamins, minerals and other specialty nutrients. These products are referred to as "medical foods."

Two categories of medical foods that may be of interest to you are those that (1) aid in detoxification, and (2) help deal with insulin and blood sugar problems.

The detoxification products are often used as part of a doctor-supervised detoxification or "metabolic clearing." The purpose is to help the body rid itself of accumulated toxins and undesirable metabolic byproducts. Detoxification medical foods typically have added ingredients that support the liver as it does its detoxification work.

Medical foods also help people with insulin resistance, or "Syndrome X," to better control their insulin and blood sugar levels. They have a protein-fat-carbohydrate ratio designed to minimize fluctuations of insulin and blood sugar. They also have ingredients to support the thyroid and adrenal glands, balance cortisol, maintain energy and avoid fatigue. Some products also contain antioxidants as well as neurological and intestinal support nutrients.

These medical foods are also formulated to be as free of food allergens as possible. The protein source is usually a rice protein. People are much more likely to be allergic to soy, dairy or egg than they are to rice.

Medical food powders may be used as:
- An occasional meal replacement
- An in-between meal snack

They can be mixed in a blender with water or vegetable juice, and whole fruit from our Recommended List. You can also blend in green powders such as barley greens, wheatgrass powder, spirulina or chlorella. Adding a green powder substantially increases the nutritive value of the meal or snack.

If you are looking for specific medical foods products, consult with your doctor or a naturopathic physician.

Section 11

More Dietary Tips

11.1 Eat Organic

Organic foods — raised without the use of chemical fertilizers or pesticides — provide several important benefits:
- They are healthier than conventional foods.
- They are lower in pesticides and other environmental chemicals.
- They have a higher level of nutrients as compared to non-organic foods.[229]

First of all, it's important to understand that organic foods are healthier for you than conventional foods grown with the application of chemical fertilizers and pesticides. The Danish Institute of Agricultural Sciences performed a study on rats showing that rats fed a diet of organic food were healthier and slimmer than rats feed the identical non-organic foods.[230] Although this was a dietary experiment with lab animals, it's reasonable to think the same benefits apply to humans.

Secondly, it's very important for you to minimize your exposure to environmental chemical substances and other toxins, for the reasons we discussed in the chapter entitled *What Causes PCOS?*

You can take a major step to reduce your exposure by switching to organic foods. Organic foods are those that are grown without the application of pesticides, artificial fertilizers or other chemicals.

Pesticides in foods are probably your biggest concern. Many crops are heavily sprayed with pesticides in order to increase crop yields, improve appearance of the food, and increase profits. However, chemical pesticides are not only toxic to bugs, they are also toxic to you.

When pesticides and other chemicals are sprayed on food crops, some of the chemical is absorbed directly from the spraying, while some is absorbed into the plant from the soil via the plant's roots.

To find out more about pesticides and other toxins in your vegetable, fruits and other foods, you can visit these websites:

1) Environmental Working Group: www.ewg.org/issues/siteindex/issues.php?issueid=101

The above site contains a collection of articles describing the pollutants that are found in your food supply and in your body.

2) FoodNews (also provided by the Environmental Working Group): www.foodnews.org

The foodsnews.org site will give you the pesticide levels for commonly purchased produce. For example, you may think that fresh spinach is very good for you. Well, it is, except that 83% of spinach contains pesticides. At least one-half of spinach tested had at least two pesticides, and one sample contained 10 pesticides. In this case, you may wish to switch to organic spinach, which has fewer pesticides.

Even though the use of some pesticides such as DDT are banned or limited in the U.S., many of the foods we eat are imported from foreign countries that have few or no limitations on the application of pesticides to crops. Foods from other countries are much more likely to contain higher levels of pesticides than foods grown in the U.S. Since it's almost impossible to tell the difference between domestic and foreign produce, you could be exposed to more pesticides than you think. This a good reason to choose organic foods.

Are Organic Foods Really Free of Pesticides?

A recent study of 94,000 food samples has shown that organically grown foods (without the application of pesticides) still contain pesticides, but only 1/3 as much as regular foods.[231] Moreover, organic foods are only 1/10 as likely to contain residues of more than one pesticide.

A significant proportion of pesticide residues in organic foods come from long-banned but environmentally stubborn chemicals such as DDT, which plants can absorb from the environment years after farmers have stopped using them. It is also possible that pesticides may have drifted from a non-organic field onto an organic field.

Nearly all of our food, water and air is polluted. Your goal is to do your best to minimize your exposure. Organic produce has lower levels of pesticides and higher levels of nutrients than ordinary produce.

Grow Your Own Vegetables

The best way to "eat organic" is to grow your own food.

If you have the space, and if you have the time, we strongly recommend you start your own organic vegetable garden. Doing so confers several important benefits:
- You can eat plant foods that were picked minutes or hours earlier. Most produce in the market is several days to weeks old and has lost most of its more fragile nutrients.
- Organic produce is much richer in nutrients.
- Working in your garden is pleasurable, good exercise and a way to reduce stress.
- You have the satisfaction of creating some of the food that you eat.

Get yourself a gardening book, buy some organic seeds and get started!

11.2 Eating in Restaurants

If you find yourself frequently eating out at restaurants, you're in trouble. A study conducted at Tufts University showed that people who consumed food from restaurants more often were fatter and conversely, people who consumed food from restaurants less often were leaner.[232]

In addition, people who frequently ate restaurant food consumed more calories and fat, and less fiber, in their diets than those who ate in restaurant less often. For example, people who ate restaurant food 13 times a month or more consumed 18% more calories per kilogram of body weight, 12% more total fat and 36% less fiber than people who ate restaurant food less than 4.3 times a month. Eating restaurant food 13 times a month versus 4.3 times a month corresponded to a difference in body fat of about 5%. According to this study, the simple avoidance of restaurants could result in a 5% weight loss.

However, we don't live in a perfect world. You will be eating out occasionally. This chapter outlines some guidelines to help you get a healthier meal.

Restaurant Food Selection

To minimize blood sugar fluctuations, have some protein in the meal, such as grilled fish. Avoid high-glycemic carbohydrates such as bread, crackers, baked potatoes and white rice. Instead, have a salad and a vegetable dish.

Avoid foods to which you are allergic.

Make sure no MSG (monosodium glutamate) is in your food. If you are in a Chinese or Japanese restaurant, be sure to ask.

The meal portion you are served may be much larger than you need. Eat slowly. Leave something on your plate when you are finished.

Listed below are some recommendations when eating out in restaurants. They are not "ideal" recommendations, but at least they give you some guidelines.

Soup & Salad Restaurant
Avoid
- Salad with dressing or mayonnaise already mixed in
- Frozen yogurt, puddings, whipped cream
- Pizza
- Salad dressings that have oil
- Muffins and bread
- Margarine, butter and butter spreads

Better Choices

- Cafeteria style (you get to control choice of food)
- Olive oil for salad dressing
- The fatty things are grouped in separate areas, so you can easily avoid them

Seafood Restaurant

Avoid

- Deep fried seafood
- Seafood dunked in butter or batter
- Stuffed seafood
- Combination plates, which usually have something fried

Better Choices

- Manhattan clam chowder better than creamy New England version.
- Clear seafood gumbo better than creamy seafood bisque
- Poached or grilled seafood better than fried
- Lemon juice better than tartar or white sauce
- A favorite: poached fish with vegetables and salad

American Steak House

Avoid

- Almost all cuts of red meat
- Ribs
- White rice

Better Choices

- Grilled chicken
- London broil (flank steak)
- Trim away all visible fat from meat serving
- Medium-well done, so fat has a chance to be cooked out
- Focus on salad and vegetables

American Diner

Avoid

- Almost everything

Better Choices

- Soups, although they may be too salty or contain wheat and dairy
- Tossed salad, dressing on the side
- Steamed vegetables
- Roast turkey
- Grilled chicken

Pizza Place

Avoid
• Almost everything

Better Choices
• Salad

Delicatessen

Avoid
• Almost everything

Better Choices
• Roast turkey
• Some delis have good soups, although they may be salty or contain wheat

Mexican Restaurant

Avoid
• Deep fried corn tortillas
• Cheese and sour cream
• Go easy on the refried beans and rice

Better Choices
• Chicken or fish taco
• Salad
• Guacamole and salsa
• Soup

Italian Restaurant

Avoid
• Any dish that is very oily
• Pasta, spaghetti, cannelloni or any other dish containing mostly wheat products
• Tortoni, spumoni or other desserts

Better Choices
• Minestrone (eat around any pasta in the soup)
• Chicken cacciatore (eat around the pasta or spaghetti)
• Green salad with vinegar dressing
• Any dish with minimal wheat or rice

Chinese Restaurant

Avoid
- Stay away any food that has MSG
- White steamed rice
- Fried rice
- Egg rolls
- Fried wontons
- Fried noodles
- Most meat dishes
- Sweet and sour dishes
- Most Chinese food

Better Choices
- Chop suey better than chow mein
- Stir-fried dishes in moderation
- Some seafood dishes
- Some vegetable dishes

Appetizers

Avoid
- Deep fried
- In a sauce

Better Choices
- Vegetable sticks
- Tomato or V8 juice

Salads

Avoid
- Potato salad
- Macaroni salad
- Greek
- Chef (unless you hold the ham and cheese)

Better Choices
- Caesar salad
- Tossed green salad
- Garden salad
- Spinach salad
- Ask for dressing on side

Salad Dressings

Avoid
- Cheesy
- Creamy

Better Choices
- Lemon juice & olive oil
- Vinegar & herb
- Salsa
- Oil-free dressing

Entrée

Avoid
- Gravies or sauces on the entree
- Deep fried

Better Choices
- Roasted, baked, broiled, boiled or stir-fried
- Trim all visible fat
- Remove skin from poultry
- Sauces served on the side - use sparingly

Potatoes

Avoid
- All potatoes

Breads

Avoid
- All bread, muffins, croissants and other baked goods

Cereals

Avoid
- Almost all cereals

Better Choices
- Hot oatmeal (**not** instant)

Vegetables

Avoid
- Served in a cream or sauce
- Deep fried and breaded

Better Choices
- Stewed
- Steamed
- Boiled
- Baked
- Raw

Breakfast

Avoid
- Bacon
- Ham
- Hash browns
- Omelets
- Fried eggs
- Eggs Benedict

Better Choices
- Poached or hard boiled egg
- Low-fat cottage cheese (if necessary)
- Vegetable side dish if available
- Hot oatmeal (not instant)

Beverages

Avoid
- Ice
- Coffee
- Milk
- Soft drinks
- Fruit juice or fruit drinks

Better Choices
- Water (add slice of lemon for flavor)
- Mineral or sparkling water
- Tomato, V8 or other vegetable juice
- Tea

Desserts

Avoid
- There are no healthy prepared desserts

Better Choices
- Small amount fresh fruit (not melon)
- Small amount of raw nuts or seeds - ask your server, they may have some on hand

Food Safety

It's not likely you'll get sick from eating restaurant food — but it's possible.

When eating out, try to only eat food that has been cooked just before it is served to you. It's a good idea to ask your server whether your food will be freshly prepared and cooked. To save money, some restaurants have their food prepared ahead of time by outside vendors, or they store foods for too long without throwing them out. The result is possible contamination with pathogenic bacteria.

In some restaurants and delicatessens, soups, sauces and stews are stored in large containers, often uncovered, to be quickly reheated in a microwave when an order is placed. Microwave cooking may not kill Salmonella or other strains of pathogenic bacteria.

Be cautious with salad bars. At first glance, salad bars seem like a good place to get healthy food in a hurry. But look again. Some years ago the Wall Street Journal sent a reporter to investigate the cleanliness of salad bars in different parts of the country. Problems were observed with both the restaurant but with the clientele. People are unsanitary in their use of salad bars. They sometimes sample food and put it back. The handles of the serving utensils frequently fall into the food trays, providing an opportunity for contamination.

Do not eat food that has been prepared by a street vendor. You have no way to evaluate the safety of the food.

Avoid restaurants where there are flies. Flies can spread parasitic cysts and pathogenic bacteria, and suggest the owner may not be concerned about cleanliness.

Recommended Reading

For additional reading about restaurant food, take a look at *Restaurant Confidential* by Michael Jacobson and Jayne Hurley. The tone of the book is a bit snippy, but the content is informative.

11.3 Eating Away from Home

Most women are on the go, whether for business or social reasons. Here are some guidelines and ideas for those times when you are away from home.

Eating in the Office

By far the best approach is to bring your lunch from home. That way, you have total control over what you are eating.

You can bring leftovers from last night's dinner (such as salmon, salad, vegetables). Or bring homemade soup such as beef and vegetable soup.

Bring a piece of fresh fruit and some nuts for dessert.

To drink, you can have herb tea, green tea or sparkling water instead of coffee or soft drinks.

Parties

If you're going to a party that does not include a sit-down dinner, we suggest you have a meal at home before you go.

If you intend to consume alcohol, beer or wine would be the preferred drink. Hard liquor is not recommended. However, if you do plan to drink hard liquor, please take a B-complex tablet and a multivitamin tablet beforehand so that you can help your system keep your blood sugar in balance.

At the party, eat as many vegetable items as you like. If vegetables are not available, look for fresh fruit. Stay away from snack crackers, potato chips and other junk food.

Busy yourself with conversation and make an effort to keep at least six feet away from the food table.

Drink plenty of non-alcoholic beverages such as sparkling water.

Visiting

Visiting a relative or friend can be a touchy thing when it comes to food.

Explain to your host in advance that you are on a special diet and you won't be able to enjoy his or her wonderful desserts and fried foods.

If offered a fatty, sugar-loaded or high-glycemic food that was especially prepared for you, have some but leave some (or most) on your plate.

If you know in advance that the host will not have any healthy food in the house, offer to prepare a healthy dish and bring it with you. Or, offer to bring some healthy ingredients and help your host to prepare the meal, using your ingredients as part of the meal.

If your host offers you bacon, fried eggs and English muffins for breakfast, don't worry. Have some breakfast and enjoy the conversation. You don't have to eat everything on your plate.

On the Road

Hotels
Hotels are like islands. It's sometimes not feasible to go to another location outside of the hotel to obtain food or eat a meal. So you may need to plan ahead.

Prepare healthy snacks at home and bring them with you. For example, you might bring a couple of apples and some nuts.

Or you could bring a high-protein meal replacement powder and a plastic shake mixer with you. To that you would add water or possibly some fruit juice (diluted 50/50 with water) and yogurt. Blend and enjoy.

Another alternative is to stop at a health store in your destination city to get healthy snacks. If there's no health store handy, go to a large supermarket to hunt out something that is fairly healthy.

At breakfast, see if the hotel offers a buffet. Look it over; you may find it allows you a better choice of food than what is on the menu. In any case, a reasonable breakfast would be hot oatmeal, eggs and beverage of your choice (not orange juice).

Many hotels offer an excellent lunch buffet featuring a salad bar, soup bar and several hot dishes. Have some chicken or fish, along with a couple of vegetable dishes and possibly a salad.

For dinner, keep it light, especially if it's late. Sliced turkey or fish with steamed vegetables is a possibility. Or a chicken salad.

In Your Car
Preparation before you leave on your trip is the key to healthy eating! Having to stop at a convenience store along the way guarantees you'll be eating poor quality food. Before you leave, prepare an assortment of snacks. Bring a small cooler if they need to be kept cold.

If you're planning to go car camping, fill your cooler with several prepared or pre-cooked meals to make your camp cooking easy and healthy.

On Campus

If you live in a college dorm or boarding or sorority house where meals are prepared for you, you have little say about what is provided. Your options are even more restricted than in a restaurant. Most "institutional" food is too high in refined carbohydrates, which is exactly the type of food you want to avoid.

When a meal is served, have the animal protein and vegetables. Minimize grain dishes and avoid all baked products. Don't have dessert unless it is fresh fruit.

In some cases, the meal preparation staff may be able to prepare meals for people with special needs, such as diabetics. If your meal preparation staff can make special meals, show relevant portions of this book to the staff and see if they are able to prepare meals that meet our guidelines.

If you cannot get enough high-quality protein in the meals that are provided to you, then perhaps you can prepare protein shakes in your room, even if you don't have a refrigerator. For example, you could have a blender, some whey protein concentrate protein powder, and fresh fruit on hand. As a snack or meal supplement, you could blend protein powder, water and fresh fruit.

Another option is to get an occasional meal at a good restaurant or have a meal at a friend's house.

You may also be able to go to the student union or on-campus food court and find salads, soups or other foods that may meet the healthy guidelines in this book.

If you live on campus, it may be especially hard to control your diet according the high standards we've outlined in this book. Just do the best you can. You won't be living on campus forever.

11.4 Healthy Eating Habits

What you eat is most important. But *how* you eat is also very helpful for improving your health. Creating the best physical and emotional environment helps you to optimally digest and assimilate the food you are eating. It also reduces potential increases in cortisol, the stress hormone that causes problems for women with PCOS.

Here are some tips for how to eat in best possible way.

- Briefly meditate, or at least take a deep breath to relax before starting to eat.

- Don't read the newspaper, watch TV or discuss unpleasant subjects while eating.

- Eat slowly. You'll eat less and enjoy your meal more if you don't hurry. Eating slowly also improves your digestion.

- Chew your food well. If you can't chew it well, don't eat it.

- Finish what you're chewing before you put more food into your mouth.

- After eating, don't eat again until the food has been digested.

- Avoid any food that causes unpleasant feelings no mater how healthy it is presumed to be. You may be intolerant or allergic to it.

- Don't drink ice water or cold beverages with a meal. The cold will stop digestion.

- Don't eat when in pain, emotionally upset, tired, or immediately after hard work.

- Eat foods that are close to room temperature (not refrigerated, not piping hot).

- Eat less than you think you need. If you're not sure you've had enough, wait 5-10 minutes before deciding eating more.

- Don't skip breakfast. Eat something 4-5 times a day. This keeps your blood sugar more balanced.

- Have some protein each time you eat. This keeps your blood sugar balanced.

- Skip desserts. As soon as you've finished, get up from the table and brush your teeth. Brushing your teeth gets the taste of food out of your mouth and signals to you that you won't be eating any more food for a while. If the weather is good, take a walk around the block or involve yourself in some other activity to take your mind off of any desire to have dessert or eat more food.

11.5 When Should You Eat?

Some women who are concerned about their weight, or live a rushed life, often skip breakfast and don't each much during the day. But when they get home, they have a big dinner and snack into the evening. This is not what you want to do!

Have Breakfast

Research suggests that consumption of high quality protein at breakfast will help to balance your insulin, control weight, sustain your energy and help you to control your appetite during the day.[233] Breakfast should not be all carbohydrates. It should be a combination of protein, carbohydrate, fat and fiber.

You may find that you are not hungry in the morning, especially if you are accustomed to skipping breakfast. We recommend that you have breakfast anyway. If you start to regularly have breakfast, you may be able to develop the habit of consuming the majority of calories earlier in the day.

Remember that during the day you are most active and are most likely to be burning off calories rather than storing them. So the time to bring calories on board is earlier in the day, not later.

Meal Frequency

Although there is some disagreement, most clinicians recommend smaller, more numerous meals for those who have blood sugar problems.

In this case, you might consider having breakfast, a mid-morning snack, lunch, a mid-afternoon snack and dinner. Only if necessary and if you are not overweight would you have a small snack in the evening.

Whether you eat 3, 4, 5 or 6 times a day, try to eat on a regular basis. A study of ten overweight women at the University of Nottingham in the U.K. showed that regular meals resulted in mildly reduced calorie intake, reduced insulin after a meal, reduced cholesterol, and increased burning of calories.[234]

Choose your in-between meal snacks carefully. They should be small and should exclude refined, processed foods as much as possible. A study from Goteborg University in Sweden showed that overweight people did more snacking than normal-weight people, but they favored sweet, fatty foods.[235] In other words, it's OK to snack, provided you avoid unhealthy, fattening foods.

Dinnertime

Dinner should not be your largest meal of the day. Mostly likely, you'll be inactive after dinner and then go to bed. Few of the calories you eat will be burned off by physical activity, so there's no need for a large, calorie-laden dinner meal and late night snacking.

11.6 Tips for Increasing Your Fertility

Here are some quick dietary tips for improving your chances of becoming pregnant and having a successful pregnancy. Many of these points are reviewed in more detail elsewhere in the book.

Stop the Junk Food

Junk food is any food that is high in calories but low in nutrition. These calories are called "empty calories." Junk foods are typically high in refined carbohydrates, sweeteners and poor quality fats. They are attractively packaged and presented, and are easy to consume. They also taste good.

Before eating any highly processed food, look at the label and ask yourself, "Do I really need to eat this?"

Eat Whole Foods

The converse of stopping junk foods is to increase consumption of whole foods. Whole foods are the essence of the diet in this book. Whole foods give you the nutritional factors you need to bring your hormones closer to normal and allow yourself to become fertile.

Whole foods are those that have not been processed. If you went to a friend's house and she offered you a glass of apple juice, a cup of applesauce or an apple, which would you choose? Even if the apple juice or applesauce were more appealing, you would choose the apple. The apple provides the best nutritional return for your body.

Regardless of where you are or what you are doing, opt for whole foods whenever possible.

Go Organic

Every year, huge quantities of chemical pollutants are added to our environment. Some of it inevitably ends up in our food supply. Nearly all of these chemicals are toxic to your body. Some are "hormone mimics" or "hormone disrupters" that can reduce fertility.

In addition, monoculture has depleted our soils of nutrients. Food may appear the same but actually contains lower quantities of nutrients.

You can minimize these problems by buying organic foods, or by growing some of your own foods.

Avoid Genetically Modified Foods

Over the past few decades, crops have been genetically modified in order to increase crop yields and to improve their processing and marketing characteristics. This increases profits for food growers, processors and distributors. You can rest assured that genetically modified foods were not created in order to improve your health.

Genetically modified crops have been introduced on a truly massive scale. It's too early to know how these altered foodstuffs will affect your fertility. Until the food industry can prove to you that genetically modified foods do not impair your fertility, it's best to avoid them.

Balance Your Essential Fats

People who consume a "modern" diet of processed foods have an imbalance of EFAs (essential fatty acids). These fats are essential because you cannot live without them, and you must get them from your food. There are two groups of essential fats: omega-6 and omega-3. Most people consume too much omega-6 and not nearly enough omega-3.

Until you restore this dietary balance, it will be next to impossible for your hormones to get themselves back into a healthy balance so that you can conceive.

Minimize Gluten Grains

A large segment of the population cannot tolerate gluten, a substance found primarily in wheat, rye and barley. Some women with gluten intolerance have impaired fertility.

Wheat is by far the biggest source of gluten, since wheat is found in nearly all baked goods as well as thousands of processed foods. Gluten's effect may be indirect in that it damages the lining of the intestines and thus reduces absorption of essential nutrients from food. The gluten itself may trigger an undesirable immune response.

Have Plenty of Fiber

Dietary fiber is necessary for optimal excretion of hormones (such as estrogen) via the stool. It also slows down absorption of foods so that blood sugar is more stable.

If you eat whole foods, you will get all the fiber you need. If you eat refined or processed foods, you may need to add supplemental fiber to your diet. However, adding fiber to a processed food diet is not nearly as beneficial as simply eating whole foods.

Reduce Saturated Fat

A diet high in saturated animal fats tends to increase estrogen. Women with PCOS may already have an estrogen level that is too high relative to progesterone and thus have difficulty ovulating. In addition, a diet that is too high in saturated fats impairs the metabolism of EFAs (essential fatty acids), creating disordered cell function that can perpetuate hormonal imbalances.

Women who are on popular "low carb" diets to lose weight may be consuming too much saturated fat.

Change Your Carbs

Notice that we did not say "cut the carbs." We said "change the carbs." You have a better chance of restoring fertility if you get rid of processed carbs and rely more on unprocessed carbs.

You can find unprocessed carbs mostly in whole vegetables and whole fruits as well as nuts and seeds. They are also found in grains and legumes, although we recommend you restrict consumption of them.

You will find undesirable carbs in nearly all processed, manufactured foods.

Reduce Alcohol

While trying to conceive, studies suggest you can improve your fertility by sharply curtailing your consumption of alcoholic beverages.

Reduce Stress

Stress hormones disrupt your other hormones, including your reproductive hormones. They also cause you to gain weight and worsen insulin resistance. To become fertile, focus on reducing sources of stress in your life.

Exercise

Exercise reduces insulin resistance, reduces body fat and provides a host of other health benefits. Regular exercise can enhance fertility for most PCOS women.

Lose Weight

If you follow the advice above, you should lose fat weight. It's hard to say how much weight you will lose, but studies show that even a 5%-10% reduction in weight significantly improves the ability to become pregnant.

Reduce Insulin Resistance

If you follow the advice above, and throughout this book, your insulin problems should substantially diminish. As insulin resistance declines, your testosterone should also decline and your reproductive hormones will be more able to establish their proper relationship so that you can ovulate and become pregnant.

Is Your Partner Fertile?

Don't overlook your partner. Over the past 60 years or so, there has been a significant decline in the fertility of many mammals on the planet, including humans. Male and female fertility have both declined. Male sperm counts and motility have dropped dramatically.

If you haven't been able to conceive, but you are ovulating, it would be wise for your partner to have his sperm checked for quantity and viability.

Consider Nutritional Supplements

Nutritional supplements are one way to help tip the balance of your hormones in the right direction. For example, there are a considerable number of supplements that improve insulin sensitivity to some degree. There are other supplements that may help directly with balancing your reproductive hormones.

Consult with a licensed health professional who knows about nutritional supplementation and how to use it to improve hormone function and increase your fertility odds.

11.7 Advice for Vegetarians

Vegetarian diets, increasingly popular, have made people more aware of the benefits of dietary fiber and increased consumption of fresh fruits and vegetables.

The widespread practice of vegetarian eating has led to an accumulation of research and experience that improves our understanding of its advantages and disadvantages.[236] [237] A review of nutrition science literature as well as over 20 years of experience treating patients who have been long-term vegetarians has convinced the authors that vegetarianism is not the optimal diet for anyone, and particularly not for women with PCOS.

Although the fiber and essential nutrients in fresh plant foods are beneficial and essential for health, humans are in fact designed to be omnivores.[238] Omnivore means "eats everything." The human body requires a diet of plant foods as well as the proteins and fats specific to animal-derived foods.

Well-informed and disciplined food choices can minimize the nutritional deficiencies that are inevitable from a diet consisting only of plant foods. Casual or uninformed food choices that exclude protein from animal sources will lead to nutritional deficiency with adverse health consequences.

Vegetarianism for Philosophical Reasons

For some, the choice to avoid meat is because of legitimate concerns about the quality of products from the meat industry. Conventional sources of beef, pork, poultry and dairy products provide the consumer with food containing herbicide, pesticide, hormone and antibiotic residues. Ocean fish are often contaminated as well. Environmental contamination of our food supply contributes to increased rates of cancers, autoimmune diseases and hormone derangement, to name just a few complications. Vegetarianism would seem to be a sensible and healthy choice. Unfortunately, human beings cannot be optimally healthy without the nutrition available only from animal sources.

For many women, vegetarianism is a moral, spiritual or ethical choice. This choice sacrifices physical well-being to some extent, but it's a choice an informed person has every right to make. Some of these vegetarians have eventually felt burdened by the undesirable health consequences of the inevitable protein and nutrient malnutrition.

These women who are vegetarians for spiritual or ethical reasons often direct their energy towards improving the food supply system. They become a force in the marketplace by buying only organically raised foods. By their market choices and consumer activism, they support food manufacturing practices that provide clean, safe, humanely raised and killed animal foods as well as fresh, nutritionally rich plant foods. Their message is that livestock must be respected and gratitude be given for their contribution to the well-being of humanity.

PCOS and Vegetarianism

Most overweight PCOS women will benefit by decreasing body weight at least 7% to 10%. This is at the heart of any successful treatment for PCOS. Obesity, especially excess body fat around the middle, is associated most of the symptoms and all of the long-term risk factors of PCOS. Weight loss is an essential aspect of effective treatment.

This book describes a basic therapeutic diet for treating PCOS, a condition related to your response to insulin levels and carbohydrate consumption. Weight loss can be achieved by any low calorie diet, including a high carbohydrate, low-fat vegetarian diet. However, such a diet will not relieve your body of the metabolic damage created by chronic excess insulin.

Therefore a ketogenic diet that minimizes carbohydrates and efficiently uses up stored fat to provide fuel for activities of daily living is most effective for treating PCOS. Research supports a ketogenic diet as safe and effective for all carbohydrate-related diseases including insulin resistance, diabetes, atherosclerosis and high blood pressure. Meals providing sufficient protein from meat are more satisfying and prevent overeating in subsequent meals — an important factor important in your weight loss efforts.

Vegetarians and Protein Adequacy

Many vegetarians look to soy products in particular to provide what they presume is adequate and appropriate protein. However, plant protein is not the same as animal-derived protein and does not perform identically in the body. In addition, there is concern about the impact of large amounts of soy consumption on thyroid function, as we discussed in the *To Soy or Not to Soy* chapter. Since soy is not an "ideal" protein and because many PCOS women have depressed thyroid function, we do not include soy as part of the Recommended Level of our diet.

If you are a vegetarian, occasional soy meals can be incorporated into your weight loss regime but soy should not be your sole source of protein.

Some popular health literature asserts that a combination of rice and legumes such as soy will provide all of your protein requirements. While this combination provides a wider array and amount of amino acids (protein components), rice is quite high in carbohydrate. Grain and legume carbohydrates may cause problems, as we discuss below.

Vegetarians and Carbohydrates

All vegetarians don't eat meat, poultry or fish. Some also do not consume eggs or dairy products. These foods are the primary source of protein in the human diet. Since protein is necessary for life, vegetarians turn to plant proteins.

One of the problems with proteins in plants such as legumes and grains is that they also come with a substantial amount of carbohydrate. Therefore, vegetarians typically consume a disproportionately high amount of carbohydrates compared to protein.

In addition, the carbohydrates consumed are often refined grain and/or legume products. These carbohydrates are usually processed or cooked, thus causing the starch in them to be more readily and quickly digested, which leads to blood sugar and insulin problems.

A diet high in starchy refined or cooked carbohydrates is precisely the type of diet that exacerbates PCOS symptoms in the majority of women who have PCOS.

Vegetarians and Vitamin B12

There is also the issue of vitamin B12 adequacy. B12 is not abundant in plant foods. It is found primarily in animal foods. However, B12 is essential for life. Assuming you cannot get all the B12 you need from plant foods, where will you get it? B12 insufficiency is a "stealth disorder," meaning it can worsen for years or even decades before frank symptoms appear. By the time symptoms appear, you have a serious health problem. If you're a strict vegetarian, you may need to take a vitamin B12 supplement.

The Vegetarian's Choice

Among all of the factors that create the metabolic syndrome that includes polycystic ovaries, food, drink and exercise are the factors fully under your control. You cannot choose your genetic make up and you cannot erase the consequences of past habits or medical conditions that contributed to PCOS. But you can choose what you eat and how you move.

A vegetarian diet can be a therapeutic health recovery approach in certain circumstances. It is not appropriate for lifelong well-being. If you have PCOS but are intent on being a vegetarian, you will need a precise, disciplined and individually designed and supported food plan that is beyond the scope of this book. If you are or intend to be a complete vegetarian, we urge you to consult with a licensed naturopathic physician or other licensed health professional who is very knowledgeable about nutrition.

11.8 If You're Pregnant

For many women with PCOS, being blessed with the birth of a healthy child is the driving force behind all the disciplined lifestyle adjustments they make with the help of this book.

The recommendations in this book are designed to help you resume normal ovulation and to become pregnant. But what should you eat and do once you know that you are pregnant?

If you are pregnant, you will eat to support your baby through nine months of gestation and hopefully also at least six months of breast feeding. This requires a very different eating pattern. *It is not appropriate to continue to eat a ketogenic, weight loss diet once you have become pregnant.* Pregnancy has many unique requirements, including more vitamin and mineral nutrition and more calories than a healthy pre-pregnant woman needs.

It is beyond the scope of this book to give detailed and precise instructions for healthy eating in pregnancy. However there are a few points that should be kept in mind by all women with PCOS who become pregnant.

You should continue to eat preferably organic, fresh, nutrient-dense whole foods. Continue to avoid processed, prepackaged foods. You will not be counting calories or restricting portion sizes as you would in a weight loss plan. Just eat freely of what you know is good for you, keeping in mind that because of your PCOS metabolic tendency, you will continue to have little or no slack when it comes to the harmful effects of refined carbohydrates, industrial additives, insufficient protein and the wrong kinds of fat.

You should welcome the natural and necessary weight gain that comes with pregnancy. Exactly how much weight you should gain with a pregnancy is very individual, depending on pre-pregnant starting weight and other factors. You will have guidance from your prenatal care provider regarding proper amounts and rate of weight gain during your pregnancy.

The idea of gaining weight while you're pregnant may feel like you're retreating from all your hard work to lose weight in the first place. Nevertheless, it's normal and necessary for a healthy woman's body to gain, and then lose, weight associated with healthy pregnancy. If you have lost weight with our recommended diet in order to enhance your fertility, you already know everything you need to do to "re-lose" any excess weight after you have weaned your baby from breastfeeding.

PCOS Pregnancy Cautions

Women with PCOS may be more susceptible to two complications of pregnancy, gestational diabetes and preeclampsia.

Gestational diabetes is a temporary, pregnancy-related increase in blood sugar that is linked to a poor quality diet. Most women have some risk. You can minimize your risk of gestational diabetes by following the basic dietary principles outlined in this book.

20%-30% of women who have gestational diabetes have ongoing diabetes after a pregnancy. You have the advantage of already knowing how to eat to avoid elevated blood sugar and insulin excess.

Preeclampsia is a condition that only occurs during pregnancy. It includes potentially dangerously high blood pressure, fluid retention, and strain on the liver and kidneys. If untreated, it can lead to maternal seizures and severe threat to an unborn baby.

Protein and vitamin/mineral deficient diets are associated with increased risk for preeclampsia. If you have been following the eating style described in this book, you know how to eat to insure you have adequate protein and you will be eating the fresh fruits, vegetables, nuts and seeds that make up a nutrient-rich diet. In addition, all pregnant women should take a specially formulated prenatal vitamin/mineral supplement.

Pregnancy Guidelines

Here are some basic guidelines for a healthy pregnancy and breastfeeding experience, using the principles described in this book:

- A ketogenic weight loss diet is not appropriate during pregnancy and breast feeding. If you're not sure what a ketogenic diet is, see the *Diet and Long-Term Weight Management* chapter.

- A pregnant woman should gain weight and maintain an increase through weaning. Exactly how much gain is right is an individual matter, which will be guided by your health care provider.

- You can achieve the weight gain necessary for a healthy pregnancy by eating a very healthy diet without the restrictions on portion sizes, especially of plant food carbohydrates. Healthy foods include fresh vegetables and fruit, high-quality animal protein, nuts and seeds, some legumes and non-gluten whole grains. Continue to avoid refined carbohydrates, sweets, packaged foods, food additives — they are just as bad for you during pregnancy than any other time! Pregnancy is not a license to eat "junk" food. Gain the weight you need by eating more of the best food, more often.

- Human beings did not evolve eating grains or dairy foods. Our ancestors had healthy babies on a diet much like what is described here. We do not need grains or dairy foods. Some cases of habitual miscarriage are linked to autoimmune processes that are made worse by grain consumption, especially wheat. Maternal diets with adequate protein and fat, especially from deep sea fishes, fresh nuts and seeds, are associated with healthy pregnancy, successful breast feeding and babies with well developed nervous systems and general well being.

- Find fulfilling, nutrient-dense whole food carbohydrates in foods like berries, pears and apples, squashes, yams and sweet potatoes. Brown rice and quinoa and other non-wheat grains are also good during pregnancy and breast feeding.

Section 12

Getting Started

12.1 Prepare for Success

A primary secret to any successful endeavor is preparation. Preparation means planning ahead, thinking positively and developing a willing attitude that will allow you to make some changes in your life. Preparation is half the equation; follow-through is the other half.

Menu Plans & Recipes

As you know, there are two levels of the healthy PCOS diet:
- Recommended Level
- Maintenance Level

Most women will start at the Recommended Level and continue with it until their symptoms improve. Only those with minimal problems may decide to start at the Maintenance Level.

Since you'll probably be starting at the Recommended Level of the diet, we've laid out a Recommended Level 30-day meal plan, plus a lot of Recommended Level recipes to go with it. We understand that this level of the healthy PCOS diet will be a huge change for you. To improve your odds of success, please review our 30-day meal plan and its recipes. Use it as a guideline for the foods you will be preparing and eating.

The Recommended Level food lists and recipes include some foods that may not be easily available to you. We have provided a variety of recipes that include different foods, so chances are you'll find a recipe to your liking. Also, you can substitute foods in our recipes, so long as the substitute food is on one of our Recommended Level food lists.

You can see the meal plan and recipes a little later in this book.

Shopping

Since the PCOS diet is primarily comprised of unprocessed, wholesome foods, you might take a field trip to your local food co-op or health food store. Although the PCOS diet does not *require* you to shop anywhere but your local market, it's a worthwhile adventure to familiarize yourself with other sources of supply.

Many natural food providers are dedicated to supporting individuals with special dietary needs. To that end, they supply free-range, organic meats, fish and poultry, organic vegetables and fruits, salt-free herb and spice combinations, organic teas and deli foods that fall well within the range of our diet recommendations.

If you live in the United States, there are many to choose from (Whole Foods, Wild Oats, New Seasons and community food cooperatives, to name a few). There are also a number of trusted providers from whom you can purchase some items online.

Wherever you shop, be sure to plan ahead. If you shop once a week, plan your menus the night before so you'll be sure to get everything you need. It's also useful to plan your menus so you'll have leftovers of your favorite recipes to eat as snacks, breakfasts and lunches.

A special note about fresh produce: it rapidly loses its nutrient value after it is harvested, even if it "looks" fresh. If you can, we suggest you shop for produce twice a week, or no less than once a week. If you have unused produce that's over a week old in the refrigerator, think about using it up quickly or discarding it.

Your Shopping List

Before you go the supermarket or health food store, plan out your meals for the next few days and make a list of everything you want to get. Doing so will make sure that you don't overlook something. Remember that preparation is half of the equation for success.

Also, shopping with a list will save you money because you won't be as tempted to purchase impulse items.

In the next chapter, we've provided you with a list of all the foods that are for the Recommended Level of the PCOS diet. The Recommended Level is the most strict level. You can print out the next chapter and use it as your master shopping list. If you are at the Maintenance Level instead of the Recommended Level, you can add other items to this list.

It's a good idea to keep a list of items you are low on posted on the refrigerator and add to it as the week goes by.

On-the-Go Meals

Life doesn't always lend itself to healthy and leisurely meal preparation. That's one of the main reasons the fast food and restaurant industries have become so popular with the general population. Working long hours, lack of information or just a busy schedule can sabotage the best intentions.

So when your dietary needs are outside of the mainstream, you get to be a little more creative than usual. We've included a few quick 'portable food' recipes that we think you'll find both handy and delicious. And here are a dozen suggestions for 'make ahead' cooking that will go a long way towards insuring your success:

1. Make one animal protein loaf using range-fed, organic beef, Diestel turkey, free-range ground chicken or game meat.

2. Roast or crockpot a chicken or a red meat roast.

3. Make one or two soups that can be frozen and used when time is especially tight.

4. Wash and cut vegetable sticks (celery, carrot, jicama, peppers, cucumbers) and refrigerate in plastic bags and containers. Remember to store cucumbers in their own bag and use them quickly because they don't have the 'staying' power of the other vegetables.

5. Make up your salad dressings, dips and condiments. As you go along, you'll get a sense of how much you'll use in a week's time and you can adjust the recipes accordingly.

6. Soak seeds for sprouts, enough for a few days at a time.

7. Roast a cookie sheet full of vegetables. Cool and store in plastic containers.

8. Make one or two high quantity vegetable dishes (Ratatouille, Chopped Salad, etc.) every few days so you'll always have plenty on hand.

9. Make a salad of organic, leafy greens (enough for a couple of days). Wash greens and dry them thoroughly (in a salad spinner). Keep the leaves whole for recipes like Lettuce Wraps or Cabbage Wraps, or tear into fork size pieces for salad. Toss together and put into a plastic bag. Greens will stay fresh for a couple of days and will be ready and waiting for you to add whatever garnishes you wish. Or, you can buy pre-mixed greens in bulk at produce counters. Wash and dry thoroughly before storing. Greens need to be thoroughly dry and their storage container ventilated in order to stay crisp and palatable.

10. Make at least one snack recipe (Tomato Cups, Stuffed Mushrooms, Sardine Sushi).

Kitchen Tools

When you begin with fresh ingredients and the right tools, almost anything can come out tasting delicious. Most of our recipes can be made quite successfully using only the tools found in most kitchens. However, we thought you might like to have a list of kitchen tools that will add versatility and convenience:

1. Bamboo or stainless steel steamer
2. Crockpot
3. Large (10" or 12") non-stick skillet with tight fitting lid
4. 6" non-stick sauté skillet
5. 16 qt. stockpot with lid
6. 9 x 13" non-stick or glass baking pan

7. 8" chef's knife
8. Kitchen scissors
9. Blender (hand-held Braun, mini-blender or counter model)
10. Food processor
11. Coffee grinder (for grinding herbs, nuts, etc)
12. Juicer
13. Dehydrator
14. Salad spinner
15. Jars and tops (or cheesecloth) for sprouting
16. Misto gourmet olive oil sprayer
17. Plenty of extra containers to make storage of leftovers easier

A Note about Food Dehydrating

You'll notice we listed a food dehydrator. When it is harvest time and fresh vegetables are abundant and inexpensive, you may wish to dehydrate some and use them later for snacks or soups. Or, you may also decide to make your own fish or meat jerky for snacks. Salmon jerky is good snack possibility.

We suggest that you do not dehydrate fruits. Dehydrated fruit will have concentrated amounts of fruit sugar, which is not helpful to some women with PCOS.

Although dehydration is a great way to preserve foods or create snacks, dehydrated foods should not be a primary element of your diet. Preferably, you will consume fresh, whole foods. Fresh, whole foods have a lower calorie density than dehydrated foods.

When dehydrating foods, don't soak in sugar or salt brines first. Rinsing in lemon juice and water is acceptable and helps retain color.

If you use dehydrated vegetables in a recipe, you'll have to add more liquid than if you're using fresh or frozen vegetables.

Timesaving Tips for the Cook

1. After you have determined your menu plan for the next few days or for the week, think about how to use leftovers from certain meals for lunches or future meals.

2. Do your cooking in batches. Plan 2 or 3 times per week to do a couple hours' worth of cooking (possibly a weekend afternoon and 1 or 2 evenings during the week).

3. Identify which evenings you need "quick prep" meals and then relax. Use foods you have previously prepared, use leftovers or try "quick" recipes such as a stir-fry. If you're really pressed for time, consider a meal replacement shake.

4. Cook larger quantities than you need for 1 meal. You then use the leftovers for the next day's lunch or perhaps even another meal. It's easy to season foods, add 1 or 2 new simple ingredients or simply make a soup out of leftovers.

5. Make a very large salad to last for 2-3 days. Keep the sliced tomatoes or cucumbers in a separate container and add when ready to eat some salad.

6. Keep your kitchen stocked with "emergency" quick meal items (tuna, healthy canned soup, etc.).

7. When you have extras left over, consider freezing certain items (such as soups).

8. Keep utensils handy. Don't tuck kitchen tools away in cabinets and drawers; you'll waste time digging for them. If you have the room, put utensils - spatulas, wooden spoons and tongs - in a container on the counter and organize other items by use.

9. Wash and dry your produce and greens as soon as you get home from the store. Then, when you're cooking, you can just throw things together. Washing salad greens won't make them spoil faster — but you must dry them thoroughly in a salad spinner, then put them into a zip-lock plastic bag.

10. Minimize mess and simplify. Use cookware that doubles as serving pieces. Also try a hand blender. You can puree soups and sauces directly in the pot, which saves the tedious transfer from a food processor.

11. Delegate. If you're the designated cook, assign your partner or family member a task, like chopping vegetables. Let the kids set the table and pour beverages. After dinner, they can help wipe the counters and wash dishes. Delegation saves you at least half an hour in the kitchen.

12.2 Shopping List for Recommended Diet Level

Here's a list of foods for the Recommended Level of the healthy PCOS diet. You can use it as a checklist when you go shopping, or use it to get ideas for your shopping list.

Vegetables

alfalfa sprouts
artichoke
asparagus
avocado
beet tops
bell peppers
bok choy (pak choi)
broccoflower
broccoli
broccoli raab (rapini)
Brussels sprouts
cabbage
cauliflower
celery
chicory
chili peppers
Chinese lettuce
chives
cilantro
collard greens
cucumber
daikon radish
dandelion greens
eggplant
endive
escarole
fennel
garlic
kale
kohlrabi
leeks
lettuce (green, Romaine)
mushrooms
mustard greens
okra
onions
parsley

Vegetables (ctd.)

pea pods, pea vines
prickly pear
purslane
radish, radish sprouts
scallions
shallots
seaweed, kelp
spinach
string beans, wax beans
summer squash (crookneck, patty pan)
Swiss chard
turnip greens
water chestnuts
watercress
zucchini squash

Fruits

apples
apricots
bananas
blackberries
blueberries
cherries
coconut
cranberries
figs
grapes
kiwi
kumquats
lemons
loganberries
mangos
nectarines
papayas
peaches
pears
plums
prunes

Nuts and Seeds *(raw)*

almonds
brazil nuts
cashews
chestnuts
filberts (hazel nuts)
flax seeds
macadamias
pecans
pine nuts
pistachios (unsalted)
walnuts

Legumes

bean sprouts
pea sprouts

Grains

Dairy Products

Meat

beef, lean
buffalo
lamb, lean
liver
pork, lean
rabbit
wild game

Poultry

chicken
Cornish game hen
Eggs (omega 3 preferred)
game birds
ostrich
pheasant
turkey

Fish

bass
clams
cod
crab
haddock
halibut
mackerel
mahi mahi
mussels
pollack
salmon
sardines (in water)
scallops
shrimp
snapper
sole
tilapia
trout
other Recommended fish

Beverages

green tea
herb tea
purified water
sparkling water

Oils

flax seed
hemp
macadamia nut
olive
walnut

Herbs and Spices

allspice
anise
basil
bay leaf
cardamom
caraway
cayenne
celery powder
chili powder
cinnamon
cloves
coriander
cumin
curry
dill
dry mustard
fennel
garlic
ginger root
marjoram
nutmeg
oregano
parsley
pepper
peppermint
rosemary
saffron
sage
savory
tarragon
thyme
turmeric
vanilla

Condiments

dark chocolate chips (milk-free)
Dijon mustard
lime or lemon juice
seasonings (Mrs. Dash, etc.)
seaweeds
tamari (low sodium, wheat-free)

12.3 Handy Cooking Tips

These are some of our thoughts about cooking. There are dozens of cookbooks you can consult for additional information, tips and recipes.

Cooking Vegetables

Try not to microwave. We know it's a quick and easy method of cooking that helps get a meal on the table fast, but you need to know that microwaving your vegetables destroys their nutritional value more than any other method of cooking. Microwaving appears to be especially destructive to flavonoids and pigments in vegetables that are so important to your good health.

Contrary to popular belief, boiling or pressure cooking food is much less destructive than microwaving.

Quickly steaming vegetables is the best way to get the most food value from your vegetables. It's better than boiling or pressure cooking and is vastly better than microwaving.

How To Steam Vegetables

Use a stock pot that has a tight fitting cover. Put your vegetables into a bamboo or stainless steel steamer basket and cover the bottom of the pot with enough water so that it does not boil dry but not enough to cover any of the vegetables when at a boil. Bring water to a low boil and cook until their color brightens and they are still a little crunchy, checking them periodically with a fork. Steaming only takes a few minutes.

Cooking Leafy Green Vegetables

There are several ways to cook leafy green vegetables. With any of these cooking methods, begin by washing and stemming your greens. You can wash them by breaking off each leaf and washing it on both sides, or placing a quantity of vegetables in a clean bowl or tub with water and 15 - 20 drops of grapefruit extract (purchased at any health food store) to disable microbes. Allow them to soak for 5 minutes, then rinse thoroughly.

Stem large leafy vegetables by breaking off the tough stem if it's a tender green. If it's a tougher green, cut out the center rib from the leafy portion and discard along with the stem.

Blanched Greens (see recipes)
- Chop into strips
- Bring water to boil in pot
- Put vegetable into boiling water and stir for about 20 seconds, or until tender
- Remove from water and drain
- Add minced garlic, chopped onions and olive oil to taste

Steamed Greens
- Chop into strips
- In a frying pan, sauté some garlic and/or onions, adding 1-2 tablespoons of olive oil
- When onions or garlic are soft, add your leafy greens
- Add a little water and cover; let simmer on moderate heat; stir and check for tenderness every 3-5 minutes
- Remove when tender and color is bright green

Some greens, especially the hardy, thick-stemmed ones (such as mustard, broccoli rabe, or collards) may taste and look better when boiled or blanched rather than steamed.

Sautéed Greens
- Chop into strips
- Add 1-2 tablespoons water in frying pan; turn on moderate heat
- Add 1-2 tablespoons of olive oil
- Add fresh minced garlic or minced ginger, and brown it very lightly
- Add chopped onions
- Add 1/4 cup water, cover and simmer for one minute
- Add tamari to taste
- Remove from pan

Other Ideas for Cooking Greens
- Add torn greens to soups and stews for color and improved nutrition. Add greens about 10 minutes before the dish is finished. Blanch stronger tasting greens briefly before adding to soups.
- Use sautéed spinach, beet greens, watercress, or chard as a bed for baked or grilled fish.

Stir-Frying

Stir-frying is a great alternative to pan or deep frying. It's a quick one-dish meal that is both tasty and convenient.

Almost anything can be stir-fried. You can use a wok if you have one; otherwise a deep-sided non-stick skillet will do. Begin with equal amounts of oil and water (not just oil) to heated pan. Add chopped meat, poultry or fish, stirring quickly until well coated with oil/water mixture. Cook until almost done and then add chopped vegetables. Continue stirring; once you add the vegetables, turn down the heat, cover tightly and pan-steam.

Cooking Flesh Foods

Do not pan fry, deep fry, smoke or barbeque flesh foods. These cooking methods create carcinogenic substances in your food.

Flesh foods may be broiled, baked, steamed, stir-fried or cooked in soups.

Always remember to remove skin from poultry before eating.

Eggs

Eggs should be poached or boiled until the yolk is somewhat hard. Undercooked eggs (very soft yolk, runny eggs) may still contain viable microorganisms (such as viruses) that are detrimental to health.

Do not fry or scramble eggs or make an omelet. Frying and scrambling exposes the cholesterol in the egg to excessive heat and oxygen. The result can be cholesterol oxide, the kind of cholesterol that causes damage in your body.

Cooking with Fats & Oils

Temperature
When cooking a fatty food, or cooking with oil, use a low or moderate level of heat, in order to minimize degradation of the fats and oils and creation of carcinogenic substances.

Use Water + Oil
The safest way to fry is to add some water first. This cools the surface of the pan and creates steam, which protects the oil from the air. After the water, add the oil.

If you're cooking vegetables and you refuse to use water, put the vegetables in the pan before adding the oil. This will cool the surface and create some water vapor, thus protecting the oil to some extent.

Use low heat if possible. Cover pan to contain water vapor.

Acceptable Cooking Oils
For cooking, the oils most tolerant of heat are those that are the most saturated: butter, lard, coconut or palm kernel oil.

Monounsaturated fats such as olive oil are not as quite as safe as saturated fats but are still acceptable.

For cooking with oil, we suggest using extra virgin olive oil or butter.

Worst Oils for Cooking

Bottled polyunsaturated oils in general are not suitable for frying, baking or cooking. Examples include flaxseed, corn, canola, safflower, peanut, almond and similar oils.

Common supermarket bottled oils are not suitable for consumption by people who want to be healthy, regardless of whether you use them for cooking or uncooked in salad dressings or sauces.   They are made from questionable ingredients, are highly processed and are high in trans-fats.

Bottled oils that say "for cooking, frying, and baking" are misleading you, since by definition, all of them are unsaturated oils and are subject to oxidation and destruction when they are heated. Examples are cottonseed, peanut or canola oils. This is marketing terminology, with no reference to health concerns.

Re-Use of Cooking Oils

Never re-use cooking oils. Always discard any oil or fat used in cooking.   Re-heating and re-using any oil or fat enormously increases the amount of free radical molecules it contains. These unstable free radical molecules seriously damage your cells and cause chronic health problems such as high blood pressure, cardiovascular disease and more.

By the way, oil re-use is a major reason why you should **never** eat French fries in a restaurant. Nearly all fast-food outlets re-use their French fry cooking oil over and over again.

Food Dehydration

If you have the time, using a food dehydrator may be useful, especially for creating healthy snacks. For example, you could dehydrate vegetables such as zucchini squash or tomatoes. Or you could dehydrate salmon or buffalo strips to create your own jerky. Dehydrating allows you to take advantage of seasonally low prices for produce, fish or meat — you can buy a larger quantity and dehydrate much of it for use at a later time. Dehydrated foods can be used in soups, or soaked and then prepared as a dish.

We recommend that you not dehydrate any fruits. Dehydrated fruits contain concentrated amounts of fructose. In a concentrated form, fructose is undesirable.

Dehydrated vegetables or fish or meat make a good snack or meal substitute if you are traveling or in a situation where you're not able to get a regular meal.

Hygiene

Good kitchen hygiene will go far to prevent illness in you and your family. Raw produce and raw flesh foods all have bacteria or other microorganisms on them. So take steps to keep your food and your kitchen clean.

Microbial infections do not cause PCOS and infertility, but they can contribute to systemic inflammation, gastrointestinal malabsorption of needed nutrients, liver stress or possible disturbance of some hormones.

Moreover, unbalanced sex-steroid levels in women with PCOS could adversely influence the competency of the immune system and alter genes that influence susceptibility and resistance to infection.[239]   Therefore, good hygiene should not be disregarded.

- Wash your hands any time they may have been exposed to microorganisms. Self-inoculation (from hands to face and mouth) is the most common way of becoming infected by bacteria, viruses or parasites.

- Carefully wash your hands with soap after using the bathroom or changing your baby's diapers. Not doing so is a common way of contaminating your food with pathogenic microorganisms.

- After handling raw flesh or eggs, wash your hands with soap.

- Germs can accumulate on sponges, dishcloths and dishtowel. Replace your used dishcloth and dishtowel with a clean one daily.

- If you use a dishwashing sponge, thoroughly rinse it daily and remove any trapped food particles. Let your sponge dry out every night, or run it through your dishwasher along with your dishes. Soak your dishwashing sponge in diluted bleach once or twice a week if you don't run it through your dishwasher. Discard any sponge that looks old or dirty.

- Using a clean washcloth, wash off your cutting board with a dilute solution of bleach, hydrogen peroxide or vodka at least once a week, or after you have used it for cutting raw flesh foods. Cutting boards are full of microscopic crevices that harbor bacteria.

- Keep flesh foods refrigerated or frozen at all times to retard proliferation of microorganisms. However, even refrigeration or freezing will not protect you from virally infected flesh because some viruses can withstand temperatures of -30°F or lower. Only cooking will destroy viruses.

- Use paper towels to swab up juice on your kitchen counter from raw flesh foods. Don't use a dishcloth, which just spreads the germs around.

- Wash produce in a bowl of water to which you've added a small amount of grapefruit extract, pure vodka, hydrogen peroxide or bleach. Let it sit a few minutes, then rinse the produce off with fresh water. These products will kill many microbes on the surface of produce.

- When preparing your meals, keep raw flesh foods away from other food that will be eaten raw, like salad. Wash the utensils you use to cut or handle raw flesh foods.

Section 13

Meal Plans and Recipes

13.1 Daily Meal Plans for 30 Days

A one-month meal plan is laid out for you on the following pages. This meal plan is for those of you who aren't sure about what to eat or are looking for meal ideas that meet the Recommended Level dietary guidelines in this book.

You are not "required" to follow this meal plan as we've laid it out. This is not a diet that you must exactly and slavishly follow.   Please let your own preferences and creativity play a role in the foods you prepare and eat.

We expect that your biggest challenge will be what to eat for breakfast. We understand that you are probably accustomed to eating grain-based foods such as breakfast cereal or bagels for breakfast. Grains are not part of the Recommended Level of our diet, so you will need to try some alternative foods. We've given you breakfast suggestions for 30 days. If you don't like what we've suggested, then make up your own breakfast from the approved lists of foods in this book.

In any case, you should not skip breakfast and you should always be sure to have some protein as part of your breakfast meal.

Food Portions

We are not dictating to you the amount of food you can eat at a meal. From time to time we make suggestions on the amount of a specific food. But generally, you will have to be the judge of what you need.

For example, if you have "baked trout" for dinner, should you eat 1/4, 1/2 or a whole trout? It depends on the size of the trout. It also depends on whether you are active or sedentary, lean or overweight, insulin resistant or not, have a large body frame or not, whether your metabolism is sluggish or not, and how much other food you have been eating that day.

Be moderate and use good judgment. As a general guideline, we suggest approximately 4-5 ounces of animal protein at a meal.

If you need more specific guidance about meal portions or components, we recommend you consult with a licensed naturopathic physician or registered dietician.

For more information about portions, see the *Portion Control* chapter.

Recipe Portions

Some of the recipes are intended to provide for more than one meal or for more than one person.

Suppose, for example, that you're going to have Turkey Meat Loaf for dinner. Our Turkey Meat Loaf recipe will provide considerably more food than you should eat at one meal. Our intention is that you share that meat loaf with your family or keep the remainder as a leftover for a future meal. We do not intend that you eat the whole thing at a sitting!

Calorie Restriction

Some of you with a weight problem may have found that "counting calories" is the only way you can control your weight. If calorie counting works for you, please continue to count. For example, if you are on a Weight Watchers program and have a maximum number of calories you may consume, there are a large number of online calorie counters on the Internet that you may use to calculate the calorie content of any meal components in this book.

However, our diet has a low calorie density, meaning that there are relatively fewer calories in a volume of food. Therefore you may find that you can eat more food than previously while keeping the total calorie count the same.

For more information, see the chapter entitled *Is Calorie Restriction a Good Idea?*

Snacks and Meal Frequency

Some individuals do well on three meals a day while others need to snack in between meals. The daily meal plans include 3 snacks in addition to the 3 daily meals. You are not required to consume 3 snacks a day (or any snacks at all).

Individuals with blood sugar fluctuations or an appetite disorder may find snacks helpful for maintaining a feeling of well-being and staying on the diet.

The Rest of the Family

The rest of the family will probably not be eating like you are, although they would almost certainly benefit as well.

Husbands, children and teenagers are accustomed to their favorite foods and may not want to make any changes. In this case, prepare your own meal but make up something extra for them.

Suppose, for example, you're having steak, steamed vegetables and a salad. Prepare for the other family members a side dish that they would like. Maybe it would be baked potato, or rice or some French bread. They can use a variety of commercial sauces or dressings to make their vegetables and salad more suitable to their tastes.

We recommend that you sit down with family members and explain why you are eating the way you are. Ask the adults and older children to review the early chapters of this book so they understand the need for your changes.

If you have family members (such as husband or older children) for whom creating additional elements for a meal is not enough, work out a plan with them by which they become responsible for their own meals.

With younger children, you have the opportunity to teach them what you are learning, including that you want to help them avoid developing eating habits that are not good for them. Bear in mind that your children may have the same genetic tendencies that you do. This means they have a higher risk of developing serious future health problems unless they start eating a healthier diet at a young age.

You can frame this as your job as a loving parent and partner. Having learned about new habits that affect health, it is your job, your loving commitment to them, to share it with them. You tell the little ones not to run out into the street; you tell the older ones to avoid alcohol and drugs – why not help them understand what you are learning about food and optimal nutrition, because you love them and want them to be well?

Binge Eaters

We know that some of you eat too much food or are compulsive binge eaters. We know this because you have told us so.

The healthy PCOS diet is designed to gradually reduce the urges to consume lots of food. But until your hormones are balanced and other issues in your life resolved, what should you do when you know you are going binge out?

The first absolutely necessary step is to have no tempting processed foods in the house or anywhere in your proximity. Please stay with the foods on our diet; otherwise you are just spinning your wheels.

If you have a compulsion to eat until your stomach is bursting, and you know nothing is going to stop you, start eating vegetables from our Recommended or Maintenance Level list for vegetables. Make them taste better with one of the sauces or dressings in our Recipe section.

Example: Instead of eating a gallon of ice cream and a bag of cookies, have on hand one container of salsa and one container of guacamole. Mix the two containers. Prepare a huge salad or steamed vegetables. Add some chicken slices if you have any on hand. Put the salsa/guacamole mix on top and mix it in a bit. Then start eating. The guacamole mix will provide the fat and the smooth mouth feel you like. The vegetables will have some of the carbs you crave. The chicken will help you feel fuller and provide nutritional balance. If you are compelled to binge, this is a much healthier way to do it.

If you're a binge eater, it's important to get help to change that behavior. We are not recommending the above guacamole-and-salsa meal as a healthy solution, only as a slightly healthier behavior in a moment of need. Binge eating indicates an unmet need that you deserve to have addressed. Binge eating and other eating disorders are complex behaviors with many causes — some may be emotional, while some may be chemical. All of these issues can be addressed with expert help. We urge you to seek professional counseling to help you through any disordered or extreme eating behaviors.

Recommended vs. Maintenance Level

The healthy PCOS diet has two levels: Recommended and Maintenance.

The Recommended level is for those who have troublesome PCOS symptoms, weight challenges, fertility problems or abnormal hormone lab test findings.

The Maintenance level is for those whose PCOS problems have significantly diminished or whose problems are mild. The Maintenance level includes foods that are not allowed at the Recommended level.

The following one-month meal plan consists almost entirely of foods from the Recommended level of the healthy PCOS diet, which is the most stringent.

At some point, you may decide to add foods from the Maintenance level of the diet. When this happens, you can still use the meal plans, but now you can include additional foods. You can also modify the recipes to include the additional foods.

Menu Items With an Asterisk (*)

When you encounter an item in your daily meal plan that has as asterisk after it, that means there is a recipe for that item in the Recipes section of the book.

Day 1

Breakfast
Spinach and Eggs*
Tea (green or herbal)

Morning Snack (optional)
Cherry tomatoes and 1/4 handful of walnut pieces

Lunch
Chicken Salad,* enough so that you feel satisfied
Tea (green or herbal)

Afternoon Snack (optional)
1 tangerine and 5-8 almonds

Dinner
Basic Stir-Fry*

Dessert or Evening Snack (optional)
5 thin slices of jicama and 6-8 cashews

Preparation for Tomorrow
Put flank steak in Meat Marinade No. 1 or No. 2* and refrigerate overnight.

Day 2

Breakfast

2-4 Cabbage Roll Ups*
Tea (green or herbal)

Morning Snack (optional)

1 piece fruit from Recommended Level list and 4-6 filberts

Lunch

1 Ostrich Burger* (substitute with turkey if you wish)
Chopped salad* (as much as you wish)
Tea (green or herbal)

OR

Leftover Stir-Fry
Tea

Afternoon Snack (optional)

2-3 small sardines (pat dry if packed in oil)
or
1/4 handful walnuts

Dinner

4-6 oz. Marinated Flank Steak*
Swiss chard & sliced zucchini squash, steamed (as much as you wish)
1/4 cup daikon radish, sliced

Dessert or Evening Snack (optional)

6-10 baby carrots

Preparation for Tomorrow

Cole slaw for lunch.

Day 3

Breakfast
Huevos Rancheros*

Morning Snack (optional)
1 teaspoon almond butter on celery sticks

Lunch
4-6 oz. leftover Marinated Flank Steak*
Cole slaw*

Afternoon Snack (optional)
1/4 handful pumpkin seeds and 5 baby carrots

Dinner
Louisiana Gumbo*

Dessert or Evening Snack (optional)
1/2 apple and/or 6-8 raw cashews

Preparation for Tomorrow
None

Day 4

Breakfast

Frittata*
Green or herbal tea

Morning Snack (optional)

3 small slices jicama and 1/4 handful seeds or nuts (your choice)

Lunch

Louisiana Gumbo* (leftover from yesterday)
Tea (green or herbal)

Afternoon Snack (optional)

Handful of grapes
5-8 raw pecans

Dinner

Herb and Garlic Lamb Chops*
Roasted Vegetables No. 1*
Herb tea

Dessert or Evening Snack (optional)

1/2 grapefruit

Preparation for Tomorrow

Roast a turkey breast for Turkey Citrus Salad - tomorrow's breakfast.

Deviled eggs for lunch.

Day 5

Breakfast
Turkey Citrus Salad*
Green tea

Morning Snack (optional)
Sugar snap peas (or vegetable sticks) dipped in Asian Dressing*

Lunch
Deviled Eggs*
Basic Garden Salad*

Afternoon Snack (optional)
1/4 cantaloupe and 1/4 handful walnuts

Dinner
Herb and Garlic Petite Sirloin*
Mango Salsa
Steamed Asparagus*
Small garden salad

Dessert or Evening Snack (optional)
Carrot sticks and 4 macadamia nuts

Preparation for Tomorrow
Soak flax seeds for Berry Nut Shake*

Day 6

Breakfast

Berry Nut Shake*

Morning Snack (optional)

1/2 Deviled Egg*

Lunch

Dijonnaise Poached Salmon*
Mixed green salad plus red peppers, red onions, raw carrots and cucumbers
2 tablespoons Balsamic Vinaigrette Dressing* or other dressing
Green tea

Afternoon Snack (optional)

1 orange
or
1/8 avocado drizzled with lime or lemon juice

Dinner

4-6 oz. Marinated Pork Loin*
Roasted Vegetables No. 1 or No. 2*
Herb tea or sparkling water

Dessert or Evening Snack (optional)

1/2 apple and 4-6 almonds

Preparation for Tomorrow

Prepare ingredients for starting Crockpot Chicken* tomorrow morning.

Day 7

Breakfast
Turkey Burger*
1/2 cup of Green Salsa*, Latin Salsa*, or Mango Salsa* (on top of burger)
1/4 cup Mexican Guacamole* (optional) (on top of burger)
Green tea

(Start Crockpot Chicken* before leaving for work).

Morning Snack (optional)
2-4 small sardines (pat dry if packed in oil)

Lunch
4 oz. pork loin, sliced from leftovers
Mediterranean Salad*

Afternoon Snack (optional)
1/4 handful pumpkin seeds and celery sticks

Dinner
Chicken Crockpot*
Spinach and Pink Grapefruit Salad* (optional)

Dessert or Evening Snack (optional)
1/2 cup berries, fresh or frozen

Preparation for Tomorrow
None.

Day 8

Breakfast

Egg-Shrimp Salad*
Hot tea with lemon slice

Morning Snack (optional)

Carrot/jicama/celery sticks with 1 teaspoon nut butter

Lunch

Curried Beef Strips*
Steamed vegetable - your choice
Tea w/ lemon slice

OR

Leftover Crockpot Chicken*

Afternoon Snack (optional)

A few cherry tomatoes

Dinner

Baked trout
Spinach Salad* with sliced red onion, tangerine sections, sesame seeds, Vinaigrette dressing
Cucumber and tomato slices

Dessert or Evening Snack (optional)

1/2 cup blueberries and 1/4 handful walnuts

Preparation for Tomorrow

None.

Day 9

Breakfast
Huevos Rancheros*
Green tea

Morning Snack (optional)
1 Tomato Cup*

Lunch
Scallion Soup*
Sardine Sushi*

Afternoon Snack (optional)
1/2 cup raspberries or blueberries and 4 pecans

Dinner
Venison Pot Roast* (or other meat)
Baked Cabbage with Dill*

Dessert or Evening Snack (optional)
1 plum or apricot
or
1/2 peach or 1/2 nectarine

Preparation for Tomorrow
Grill chicken for tomorrow's Hawaiian Chicken Salad*

Soak seeds/nuts for Aloha Smoothie* tomorrow morning

Day 10

Breakfast

Aloha Smoothie*
2-3 oz. cold venison (or other meat, poultry or seafood)

Morning Snack (optional)

1 Tomato Cup*

Lunch

Hawaiian Chicken Salad*
Tea

Afternoon Snack (optional)

5-10 grapes and 1/4 handful walnuts

Dinner

Liver and Onions*
Mashed Cauliflower* with Mushroom Gravy*
Steamed Swiss chard

Dessert or Evening Snack (optional)

4-5 olives

Preparation for Tomorrow

None.

Day 11

Breakfast

1/2 grapefruit
1-2 poached or soft/hard boiled eggs
3-4 pecans
Green tea

Morning Snack (optional)

Lettuce Roll Up*

Lunch

Broccoli with Garlic and Lemon*
4 oz. Buffalo Burger* (top with a bit of guacamole or salsa if desired)
Small chopped or garden salad
Hot lemon water

Afternoon Snack (optional)

2-3 Celery sticks stuffed with Nut Pate*

Dinner

Gazpacho
Chili Pepper Halibut

Dessert or Evening Snack (optional)

1/2 cup berries and 2-4 macadamia nuts

Preparation for Tomorrow

Soak seeds overnight for Apricot Apple Flaxseed Smoothie*

Day 12

Breakfast

Apricot-Apple Flaxseed Smoothie*
4 oz. slices of beef, turkey, chicken or seafood
Hot lemon water or green tea

Morning Snack (optional)

1 sliced kiwi and 4-5 macadamia nuts

Lunch

4 oz. cold, leftover Chili Pepper Halibut*
Mango Salsa*
Confetti Salad*

Afternoon Snack (optional)

Jicama sticks and 4-5 macadamia nuts

Dinner

Chicken Vegetable Soup*
Confetti Salad* with Lemon Vinaigrette
Herbal Tea

Dessert or Evening Snack (optional)

Daikon radish slices and a few green olives

Preparation for Tomorrow

Marinate Creole Rabbit*

Day 13

Breakfast

3-6 oz. leftover meat, fish or poultry
Confetti Salad* with dressing of your choice
Green tea

Morning Snack (optional)

4-5 cherry tomatoes

Lunch

Chicken Vegetable Soup (leftover)
Small Basic Garden Salad* with Herb Dressing*

Afternoon Snack (optional)

2-3 small sardines (pat dry if packed in oil)

Dinner

Creole Rabbit*
Walnut Watercress Stir Fry
Steamed broccoli

Dessert or Evening Snack (optional)

2 apricots, fresh

Preparation for Tomorrow

None.

Day 14

Breakfast
Lettuce Roll Ups*
3 oz. canned tuna or any leftover fish
Green tea

Morning Snack (optional)
Tomatoes Dijon*

Lunch
Salade Nicoise*

Afternoon Snack (optional)
4-6 pecans and cucumber slices

Dinner
Italian Braised Steak*
Broccoli with Garlic and Lemon*
Wild Greens Salad* or Shoestring Carrot Salad*

Dessert or Evening Snack (optional)
2-5 olives

Preparation for Tomorrow
None.

Day 15

Breakfast

1 or 2 boiled eggs on bed of dandelion or other greens
(add any sauce or dressing from Recipe list if desired)
1 tangerine
Green tea

Morning Snack (optional)

1/2 apple and 1/4 handful nuts

Lunch

Grilled Turkey with Lemon Mustard*
Leeky Carrots*

Afternoon Snack (optional)

1/8 avocado plus 2 sections pink grapefruit

Dinner

Ratatouille*
Lemon Parslied Fish*
Herb tea

Dessert or Evening Snack (optional)

1/2 cup fresh strawberries

Preparation for Tomorrow

Soak seeds/nuts overnight for Raspberry Coconut Slush*

Day 16

Breakfast

Raspberry Coconut Slush*
3 oz. sliced leftover meat, poultry, or fish

Morning Snack (optional)

Celery sticks or cherry tomatoes with 1-2 teaspoons Nut Pâté*

Lunch

Ostrich Burger*
Spinach and Pink Grapefruit Salad* with Grapefruit Vinaigrette*
Tea

Afternoon Snack (optional)

6-7 baby carrots and 3-4 olives

Dinner

Turkey Meat Loaf*
Spicy Wilted Greens
Hot lemon water or sparkling water

Dessert or Evening Snack (optional)

1/2 cup berries and 2 macadamia nuts

Preparation for Tomorrow

None.

Day 17

Breakfast
Frittata*
Green tea

Morning Snack (optional)
1/2 cup berries

Lunch
Leftover Turkey Meat Loaf*
Small Raw Veggie Delight* salad

Afternoon Snack (optional)
3-4 small carrot sticks and 1 teaspoon nut butter

Dinner
Pecan Catfish*
Cauliflower with Mushrooms*
Small Basic Garden Salad* with Lime, Oil and Garlic Dressing*
Herb tea

Dessert or Evening Snack (optional)
Cucumber sticks

Preparation for Tomorrow
Prepare Curried Squash Soup*, if you wish.

Day 18

Breakfast

Curried Squash Soup*
4 oz. leftover meat, poultry or seafood

Morning Snack (optional)

Mixed sprouts

Lunch

Asian Salad*
2-4 oz. Poached Chicken*

Afternoon Snack (optional)

Tomato and cucumber rounds
1/4 handful pine nuts

Dinner

Basic Stew*
Salad of your choice

Dessert or Evening Snack (optional)

1/4 cantaloupe and 3-4 almonds

Preparation for Tomorrow

None.

Day 19

Breakfast
1-2 Deviled Eggs*
Celery sticks with Nut Pâté* or Lettuce Roll Ups*
Green tea

Morning Snack (optional)
1/2 cup blueberries

Lunch
Leftover Basic Stew*

Afternoon Snack (optional)
4-5 cherry tomatoes and 1/8 avocado

Dinner
Broiled Tilapia Pesto*
Roasted Vegetables No. 1 or No. 2*

Dessert or Evening Snack (optional)
2 fresh apricots

Preparation for Tomorrow
Soak seeds/nuts overnight for Aloha Smoothie*

Day 20

Breakfast
Aloha Smoothie*
3 oz. leftover slices of meat or poultry, or 1 egg any style

Morning Snack (optional)
Handful of sprouts and 2-3 olives

Lunch
Cabbage Roll Ups*
Green tea

Afternoon Snack (optional)
Cucumber Mint Smoothie*

Dinner
Apricot Chicken*
Mustard Greens with Vinaigrette*

Dessert or Evening Snack (optional)
1/2 cup berries and 2 macadamia nuts

Preparation for Tomorrow
None.

Day 21

Breakfast
Huevos Rancheros*
Green tea

Morning Snack (optional)
2-5 olives

Lunch
Salmon Salad*
Herb tea

Afternoon Snack (optional)
Celery sticks with salsa

Dinner
Yakitori Beef*
Vegetables in Ginger Sauce*

Dessert or Evening Snack (optional)
1 kiwi and 10-15 pine nuts

Preparation for Tomorrow
None

Day 22

Breakfast

Egg-Shrimp Salad*
Green tea

Morning Snack (optional)

Tomato Cup*

Lunch

Cajun Filets*
Celery Slaw*
Hot lemon water

Afternoon Snack (optional)

1/2 cup raspberries and 1/4 handful pine nuts

Dinner

Basic Soup*
Spinach Salad*

Dessert or Evening Snack (optional)

1/2 pear and a few macadamia nuts

Preparation for Tomorrow

Prepare for Chicken Cucumber Delights*

Day 23

Breakfast
Cucumber Delights*
1/2 grapefruit
Green tea

Morning Snack (optional)
1 kiwi or 2 apricots, and 1/4 handful walnuts

Lunch
Leftover Basic Soup*
Avocado Citrus Salad*

Afternoon Snack (optional)
Cucumber rounds and handful sprouts

Dinner
Creole Rabbit*
Cauliflower with Mushrooms*
Small Garden Salad*

Dessert or Evening Snack (optional)
1 tangerine

Preparation for Tomorrow
None.

Day 24

Breakfast

Spinach and Eggs*
Green tea

Morning Snack (optional)

A few carrot sticks with 1-2 tablespoons guacamole

Lunch

Leftover Creole Rabbit*
Warm Nut and Cress Salad*
Steamed broccoli (if you wish)

Afternoon Snack (optional)

1 piece fruit and 4-6 almonds

Dinner

Asian Flank Steak*
Stir Fried Bok Choy*
Bean Sprout Salad*

Dessert or Evening Snack (optional)

3-4 fresh strawberries

Preparation for Tomorrow

None.

Day 25

Breakfast

Cole Slaw*
3-6 oz. leftover meat, poultry or fish — or a hard boiled egg, sliced
Green tea

Morning Snack (optional)

2-4 olives and handful sprouts

Lunch

Curried Squash Soup*
Tarragon Turkey Patty*

Afternoon Snack (optional)

1-2 plums and 1/4 handful walnuts

Dinner

Herbed Salmon*
Cabbage and Cherry Salad*
Steamed cauliflower (if desired)

Dessert or Evening Snack (optional)

1/3 pear and some pumpkin seeds

Preparation for Tomorrow

None.

Day 26

Breakfast

Confetti Salad* or Raw Veggie Delight*
4-6 oz. canned tuna or salmon, added to salad
Choice of dressing from Recipes list
Green tea

Morning Snack (optional)

1/2 peach or nectarine and 2-3 pecans

Lunch

Herbed London Broil*
Shoestring Carrot Salad*
Steamed asparagus

Afternoon Snack (optional)

Raw vegetables with 2 tablespoons guacamole

Dinner

Baked White Fish*
Cooked Cabbage*
Mustard Greens in Vinaigrette*

Dessert or Evening Snack (optional)

Cucumber sticks and a few cherry tomatoes

Preparation for Tomorrow

None.

Day 27

Breakfast
3-6 oz. leftover Herbed London Broil*
Lettuce Roll Ups*
Green tea

Morning Snack (optional)
1/4 handful nuts and 6 baby carrots

Lunch
Apple Turkey Salad*
Cole Slaw*

Afternoon Snack (optional)
1/8 avocado and 2-3 sections of pink grapefruit

Dinner
Steak and Vegetable Soup*

Dessert or Evening Snack (optional)
1/2 cup berries and sprinkling of pine nuts

Preparation for Tomorrow
Gazpacho, if you don't have any on hand.

Day 28

Breakfast

Gazpacho*
3-5 pre-cooked shrimp, added to gazpacho

Morning Snack (optional)

1 orange or kiwi with 5 macadamia nuts

Lunch

Pecan Catfish*
Zucchini Sauté*

Afternoon Snack (optional)

1-2 Tomatoes Dijon* or Tomato Cup*

Dinner

Baked Buffalo Stew*
Basic Garden Salad* with Spicy Salad Dressing*

Dessert or Evening Snack (optional)

2-4 green olives and cucumber slices

Preparation for Tomorrow

None.

Day 29

Breakfast
Leftover Baked Buffalo Stew*
Green tea

Morning Snack (optional)
Celery with 2 teaspoons Nut Pâté* or nut butter

Lunch
Chicken with Grape Salad*
2 Tomato Cups* or Tomatoes Dijon*

Afternoon Snack (optional)
3-5 olives and jicama sticks

Dinner
Basic Stir Fry*

Dessert or Evening Snack (optional)
1/4 papaya and 2-3 macadamia nuts

Preparation for Tomorrow
None.

Day 30

Breakfast
Frittata*
Green tea

Morning Snack (optional)
1 kiwi and 1/4 handful walnuts

Lunch
Italian Beef Soup*

Afternoon Snack (optional)
Handful sprouts and 1/8 avocado

Dinner
Fish Filets in Red Sauce*
Spinach Salad* with Lime, Oil and Garlic Dressing*
Mashed Cauliflower*

Dessert or Evening Snack (optional)
2/3 cup fresh berries in season sprinkled with 3-4 chopped macadamia nuts and 1 teaspoon dark chocolate drops

Preparation for Tomorrow
Make a date with your partner or best friend to go out tomorrow evening to the best restaurant in town. You may order whatever your heart desires.

You've completed the first month of a very challenging diet program that has asked you to fundamentally alter what you are accustomed to eating. Congratulations on getting this far!

Continue with your progress on your new diet for a healthier life — and don't forget to have a big celebration every month.

13.2 Recipes

The Recipes section of this book is divided into these sub-sections:

1. Basic Meals
2. Meat
3. Seafood
4. Poultry
5. Eggs
6. Salads
7. Vegetables
8. Soups
9. Juices and Smoothies
10. Snacks and Handhelds
11. Sauces and Dressings

Before you dig into the recipes, we'd like to share a few thoughts with you about basic meals and sandwiches.

Basic Meals

The *Basic Meals* section contains a few "basic" recipes that are quite versatile. You can use many combinations of animal protein and vegetables to create meals for you and your family.

Like many of you, we are very busy. Often, we don't have the time to prepare a gourmet meal. Sometimes, we need to be able to fix a good meal in 15 minutes.

Stir-Fry
One of our favorites is the stir-fry. Here's a recent example of what we did with a stir-fry. It was 5:45 on a weeknight. A family member had to leave at 7:00 PM, and dinner needed to be served around 6:00 so that eating dinner wouldn't be too rushed. But we had been extremely busy and hadn't been to the grocery store for a few days. There wasn't much food in the house. What could be created in 15 minutes?

Here's what we did. We put a big non-stick skillet on stove, medium low heat, and added about 3 tablespoons of water and 2 or 3 tablespoons of olive oil. Grabbed a couple of onions and a few cloves of garlic out of the pantry. Quickly sliced and put into covered skillet and turned up heat to medium-high. An animal protein was needed. Looked in the refrigerator — there was nothing. Looked in the freezer.

Aha! There was a bag of frozen shrimp. Took 4 large handfuls of shrimp and dumped into skillet. Covered skillet. Our next thought turned to vegetables. Looked again in the fridge — there was a head of broccoli, 1-1/2 zucchinis and half a head of Chinese cabbage.

Usually we have lots of vegetables on hand, but this is all we had today. Sliced all of it and put into covered skillet.

As we let it all cook for a minute or two, we decided to add some tamari (a wheat-free soy sauce), leaving the skillet uncovered. There was some disagreement about what else to add for flavor, but we ended up adding 1-2 teaspoons of turmeric for added flavor and color. We added a dash more water as things looked a bit dry. We cooked the stir-fry in the uncovered skillet till most ingredients were somewhat tender. We started eating dinner right on time at 6:00 PM.

Soups and Stews

Hearty homemade soups or stews are quite versatile. What we do is make up a huge pot of soup or stew.

Chicken soup is one example. We may first boil a whole chicken, strip away all cooked meat and put the meat into a large soup pot with water/chicken broth. We then chop a large quantity of vegetables. We typically use whatever vegetables are on hand. We don't bother to follow a recipe — we just make it up as we go along. We may add anywhere from 3-6 different vegetables to the soup, in differing amounts depending on the type of vegetable and depending on what we had on hand. We chop them up and put them into the pot and let everything cook. Of course, we add a considerable amount of herbs and spices, depending on our mood.

When cooked, we may run about 1/3 of the soup through a blender, then put the blended material back into the pot. This makes for a more creamy soup. So now we have a hearty soup, high in protein, loaded with vegetables, with a texture that is both chunky and somewhat creamy. Or, instead of boiling a chicken, we may (to save time) just throw in 2-3 fillets of chopped fish, or chunks of leftover cooked turkey, or a cheap cut of beef. We don't always cream our soups. What we end up with is a fairly huge pot of soup. That one pot may last us a week, depending on how many times we have it.

Our soups are not thin and watery. They are thick and hearty because they have a high percentage of animal protein and vegetables. One bowl of this soup is filling. With two bowls, we feel over-full. A protein-rich, hearty soup can be an entire meal; or a smaller portion can be served as part of a meal.

We freeze what we aren't going to use during the next few days. We put it into individual meal-size plastic containers and freeze them. We now have a super-fast, back-up meal to consume at any time.

After we've finished consuming any unfrozen soup or stew, we take 1-2 containers of out of the freezer and put them in the refrigerator so they will slowly get thawed out and be available for an "instant" meal at any time. When we're feeling lazy or rushed, we just get a container of out of the refrigerator, put it into a ceramic bowl and microwave it. We now have a meal in 5 minutes.

Salads

Salads are also versatile and fast. We usually have some leftover meat, poultry or fish in the refrigerator. We simply get some lettuce, spinach or other greens out of the refrigerator, wash them (if not yet washed), cut or tear them, and put them into a salad bowl. To that we may add something crunchy like chopped celery or sliced zucchini. We also add any accent vegetables we have on hand, such as green onions or parsley.

We then add our animal protein, either chopped or sliced. If we don't have fish, poultry or red meat on hand, we may quickly boil a couple of eggs and make it an egg salad.

Finally, we'll drizzle some salad dressing on top, then mix or toss the salad lightly. We use one of the dressings in the *Sauces and Dressings* section of the recipes in this book.

To finish it off, we often sprinkle the salad raw cashews, walnuts or some other nut or seed.

We can generally make a nice salad in about 10 minutes.

Sandwiches and Roll-ups

You may have discovered by now that no bread is allowed on the healthy PCOS diet. This means no sandwiches, and no toast and jam. These are modern-day foods that may not mesh well with your genetic makeup. One could imagine that the sandwich has been around since the dawn of history. But this is not the case.

Contrary to what you may have heard, the sandwich was not invented by the Earl of Sandwich in 1765. The first recorded sandwich was by the famous rabbi, Hillel the Elder, who lived during the 1st century B.C. He started the Passover custom of sandwiching a mixture of chopped nuts, apples, spices, and wine between two matzohs to eat with bitter herbs.

During the Middle Ages, thick blocks of coarse stale bread called trenchers were used in place of plates. Meats and other foods were piled on top of the bread to be eaten with fingers and sometimes with the aid of knives. The trenchers, thick and stale, absorbed the juice, the grease, and the sauces. At the end of the meal, one either ate the trencher or, if hunger had been satisfied, tossed the gravy-soaked bread to their dogs or gave it to a less fortunate human.

The sandwich was introduced to America by Englishwoman Elizabeth Leslie in 1840. In her cookbook, *Directions for Cookery*, she had a recipe for ham sandwiches that she suggested as a main dish. Since then, we have embraced the sandwich as a mainstay of our diet. So the sandwich has been with us for less than two centuries. Even today, the majority of the world's population does not habitually eat sandwiches.

But since the healthy PCOS diet does not include sandwich bread, what can you use instead?

We would suggest you use wraps to create "roll-ups."

Wraps consist of any allowed food within which you can wrap other foods. Examples of possible wraps are:

- Lettuce leaves
- Cabbage leaves (lightly steamed)
- Collard leaves (lightly steamed)
- Kale leaves (lightly steamed)
- Steamed eggplant slices
- Pickled grape leaves
- Thin omelets
- Nori seaweed sheets
- Meat slices
- Vegetable leathers

There are several types of wrapping methods:

- *Enchilada style* - lay wrapper flat, spread with 2-3 tablespoons of filling, fold wrapper over filling, roll up tightly
- *Burrito style* - lay wrapper flat, spread with filling, fold opposite sides inward 1/4 - 1/3 of the way on each side, fold wrapper over filling, roll into tight bundle
- *Tostada style* - lay wrapper flat on plate, spread with vegetables, sprouts, meats, topping

So it's possible you can have something that resembles a sandwich. You're just using something other than bread.

Serving Sizes

Please note that the number of servings in the following recipes vary from recipe to recipe. We have no way of knowing how many are in your family, so please adjust ingredient amounts to the number of people you are feeding and the amount of leftovers you wish to create.

The serving sizes in each recipe are only broad suggestions. While some PCOS women are overweight and insulin resistant, others are lean and may not be insulin resistant. Therefore, the serving size that works well for you may be too much or too little for another woman. It's up to you to exercise good judgment regarding meal portion sizes. We cannot tell you the exact meal portion sizes you should consume — everyone is unique. However, in general, most people eat more food than they need.

If you are on a Weight Watchers program and have a maximum number of calories you may consume, there are a large number of online calorie counters on the Internet that you may use to calculate the calorie content of any recipe in this book.

13.2.1 Basic Meals

Recipes in This Section:

Basic Garden Salad
Basic Soup
Basic Stew
Basic Stir Fry

~

Basic Garden Salad

2 cups any combination of leafy greens on Recommended List, such as lettuce, endive, escarole, radicchio, spinach, dandelion greens, plus any of the following ingredients:
1/2 cup watercress, broken into 1" pieces
1/2 cup broccoli, small spears
1/2 cup bean sprouts
1/2 cup jicama, diced or thinly sliced
1/3 cup radish or daikon radish, thinly sliced
1 stalk celery, chopped
1 carrot, diced, shredded or thinly sliced
1-2 green onions, cut into 1" pieces
1/4 cup pine nuts, walnuts or slivered almonds

Dress with any dressing listed in the Sauces and Dressings section of the Recipes.

Note:
You may add or substitute any other vegetables from the Recommended list.

Yield: approximately 4 servings

Basic Soup

2 cloves garlic
1 medium onion
1 tablespoon extra virgin olive oil
2 quarts low-salt chicken broth
2 chicken breasts, bone and skin removed
6 tomatoes (or 24 ounces canned tomatoes if fresh not available)
2 zucchini, chopped
2 carrots
1 cup string beans, chopped into 1" pieces
1/2 cup fresh parsley
1/2 tablespoon turmeric
Pinch of pepper (optional)

Sauté garlic and onion in a little olive oil in a soup pot. Add broth and bring to a boil.
Add chicken. Simmer 30 minutes. Remove chicken, cool and dice. Add vegetables and spices.
Simmer another 15 - 20 minutes. Return chicken to pot and serve when chicken is reheated.

Variation:
Substitute a boneless turkey breast for the chicken, or 16-24 oz. of any meat or fish.
Add or substitute other vegetables from Recommended List, as you wish.

Yield: approximately 5 servings

Basic Stew

1 pound stew meat, cut into 1 inch cubes
1 teaspoon salt
1/2 teaspoon ground pepper
2 tablespoons extra virgin olive oil
3/4 cup chopped onion
5 cloves garlic, crushed
1 bay leaf
1 tablespoon dried thyme leaves
1 medium-large tomato
3/4 cup carrots, sliced
4 stalks celery, sliced
1/4 cauliflower or cabbage
1 pound mushrooms (any kind), sliced
3 cups pure water
32 ounces beef or chicken stock
1/2 cup chopped parsley

Season meat with salt and pepper. Heat heavy kettle or crockpot to medium, then add 2 tablespoons water and 2 tablespoons oil to pan. Steam-sauté beef until browned, about 8 minutes. Add all remaining ingredients except parsley. Simmer for several hours and serve with sprinkle of chopped parsley.

Notes:
You can substitute other meats, poultry or vegetables from our Recommended lists.

Yield: 5-8 servings

Basic Stir Fry

1/4 cup olive oil
2 pounds lean meat or chicken, cubed or sliced
2 medium onions, sliced
4 cloves garlic, chunks
1/3 Chinese cabbage (or any cabbage), sliced
4 carrots, chopped
2 cups tender snow pea pods
1-2 small Japanese egg plant or 1/4 regular egg plant, cubed
1 medium size bok choy, sliced crosswise
1 cup water or stock
1/2 pound bean sprouts
2 tablespoons tamari
1/3 cup pine nuts

In large frying pan or wok, add 3 tablespoons of water, then add olive oil and heat. Brown meat and remove from pan. Add onion and garlic. Sauté until soft.

Increase heat to medium high. Add cabbage and carrots. Sauté about 5 minutes. Add eggplant, then pea pods and bok choy. Sauté a few minutes. Add water or vegetable stock. Add meat to pan. Stir and cover. Simmer 10 minutes. If liquid evaporates, add more water or stock.

Add tamari and bean sprouts. Stir and simmer 30 seconds. Garnish with pine nuts and serve.

Variations:
You may used beef, pork, turkey or fish instead of chicken. Even a combination of meats is OK if you have them on hand. If you're using leftover meat that is already cooked, don't brown it — just add it 3 minutes before you're finished cooking.

If you don't like any of the above vegetables, try other vegetables. Always add densest vegetables first, followed by the leafy ones.

Yield: 3 - 4 servings

13.2.2 Meat

Recipes in This Section

Asian Flank Steak
Baked Buffalo Stew
Beef and Pepper Fajitas
Beef, Mushroom and Spinach Eggs
Beef or Buffalo Chili
Beef or Wild Sirloin with Mushrooms
Beef Sukiyaki
Buffalo Burgers
Creole Rabbit
Curried Beef Strips
Grilled Venison
Herb and Garlic Sirloin or Lamb
Herbed London Broil
Italian Braised Steak
Liver and Onions
Marinated Flank Steak
Marinated Pork Loin
Mushroom Cube Steaks with Wine
Rabbit Stew
Venison Pot Roast
Yakitori Beef

Asian Flank Steak

1 pound flank steak
2 tablespoons tamari
1 tablespoons ginger root, peeled and minced
1/4 cup teaspoon olive oil
2 cloves garlic, crushed

Trim fat from steak. Combine tamari, ginger, oil and garlic in a large heavy-duty zip-top plastic bag. Add steak and seal bag. Marinate in refrigerator 8 hours, turning bag occasionally. Remove steak from bag. Reserve marinade for basting.

Prepare grill or broiler. Place steak on grill rack or broiler pan coated with cooking spray and cook 8 minutes on each side or until desired degree of doneness. You may baste meat with reserved marinade when you turn it. Cut steak diagonally across the grain into thin slices.

Yield: 4 servings

Baked Buffalo Stew

1 pound buffalo stew meat, cut into 1-1/2 inch cubes
1 large carrot, cut in large chunks
1 large onion, cut in large chunks
6 Brussels sprouts, cut into quarters
3 cloves garlic, sliced
3 stalks celery, chopped
1 green pepper, chopped
2 large tomatoes, chopped
1 teaspoon tamari
1/4 teaspoon freshly ground black pepper (optional)
1/4 teaspoon salt (optional)
1 teaspoon Salt-Free All-Purpose Seasoning*
1/2 cup beef stock/broth
1 teaspoons grated fresh horseradish (optional)

Preheat oven to 275° F. Place meat cubes in a large casserole dish. Add carrot, onion, Brussels sprouts, garlic, celery, green pepper, tomatoes, seasonings, and stock. Cover tightly and bake for 5 hours. Sprinkle with grated horseradish before serving.

Yield: 2 - 4 servings

Beef and Pepper Fajitas

1 pound free-range beef steak, cut into strips
1 tablespoon extra virgin olive oil
1 medium onion, sliced
1 cup green bell pepper, cut into strips
1 cup yellow bell pepper, cut into strips
1 cup red bell pepper, cut into strips
2 medium zucchini, cut into diagonal strips
2 stalks celery, cut diagonally
2 tablespoons chili powder
1 tablespoon cumin
1 teaspoon garlic power
1 teaspoon oregano
1/2 cup Latin Salsa* (or a salsa of your choice)

Heat a large skillet over medium high heat. Add olive oil and sauté onions, peppers, zucchini, celery and seasonings until onions are translucent. Remove from pan and hold.

Add beef slices and sauté until they are no longer pink. Add vegetables back to the pan and sauté until everything is hot. Serve with Latin Salsa* or a salsa of your choice.

Yield: 4 servings

Beef, Mushroom and Spinach Eggs

1/4 pound extra lean ground beef
1/2 tablespoon olive oil
1 clove minced garlic
1/2 cup chopped mushrooms
1/2 tablespoon basil
2 cups fresh spinach, chopped
1 hard boiled egg
Tamari to taste

Brown ground beef and garlic in olive oil over medium heat. When meat is almost done, add chopped mushrooms, basil, spinach and tamari. Cook over low heat until spinach is wilted and soft. Place on plate and top with sliced hard boiled egg.

Yield: 1 serving

Beef or Buffalo Chili

1 tablespoon extra virgin olive oil
1/2 cup onions, chopped
1 1/2 cups celery, chopped
1 cup green pepper, chopped
2-3 cloves garlic, minced
1-1/2 pound ground buffalo or extra lean ground beef
1 teaspoons chili powder
2-1/2 teaspoons ground cumin
2 teaspoons dried thyme
1/2 teaspoon Morton Salt Substitute or 1/4 teaspoon regular salt
3-4 fresh tomatoes, chopped or blended in blender (If fresh tomatoes are unavailable, use about 16 ounces of canned tomatoes instead)
12 ounces Tomato Chili Salsa*

Heat oil in large skillet. Sauté onions, celery, green pepper and garlic until onions are soft and transparent (about 4 minutes). Add ground buffalo, chili powder, cumin and thyme and cook for 5 minutes, stirring frequently. Add salt, tomatoes and Tomato Chili Salsa into a pot. Cover and simmer on low for at least an hour.

Yield: 4 servings

Notes:
This recipe can be made in a crockpot. After sautéing the vegetables in skillet, add remaining ingredients to crockpot and cook on low for several hours.

Beef or Wild Sirloin with Mushrooms

1-1/2 pounds free-range beef (or wild game) sirloins or tenderloins, cut into 2x1x1 inch
strips and visible fat removed
1/2 cup scallions, thinly sliced
2 tablespoons tamari
5 tablespoons extra virgin olive oil
2 tablespoons freshly squeezed lemon juice
2 cloves garlic, minced
Black pepper to taste (optional)
1/2 teaspoon crumbled whole dried thyme leaves
1 pound Portobello mushrooms
Morton Salt Substitute or regular salt to taste
1 cup rich beef stock

In a bowl, whisk together scallions, tamari, 3 tablespoons of the olive oil, lemon juice,
garlic, pepper, and thyme. Add meat. Cover and refrigerate 2 hours or longer.

Remove mushroom stems and save them for another use. Slice the caps about 1/2 inch
thick. Heat skillet over medium heat until hot. Add 2 tablespoons water and the remaining
2 tablespoons olive oil. Add the mushrooms and stir well. Sprinkle with salt and pepper.
Cook, stirring frequently, until the mushrooms are tender (about 5 minutes).
Remove mushrooms and any liquid from the pan and set aside.

Place the pan over medium heat and add about half the meat with any marinade that
adheres to it. Separate the meat pieces, so they don't steam as they cook. For rare or
medium-rare, brown on all sides for about 2 minutes total. Remove from the pan and keep
warm. Repeat with remaining meat.

Pour off any fat remaining in the skillet, leaving any browned bits of meat. Add the beef
stock to the pan and return it to high heat. Stir well, scraping the bottom of the pan with a
wooden spoon to dislodge browned bits; boil until the liquid is reduced and slightly
thickened. Decrease the heat to medium low. Add the mushrooms and cook for a few
seconds while stirring; add the meat with any juices and cook briefly, continuing to stir,
just until the meat is heated thoroughly. Serve immediately.

Yield: 4 servings

Note:
You can use elk, deer, antelope or caribou meat in this recipe.

Beef Sukiyaki

2-3 cloves garlic, minced
1/2 cup tamari
2 tablespoons rice wine vinegar
2 tablespoons beef or free range chicken stock
1 - 1 1/2 pounds organic or free-range flank steak
1-3/4 cups beef or free-range chicken stock
1 tablespoon olive oil
2 cups celery, cut in diagonal strips
2 cups onions, sliced into thin crescents
2 cups cabbage, shredded
4 cups bok choy, Swiss chard or Chinese cabbage
2 cups mushrooms, sliced
2-5 green onions, cut diagonally
2-3 cups of fresh bean sprouts

To make marinade, mix garlic, tamari, vinegar and 2 tablespoons stock in covered container. Cut steak across the grain into thin slices with a sharp knife (this is easier if steak is partially frozen). Add to marinade mix, coating thoroughly, and marinate for several hours.

When ready to cook, cut vegetables and set aside. Drain marinade from meat, add remaining 1-3/4 cups stock to marinade and set aside. Heat wok or heavy skillet; add 1 tablespoon water and the olive oil. When hot, add meat and sauté, stirring constantly for about 2 minutes, until meat begins to lose its pink color. Remove meat from pan. Add celery and onions to pan, stirring for 2 minutes. Add 1/4 cup of the marinade, followed by the shredded cabbage and bok choy or chard. Stir fry until veggies begin to wilt. Pour in another 1/4 cup marinade and cover for 2 minutes to steam.

Reduce heat and add mushrooms, green onions and beef slices. Stir to mix. Pour remaining marinade over all and serve on a bed of fresh bean sprouts.

Yield: 6 servings

Buffalo Burgers

1/2 pound ground buffalo meat
1/2 tablespoon horseradish
1/2 teaspoon Spike vegetable seasoning
Black pepper to taste

Combine all ingredients and form into patties. Broil, grill or steam-fry until done (about 3-4 minutes on each side, or until brown throughout). Do not overcook.

Top with a bit of guacamole and/or salsa, if desired.

Yield: 1 - 2 servings

Creole Rabbit

3 pounds rabbit meat, cleaned and cut into pieces
1 teaspoon Morton Salt Substitute or 1/4 teaspoon regular salt
1/4 teaspoon black pepper
1/4 teaspoon cayenne pepper
1/4 cup onion, chopped
3 cloves fresh garlic, minced
2 tablespoons white vinegar
1 tablespoon extra virgin olive oil
1 cup sliced mushrooms
1 tablespoon fresh parsley, minced
2 tablespoons green bell pepper, minced
2 tablespoons green onions, chopped fine
1/3 cup dry white wine

Wash and dry rabbit pieces and place in bowl. Combine salt, black pepper, cayenne pepper, onion, garlic, vinegar and oil, and pour over rabbit, turning pieces to coat. Cover bowl and marinate overnight in refrigerator.

Preheat oven to 450° F. Transfer rabbit and marinade to oiled baking dish. Bake in preheated oven for 1 hour. Combine remaining ingredients and pour over rabbit. Bake 30 to 45 minutes longer, until rabbit is fork-tender.

Yield: 6 - 8 servings

Curried Beef Strips

2 tablespoons extra virgin olive oil
4 ounces lean beef, cut into 1/4 inch strips
1 apple, coarsely chopped
1 onion, coarsely chopped
1 red pepper, coarsely chopped
1/2 cloves garlic, minced fine
1 tablespoon curry powder
Tamari to taste
1/2 cup water

Heat pan gently. Add small amount of water to moisten bottom of pan, followed by olive oil. Heat thoroughly and add beef, apple, onion, red pepper and garlic. Steam-sauté until beef is brown and onion is tender. Add curry powder, tamari and water. Cover tightly and cook on medium low for 30 minutes, adding water as needed.

Yield: 1 - 2 servings

Grilled Venison

4 venison steaks (4 ounces each)
2 tablespoons chopped rosemary
2 tablespoons minced garlic
2 tablespoons chopped fresh or dried thyme
1/4 cup extra virgin olive oil
1 tablespoon tamari
Pepper to taste

For marinade, combine oil and herbs. Marinate venison for 4 hours in refrigerator, covered. Remove from marinade and shake off excess oil. Place venison on indoor or outdoor grill. Season with pepper and brush with marinade. Depending on thickness and heat of grill, cook for 5-9 minutes turning once. Serve medium to medium rare for maximum juiciness and tenderness.

Yield: 4 servings

Herb and Garlic Beef or Lamb

2 lamb shoulder steaks, chops, or petite sirloin steak
1 tablespoon minced garlic
1/4 teaspoon dried rosemary
1/2 teaspoon dried oregano
1/2 teaspoon dried tarragon
2 tablespoons lemon juice
1/2 tablespoon tamari
Pepper to taste

Preheat oven to 350° F. Place meat in a baking dish. Combine the remaining ingredients, pour over chops and bake until done (about 35-45 minutes).

Yield: 2 servings

Herbed London Broil

London broil beef (1 - 1 1/2 lbs.), trimmed of fat and cut into four pieces
1 tablespoon extra virgin olive oil
2 cloves garlic, minced
4 teaspoons Salt-Free All-Purpose Seasoning*

Place meat in a shallow dish. Rub both sides with oil, garlic and Salt-Free All-Purpose Seasoning. Let stand for up to one hour if you have the time. Prepare grill or preheat broiler. Grill about 8-10 minutes on each side, depending on thickness and your meat preference. If broiling, cook meat two inches from heat source to desired state (four minutes per side for rare).

Yield: 4 servings

Italian Braised Steak

1 1/2 pounds lean free-range round steak, cut into 1/4 inch strips
1/2 teaspoon Salt-Free All-Purpose Seasoning*
1 tablespoon extra virgin olive oil
1 3/4 cup organic beef broth
1 cup chopped tomatoes
1 medium onion, sliced
1 clove garlic, finely chopped
1 large green bell pepper, cut in strips
1 zucchini, cut in strips

Season meat with Salt-Free All-Purpose Seasoning. Moisten bottom of large frying pan and add oil. Then add meat and brown on sides, drain off any fat. Add broth, tomatoes, onion and garlic to the meat. Cover and simmer about 1 hour until meat is tender. Add green pepper and zucchini strips and stir-cook for another 5 minutes.

Yield: 4 - 6 servings

Liver and Onions

4-6 ounces free range beef liver
1 tablespoon lemon juice
2 tablespoons pure water
1 tablespoon olive oil
1 clove garlic, minced fine
1-2 medium onions
2 tablespoons tamari

Place liver on a plate and drizzle with lemon juice. Let stand while preparing the rest of the recipe.

Heat a covered sauté pan over low heat. When hot, add water; then add olive oil, garlic, onions and tamari. Steam-sauté until onions begin to turn translucent. Add liver to pan and cook 3 minutes on each side. Then cover pan tightly and allow liver to steam for 5-10 minutes, or until thoroughly cooked (time will vary depending on thickness of the liver). Remove liver to serving plate and top with onion mixture.

Yield: 1 serving

Marinated Flank Steak

1-1/2 pounds flank steak
Meat Marinade*

Wash and pat flank steak dry. Place into large zip lock bag. Add Meat Marinade.
Refrigerate for 1-4 hours if you can. Better yet, let the flank steak marinade overnight in
the refrigerator. Turn bag over from time to time to make sure all parts of the meat get
some marinade.

Set oven rack to proper broiling level. Turn oven on to "broil." Place meat on broiler pan.
Baste with marinade and broil for about 9 minutes on one side. Remove, turn meat over,
baste with marinade other side and return to broiler for another 8 minutes.

Remove and let meat sit for about 3 minutes. Thinly slice on the diagonal.

Yield: 3 - 5 servings

Marinated Pork Loin

1-1/2 pounds pork loin
Pork Loin Marinade*

Pat pork dry. Place into large zip lock bag. Add Pork Loin Marinade. Refrigerate and let it
marinate for 1-4 hours, or overnight if you have the time. Turn bag over from time to time
to make sure all parts of the meat get some marinade.

Preheat oven to 325° F. Place pork in roasting pan, and pour marinade over it.
Season with salt and pepper, if desired. Bake for 1-1/2 to 2 hours, until a meat
thermometer registers 185° F.

Remove pork from baking dish and set on cutting board. Let cool 10 minutes, then slice.

Yield: 3 - 5 servings

Mushroom Cube Steaks with Wine

4 large free-range beef cube steaks
1/2 cup red wine
12 ounces fresh mushrooms, sliced
4 cloves garlic, minced
4 tablespoons onion, minced
2 tablespoons parsley, minced
2 tablespoons butter

Place beef steaks, wine, mushrooms, garlic, onion and parsley into covered container and marinate for at least an hour (better if marinated overnight).

Remove steaks from marinade and set marinade aside. Heat skillet over medium heat and melt butter. Add steaks, 2 at a time unless pan is very large. Braise steaks for 2 - 3 minutes on each side. Remove from skillet and place steaks in single layer in shallow casserole dish or serving platter.

Add reserved marinade to pan and heat until boiling, scraping meat juices into mix. Cook for a few minutes to reduce liquid. Pour over steaks and serve immediately.

Yield: 4 servings

Rabbit Stew

2 tablespoons extra virgin olive oil
1 rabbit (about 2 pounds.), cut into serving pieces
1 tablespoons tamari
1/2 teaspoon black pepper (optional)
1 large onion, chunked
2 cloves fresh garlic, minced
2 cups chicken or vegetable broth
2 large carrots, chunked
3 stalks celery, chunked
10-12 button mushrooms, sliced
1 medium kohlrabi, chunked
1 large tomato, coarsely chopped
1/2 teaspoon fresh or dried rosemary
2 tablespoons fresh or dried parsley

Preheat the oven to 350° F. Place the oil in a large, heavy skillet over low heat. Put 2 tablespoons water and then olive oil in pan and brown the rabbit pieces (about 5-7 minutes per side). Add tamari and sprinkle with pepper. Place the browned rabbit, carrots, celery, mushrooms, kohlrabi and chopped tomato into a shallow baking pan.

Next, add the onion to the skillet and cook over low heat for 7 to 10 minutes to soften. Add the garlic and cook 2 minutes more, stirring. Add broth and bring mixture to a boil, scraping up the browned bits on the bottom of the skillet. Reduce the heat; add the rosemary and parsley, cooking for another 2 minutes. Pour the sauce over the rabbit and vegetables. Bake for 45 minutes. To serve, place rabbit pieces on a serving platter and pour remaining pan juices over top.

Yield: 4 servings

Venison Pot Roast

2 tablespoons extra virgin olive oil
3 - 4 pound venison pot roast
Black pepper to taste
2 tablespoons tamari
4-6 medium tomatoes, chopped
1 medium onion, chopped
1 cup celery, chopped
1 tablespoon parsley, minced
2 teaspoons oregano
3 cloves garlic, minced
1 cup vegetable or beef broth

Preheat oven to 325° F. In Dutch oven, add olive oil and brown roast on all sides. Add pepper and tamari to taste. Combine remaining ingredients and pour over pot roast. Cover and bake 3-4 hours.

Variation:
If venison not available, use free-range beef or any large cut of meat from a large game animal.

Yield: 6 - 8 servings

Yakitori Beef

1 pound free range beef sirloin, chunked
1/2 cup tamari
2 tablespoons lemon juice
1 clove garlic, crushed
1/2 teaspoon ginger, ground
1 tablespoon extra virgin olive oil
2 green onions, finely chopped

Combine tamari, lemon juice, garlic, ginger, oil, and onion in food processor or blender and blend well. Place in glass pan. Thread meat on bamboo skewers and place skewered meat in marinade, turn to coat all sides. Cover and refrigerate 4 hours; drain. Arrange on broiler pan and broil 5 to 8 inches from heating element. Broil 1 1/2 to 2 minutes; turn to broil 1 minute longer. Serve hot.

Yield: 2 - 4 servings

13.2.3 Seafood

Recipes in This Section

Almond Crusted Snapper
Baked White Fish
Broiled Tilapia Pesto
Cajun Filets
Chili Pepper Halibut
Dijonnaise Poached Salmon
Fish Filets in Red Sauce
Herbed Salmon
Lemon Parslied Fish
Pecan Catfish
Sardine Sushi

~

Almond Crusted Snapper

1 pound red snapper
1/2 teaspoon black pepper (adjust to taste)
1/2 teaspoon Salt-Free All-Purpose Seasoning*, Spike or Mrs. Dash
1/2 cup almonds, ground fine (or other nut or seed if you prefer)
2 tablespoons extra virgin olive oil

Preheat oven to 350° F.

Rinse the fish fillets and pat dry. Apply seasoning and pepper to both sides of fish. Grind the almonds to a fine powder in a food processor, running the machine in short bursts. Do not overgrind or the mixture will become oily.

Put 1 tablespoon olive oil in glass baking dish, then add fish. Sprinkle fish with almond meal and bake for 15-20 minutes or until fish flakes easily with a fork. Serve with lemon or lime.

Yield: 2-3 servings

Baked White Fish

1/4 cup raw macadamia nuts
2 large tomatoes
1 pound halibut, turbot or other white fish
1 small onion, minced
1/4 teaspoon black pepper
1 egg white
1 tablespoon extra virgin olive oil
1/2 teaspoon Salt Free All Purpose Seasoning*
1 medium onion, sliced
1 green bell pepper, chopped

Grind macadamia nuts in coffee grinder or food processor to a fine meal. Do not overgrind or they will become oily. Set aside.

Puree tomatoes in a food processor or blender. Set aside.

Chop the fish and the small onion in a food processor. Add the nut meal, pepper and egg white. Mix well. Shape into 12 balls.

Preheat oven to 325° F. Combine oil, sliced onion, green pepper and tomato puree in a baking dish. Arrange the fish balls in it; cover and bake for 40 to 45 minutes. Baste with the sauce before serving.

Yield: 2 - 4 servings

Broiled Tilapia Pesto

4 filets of tilapia (about 6 ounces each)
2 cloves garlic, minced
1/3 cup fresh lemon juice
1 tablespoon tamari
1 teaspoon extra virgin olive oil
2 tablespoons minced onion
Lemon slices
4 tablespoons Italian Basil Pesto*

Place fish in flat pan. Mix garlic, lemon juice, tamari, olive oil and onion together, and pour over fish. Marinate for at least 30 minutes.

Place fish on broiler pan and baste with marinade. Broil 6 inches from heat, for 3 - 4 minutes, depending on thickness of tilapia filets. Pull out broiler pan and spread 1 tablespoon of Italian Basil Pesto on each filet. Turn broiler heat off and return pan to oven for 2 more minutes to warm the pesto.

Serve with lemon slices.

Yield: 4 servings

Cajun Filets

2 tablespoon olive oil
2 tablespoons lemon juice
1 tablespoon tamari
2 1/2 pounds of fish filets - sole, trout, snapper or catfish
1/8 teaspoon crushed red pepper
1/8 teaspoon garlic powder or 1 clove minced, fresh garlic

Preheat oven to 350° F. Heat oil with lemon juice and tamari on low heat in a shallow pan. Coat both sides of fish fillets with this mix. Lay fillets side by side, overlapping slightly if necessary, in a pan. Mix dry spices together, and sprinkle over fillets. Bake for 20-25 minutes, depending on size of filets and type of fish (catfish bakes the longest). The pan may blacken, but that's okay; the liquid will keep the fish moist. Serve immediately.

Yield: 4 - 5 servings

Chili Pepper Halibut

4 halibut fillets (4 ounces each)
1/4 cup fresh lime juice
1 tablespoon fresh lemon juice
1 teaspoon tamari
1 teaspoon chili powder
4 green onions, sliced in 1/2 inch lengths
1 tomato, coarsely chopped
1/2 cup Anaheim pepper, chopped
1/2 cup red bell pepper, chopped
Cilantro for garnish

Preheat oven to 350° F. Place halibut in a shallow baking dish. Combine lime juice, lemon juice, tamari and chili powder in bowl and pour over halibut. Marinate 10 minutes, turning once or twice. Sprinkle onions, tomato and peppers over fish. Cover. Bake for 30 minutes or just until halibut flakes in center. Let stand, covered, 4 minutes before serving. Garnish with fresh cilantro.

Variation:
If halibut is unavailable, you can use snapper, cod or any other white fish.

Yield: 3-4 servings

Dijonnaise Poached Salmon

1/4 cup lemon juice
2 bay leaves
4 wild salmon filets (about 6 ounces each)
1 teaspoon Spike or 1/4 teaspoon salt
1/3 cup Omega 3 Mayonnaise*
2 tablespoons Dijon mustard

Pour about 2 inches of water into a covered skillet. Add lemon juice and bay leaves and bring to a boil. Reduce heat to a simmer. Rinse fish in fresh water, sprinkle with Spike and/or salt, and gently slip fish into water. Cover and poach for about 8 minutes.

While fish is poaching, mix Omega 3 Mayonnaise with the Dijon mustard. When fish is done (it should be opaque but still firm), remove from pan with slotted spoon or spatula. Place on serving plate and spoon sauce over each filet.

Yield: 4 servings

Fish Filets in Red Sauce

2 tablespoons extra virgin olive oil
2 medium onions, chopped
2 cloves garlic, minced
2 cups fresh or canned tomatoes
1/2 cup dry white wine or water
1 cup black pitted olives
1/2 cup basil, chopped
1 sprig fresh rosemary (or 1/2 tablespoon dried)
1 sprig fresh thyme (or 1/2 tablespoon dried)
Morton Salt Substitute or regular salt to taste (optional)
Black pepper to taste (optional)
1 1/2 pounds red snapper or other thick white fish, skinless

Add 2 tablespoons water then olive oil to deep skillet. Add onion and cook until soft. Add garlic and tomatoes. Raise heat and let some of the tomato juice evaporate as you stir occasionally. Add wine or water, cook another 5 minutes.

Add olives, part of the basil, rosemary, thyme, salt and pepper. Cook for several minutes to combine flavors. Submerge fish in sauce and cook over medium heat until fish is tender and white, about 8 minutes. Garnish with remaining basil.

Yield: 4 servings

Herbed Salmon

4 wild salmon filets (about 6 ounces each)
1 tablespoon extra virgin olive oil
2 cloves garlic
1 teaspoon ground cumin
1/4 teaspoon black pepper
1 tablespoon capers
1 cup parsley, chopped
1 cup cilantro, chopped
3 teaspoons grated lemon rind
1/3 cup fresh lemon juice
1/2 teaspoon Spike or Mrs. Dash seasoning

Preheat oven to 350° F. Rinse fish and pat dry. Place on lightly oiled cookie sheet.
In blender or food processor, combine olive oil, garlic, spices, capers, parsley, cilantro,
lemon rind and juice and seasonings. Spread over fish. Bake uncovered for 15 minutes or
until fish flakes easily with fork.

Yield: 4 servings

Lemon Parslied Fish

1 pound whitefish or sole filets
1/4 cup lemon juice
2 teaspoons extra virgin olive oil
1/4 teaspoon white pepper
1 small onion, thinly sliced
1 small lemon, washed well and thinly sliced
1/2 bunch fresh parsley (leaves only), washed and minced

Cut fish into serving-size pieces. Place fish in an ungreased 11"x 7"x 2" baking dish.
Drizzle with lemon juice and oil; sprinkle with pepper. Arrange lemon and onion slices
over fish; sprinkle with parsley. Cover and let stand for 5 minutes. Bake at 350° F for 15-20
minutes or until fish flakes easily with a fork.

Yield: 2 - 3 servings

Pecan Catfish

1/4 cup extra virgin olive oil
1/4 cup pecans, chopped fine
1 tablespoon lemon juice
1/4 teaspoon ground savory
1 teaspoon tamari
1/4 teaspoon red pepper flakes
1 teaspoon lemon rind, grated
2 pounds catfish filets

Make pecan sauce by combining 1/4 cup, less 1 tablespoon olive oil, chopped pecans, lemon juice and savory. Blend well.

Preheat oven to 350° F.

Combine tamari, pepper flakes and lemon rind. Spread evenly on fish. Heat nonstick skillet over medium heat. Add 1 teaspoon water and 1 tablespoon olive oil. Brown fillets over medium heat until light brown, turning once. Place filets in well-greased 12 x 8 x 2 baking dish. Drizzle pecan lemon sauce over fillets. Bake uncovered for 12 minutes or until fish flakes easily when tested with a fork.

Yield: 4 servings

Sardine Sushi

Several sheets of Nori (dried seaweed)
1/4 roasted red bell pepper cut into thin strips
1/2 avocado cut into thin strips
1/2 cucumber cut into thin strips
A few sprigs cilantro
1 can sardines, water-packed
A bit of ginger cut into small strips
2 tablespoons tamari
Rice vinegar (optional)

Work with one sheet of Nori seaweed at a time. Place sheet of Nori on a piece of parchment or plastic wrap. Starting about 1-1/2 inches from edge of seaweed sheet, place ingredients (bell pepper, avocado, cucumber, cilantro, sardines and ginger), forming a row running parallel to the edge of the sheet. Sprinkle lightly with tamari and rice vinegar.
Begin rolling from the edge nearest the ingredients, tucking as you go so that it forms a neat, tight roll. Using the plastic wrap or parchment, wrap the Sushi, burrito style, and refrigerate for later use. Can be eaten as a roll, or sliced into thick disks and served as a snack or hors d'oeuvres.

Suggested Serving: 2 rolls

Note:
If water-packed sardines are not available, use sardines packed in oil. In this case, pat the sardines dry with a paper towel before using.

13.2.4 Poultry

Recipes in This Section

Apricot Chicken
Baked Ginger Chicken
Chicken Cucumber Delights
Crockpot Chicken
Grilled Turkey with Lemon Mustard
Ostrich Burgers
Poached Chicken
Poultry Cutlets
Shitake Ostrich Steaks
Tarragon Turkey Patty
Turkey and Mushrooms
Turkey Breast Crockpot
Turkey Burger
Turkey Meat Loaf
Turkey Stew ala Crockpot

~

Apricot Chicken

3 free range chicken breasts
1/2 pound mushrooms, cleaned and quartered
1 cup carrots, sliced
1 medium onion, chunked
1 cup celery, sliced
6 medium apricots, fresh (dried OK if soaked for 3 hours first)
Chicken broth to cover chicken pieces

Place chicken pieces on bottom of crockpot. Cover with broth. Place mushrooms, carrots, onion, celery and apricots on top (do not cover these with broth as there will be too much liquid). Cook for 6 - 7 hours on low.

Yield: 3 servings

Baked Ginger Chicken

2-3 pounds free range chicken or chicken pieces
2 tablespoons extra virgin olive oil
2 tablespoons tamari
3 tablespoons grated fresh ginger or 1 tablespoon ground ginger powder
2 tablespoons grated fresh garlic or 1 teaspoon ground garlic powder

Preheat oven to 350° F.

Wash and dry chicken. Oil roasting pan with 1 tablespoon olive oil and place chicken in oiled pan. Mix the second tablespoon of oil with the tamari; add ginger and garlic. Stir well and pour over or rub onto the chicken. Bake uncovered for 40-60 minutes (20 minutes per pound of bird).

Yield: 4 - 6 servings

Chicken Cucumber Delights

1 cup cooked chicken breast, finely chopped
3 teaspoon Omega 3 Mayonnaise*
1/4 cup onion, finely chopped
2 tablespoons pecans, finely chopped
Salt-Free All-Purpose Seasoning* to taste
White pepper to taste
1-2 cucumbers, washed and peeled

Combine all ingredients except cucumber. Cover and refrigerate at least 2 hours. When ready to serve, slice cucumbers into 1/4 inch thick slices. Spread 1-2 teaspoons chicken mixture on each cucumber slice.

Yield: About 30 Delights

Crockpot Chicken

2 carrots, sliced
2 onions, sliced
2 celery stalks with leaves, cut in 1 inch pieces
3 pound whole free range chicken, skin and visible fat removed
2 teaspoons tamari
1/4 teaspoon black pepper
1/2 cup chicken broth
1 teaspoon fresh or dried basil
1 teaspoon Mrs. Dash

Put carrots, onions, and celery in bottom of crockpot. Add chicken. Top with tamari, pepper and broth. Sprinkle basil and Mrs. Dash over top. Cover and cook on low until done (8 to 10 hours). Remove chicken and vegetables with spatula.

Yield: 6 servings.

Note:
You can also use a high setting on your crockpot (chicken will be done in 3 to 4 hours) but you will need to increase the water to 1 cup.

Grilled Turkey with Lemon Mustard

1 pound turkey breast cutlets (about 1/4" thick)
2 tablespoons Dijon-style mustard
1 tablespoon Omega 3 Mayonnaise*
Spike, black pepper and paprika to taste
1 teaspoon fresh lemon juice
2 tablespoon fresh parsley, chopped

Preheat broiler. Coat broiler pan with non-stick cooking spray. If you don't have non-stick spray, rub some olive oil into bottom of pan. Rinse turkey and pat dry. Mix together mustard, mayonnaise, Spike and lemon juice in a small bowl. Coat one side of turkey with half of mustard mixture. Broil about 4 inches from heat source for 5 minutes. Turn and coat other side of turkey with mustard mixture and sprinkle with pepper and paprika. Broil 1 minute or until top is browned. Garnish with chopped parsley.

Yield: 2 servings

Ostrich Burgers

2 tablespoons onion, finely chopped
1 clove garlic, finely minced
1 teaspoon extra virgin olive oil
1 pound ground ostrich meat (use turkey if ostrich not available)
1 teaspoon tamari
1/4 teaspoon freshly ground black pepper

Sauté onion and garlic in olive oil. Gently mix onion and garlic mixture with meat, tamari and pepper.

To cook in a skillet: Heat a skillet over medium heat. Form three patties 1/2" thick and 3-1/2' in diameter, and sauté about two minutes on each side.

To cook on the grill: Preheat grill, brush meat with oil and grill about four minutes on each side. If you wish, serve with grilled onions, and/or sautéed mushrooms, guacamole, sliced tomatoes and lettuce.

Yield: 3 servings

Poached Chicken

Pure water
1/2 onion, chunked
2 cloves garlic, whole, peeled
1 tablespoon tamari
4-5 whole peppercorns
2 bay leaves
Sprig of fresh sage or 1 teaspoon dried sage
1 teaspoon dried rosemary
1 teaspoon dried thyme
2 free range chicken breasts, skinless (about 4 ounces each)

In bottom of covered frying pan, put about 1 inch of water. Add all vegetables, herbs and seasonings and bring to low simmer. Add chicken breasts, cover tightly and simmer on medium low heat for 15-20 minutes, or until chicken is done. Remove with slotted spoon. Serve hot or slice and serve cold.

Variation:
This recipe can be modified for poaching fish by eliminating the rosemary, sage and thyme and adding fresh dill or cilantro and summer savory.

Poultry Cutlets

1 1/2 pounds turkey or free-range chicken thighs
1 1/4 teaspoons Spike
Black pepper to taste
1 teaspoon poultry seasoning
1 tablespoon butter
1/8 cup lemon juice
1/8 cup free-range chicken or turkey stock

With a meat mallet, pound thigh pieces to about 1/8 inch thick. Sprinkle with Spike, black pepper and poultry seasoning. Heat skillet or sauté pan over medium heat. Melt butter in pan and sear the cutlets quickly on both sides until browned (about 1 minute per side). Add lemon juice and continue cooking for another 2 or 3 minutes. Remove from pan and return pan to heat. Add stock and deglaze (stirring and loosening pan residue). Turn heat up and reduce liquid to half. Pour over poultry and serve immediately.

Yield: 3 - 4 servings

Shitake Ostrich Steaks

2 pounds ostrich steaks, cut about 1/2 inch thick
1/2 pound fresh shitake mushrooms, sliced thin
1 teaspoon Spike seasoning
1 teaspoon freshly ground black pepper
4 tablespoons extra virgin olive oil
3 tablespoons onion, finely chopped
1 cup beef stock
1 tablespoon fresh thyme, chopped
1/2 teaspoon tamari

Slice mushrooms thinly. Heat non-stick skillet over medium heat. Add 1 tablespoon water and 2 tablespoons olive oil. Add mushrooms and 1/2 teaspoon tamari. Toss and cook until mushrooms are lightly browned and tender (about 2 to 3 minutes). Set aside.

Rinse and pat ostrich dry. Sprinkle both sides lightly with Spike seasoning and pepper. Heat a skillet over medium high heat and add 2 tablespoons water and 2 tablespoons olive oil. Steam-sauté ostrich steaks for 1 minute on each side. Set ostrich aside, cover loosely and keep warm while you make the sauce.

Pour off any fat remaining in skillet. Add chopped onion. Return skillet to medium-high heat and add beef stock. Cook briskly to reduce sauce by about 1/4. Reduce heat to medium and add mushrooms. Add ostrich to pan to reheat, basting it with the sauce. Sprinkle chopped thyme over ostrich and serve.

Yield: 6 servings

Tarragon Turkey Patty

1/4 pound ground turkey
2 tablespoons chopped onion
1 teaspoon fresh parsley, chopped
1/4 teaspoon dried thyme, or 1/2 teaspoon fresh thyme, chopped fine
1/4 teaspoon dried tarragon, or 1/2 teaspoon fresh tarragon, chopped fine
1 egg white
1 teaspoon extra virgin olive oil
2 tablespoons macadamia nuts, ground to fine meal

Mix all ingredients except oil and nut meal in a small bowl. Form the turkey mixture into a 3/4-inch thick patty. Heat skillet with medium heat; add 1 teaspoon water and then oil. Dredge the turkey patty in the nut meal and place into skillet. Cook for about 5 minutes on each side, or until the juices run clear when pricked with a fork. Do not overcook.

Yield: 1 serving

Turkey and Mushrooms

2 tablespoons extra virgin olive oil
3/4 pound ground turkey
10-12 button mushrooms, coarsely chopped
2 stalks celery, coarsely chopped
1-2 cloves of garlic, chopped fine
1 onion, coarsely chopped
1 tablespoon Fines Herbs*
Tamari to taste

Heat pan and add a little water. Then add oil, followed by ground turkey, mushrooms, celery, garlic, onion and Fines Herbs. Steam-fry until turkey is cooked through. Add tamari to taste. Adjust the seasonings if necessary.

Yield: 2-3 servings

Variation:
You can substitute or add any leftover vegetables in this recipe.

Turkey Breast Crockpot

4 pound turkey breast
2 carrots, cut into 1" lengths
3 celery stalks, sliced
2 onions, cut into chunks
3 cloves garlic, minced
1 cup chicken broth
1 bay leaf
A few whole peppercorns
1 teaspoon poultry seasoning
 2 teaspoons tamari

Combine ingredients in crockpot, cover and cook on low for 5 to 8 hours.

Yield: 4 - 6 servings

Turkey Burger

1/4 pound ground turkey
1 clove garlic, finely chopped
1 egg
1 teaspoon tamari
1 teaspoon onion powder
2 teaspoon extra virgin olive oil

Mix all ingredients except olive oil together and form into patty. Heat frying pan with medium heat; add 2 teaspoons water, then oil. Add patty and steam-sauté for 8-10 minutes or until turkey is cooked.

Yield: 1 serving

Turkey Meat Loaf

1/4 cup walnuts, ground fine
2 pounds ground turkey
1/2 onion, diced
1 zucchini, diced
8 mushrooms, chopped
1 medium carrot, grated
Handful of spinach, chopped fine
1 egg, well beaten
2 teaspoons Spike

Preheat oven to 350° F. Grind walnuts in blender but do not overgrind or they will get oily. Mix all ingredients together. Pat into a long loaf in a 9 x13 pan. Bake for 90 minutes.

Yield: 4 - 6 servings

Turkey Stew ala Crockpot

2 pounds turkey parts, skinless
1 medium onion, sliced
2 stalks celery, chunked
1 medium tomato, chopped
1 medium carrot, chopped
1/2 green bell pepper, chopped (optional)
2 cloves garlic, chopped fine
1 teaspoon Spike or Mrs. Dash seasoning
1 teaspoon thyme
1 teaspoon marjoram
2 cups chicken stock

Place all ingredients in crockpot and cook on low for 6 - 8 hours.

Yield: 4 servings

13.2.5 Eggs

Recipes in This Section

Deviled Eggs
Frittata
Huevos Rancheros
Spinach and Eggs

~

Deviled Eggs

6 large organic eggs
1/3 cup Omega 3 Mayonnaise*
2 teaspoons Dijon mustard
1/2 teaspoon Spike
Black pepper to taste
1/4 teaspoon dill (optional)
Paprika (optional)

Bring water to a boil over high heat. Slip eggs into water slowly with a spoon and reduce heat to simmer. Cook for 5 or 6 minutes. Pour off hot water and fill pan with cold water to immediately cool eggs.

When eggs are cool, peel them and cut them in half lengthwise. Scoop out yolks into small bowl and place whites on a serving platter. To the yolks add mayonnaise, mustard and seasonings. Mash together and mix well until fluffy. Fill cavity of each egg white half with yolk mixture and sprinkle top with dill or paprika.

Yield: 6 servings

Frittata

1 tablespoons olive oil
1/2 pound mushrooms, sliced
1 clove garlic, minced (optional)
1/2 cup onion, chopped
1/2 red bell pepper, chopped fine
2 cups vegetables, chopped (can use asparagus, broccoli, zucchini, spinach or greens)
1/2 tablespoon marjoram
1/2 teaspoon oregano
1 1/2 teaspoons Spike
1/4 teaspoon black pepper
4 eggs
1/2 teaspoon Dijon mustard
1/8 cup parsley, chopped

Add olive oil to large skillet, turn heat to medium-low. Add mushrooms, garlic and onions. Sauté until onions are soft and transparent. Add pepper, vegetables and seasonings. Stir well and continue cooking until vegetables turn bright green.

Break eggs into bowl and add mustard. Mix together well and pour over vegetable mixture in skillet. Cook until eggs are set, about 4 minutes. Serve with chopped parsley.

Yield: 4 servings

Huevos Rancheros

1 tablespoon extra virgin olive oil
4-5 tomatoes, chopped
1/4 onion, chopped
3 cloves garlic, pressed through garlic press or finely chopped
Serrano or other chili peppers to taste, chopped (optional)
Pinch of chili powder (optional)
4 eggs
6 large lettuce leaves

Set small frying pan to medium heat. Add 2 teaspoons of water and then 1 tablespoon of oil. Add tomatoes, onion, garlic, peppers, and chili powder. Bring sauce to a boil, reduce heat and simmer for about 10 minutes.

Brush bottom of larger frying pan with olive oil. Gently fry eggs "sunny side up." (Don't overcook or cook top side of eggs).

Lay out 3 lettuce leaves on each of two plates. Place 2 eggs on each bed of lettuce leaves. Cover eggs with the mixture from the other pan. The topping will partially cook the tops of the eggs.

Yield: 2 servings

Spinach and Eggs

1 hard cooked egg
2-3 cups fresh spinach or mixed greens
1 small onion, chopped fine
Salt-Free All-Purpose Seasoning* or Spike to taste

Slice egg and place over greens. Season to taste.

Yield: 1 serving

13.2.6 Salads

Recipes in This Section

Apple Turkey Salad
Asian Salad
Avocado Citrus Salad
Bean Sprout Salad
Cabbage and Cherry Salad
Chicken and Grape Salad
Chicken Salad
Chopped Salad
Confetti Salad
Egg-Shrimp Salad
Fennel, Orange and Arugula Salad
Hawaiian Chicken Salad
Leftover Fish Salad
Mediterranean Salad
Raw Veggie Delight
Salade Niçoise
Salmon Salad
Shoestring Carrot Salad
Spinach and Pink Grapefruit Salad
Spinach Salad
Turkey and Broiled Eggplant Salad
Turkey Citrus Salad
Warm Beef and Walnut Salad
Warm Nut and Cress Salad
Wild Greens Salad

Apple Turkey Salad

2 cups unpeeled apples, diced
1 1/2 teaspoons lemon juice
2 1/2 cups cooked organic turkey, diced
1 cup celery, diced
3/4 teaspoon Spike, Mrs. Dash or Salt-Free All-Purpose Seasoning*
1/4 teaspoon pepper (optional)
3 tablespoons Omega 3 Mayonnaise*

Mix apples and lemon juice lightly. Add remaining ingredients and toss lightly.
Serve on a bed of lettuce or other greens.

Yield: 2 - 4 servings

Asian Salad

1 large head Bibb lettuce
1 large head Boston lettuce
2 stalks Chinese cabbage
1 cup bean sprouts
3/4 cup jicama, thin 1" strips
3 - 4 tablespoons Asian Dressing*

Pat lettuce and cabbage dry, tear into bite-size pieces and put into wooden salad bowl.
Rinse bean sprouts and pat dry. Add sprouts and jicama. Dress with Asian Dressing.
Toss lightly until all ingredients are coated.

Avocado Citrus Salad

1 orange, cut into chunks
1/2 pink grapefruit, cut into chunks
1/2 avocado, sliced thin
Pine nuts (optional)

Combine. Sprinkle lightly with pine nuts, if desired. Add rice vinegar to taste.

Yield: 1-2 servings

Bean Sprout Salad

4 ounces fresh bean sprouts
1 fresh green chili, seeded and sliced
1 small onion, finely sliced
1 teaspoon tamari
1 tablespoon lemon juice

Wash bean sprouts thoroughly and drain well. Mix all ingredients together.
Refrigerate for several hours before serving.

Yield: 1 serving

Cabbage and Cherry Salad

2 cups cabbage, shredded
1 orange, peeled and chopped
1/2 cup jicama, peeled and chopped
1 cup pitted fresh or frozen sweet cherries
1/2 cup butter lettuce, washed, dried and torn into bite-size pieces
1/2 cup walnuts

Combine ingredients in salad bowl and top with Ginger Dressing*. Serve cold.

Yield: 2 servings

Chicken and Grape Salad

Romaine lettuce leaves, torn into bite-size pieces
1 head Belgian endive
1- 1/2 cup cooked, chilled julienne slices of chicken breast
2/3 cup green or red seedless grapes
3 tablespoons chopped walnuts
Alfalfa sprouts as garnish
Dressing of your choice from our list

To assemble salad, line a large serving platter or individual plates with romaine leaves. Quarter the Belgium endive and arrange Belgian endive, chicken pieces, grapes, and nuts on leaves. Garnish with alfalfa sprouts if desired. Drizzle with 1-2 tablespoons of dressing per serving.

Yield: 2 servings

Chicken Salad

1/4 - 1/2 cooked chicken breast, sliced or diced
1-2 cups premixed salad greens
1 stalk celery, chopped
1 green onion, chopped
Olive-Lemon Dressing*
2-3 tablespoons raw sunflower seeds or raw cashews

Mix all ingredients into bowl, except seeds/nuts. Add small-moderate amount of dressing and toss. Garnish with seeds/nuts.

Yield: 1 serving

Chopped Salad

Coarsely chop the following vegetables in any combination:

Carrots
Cauliflower
Broccoflower
Celery
Cucumber
Jicama
Scallions
Cabbage

Store in covered container. Serve with Vinaigrette dressing* or lemon juice.

Confetti Salad

8 cups of any kind of mixed greens (such as baby spinach, red lettuce, green lettuce, romaine, wild greens, cabbage (red and green), arugula, radicchio, kale, or chard). Wash, dry and chop coarsely.

Chop and add any and all of the following:
Alfalfa sprouts
Asparagus (raw)
Bean sprouts
Bell peppers (green, red, yellow)
Carrots (no more than one carrot)
Cucumber
Fennel bulbs
Herbs (dill, parsley, thyme, cilantro)
Kohlrabi
Onions (red, white, yellow or green)
Pea pods (edible)
Radishes
Tomatoes
Zucchini or other summer squash (patty pan, yellow, crookneck)

Toss together and serve with your favorite dressing.

Yield: 6-12 servings

Egg-Shrimp Salad

2 cups pre-washed spinach
2-3 teaspoons flax seed, freshly ground (use another seed or nut if you wish)
1-2 hard boiled eggs, sliced
3 precooked shrimp, tails removed
1 tablespoon Mexican Guacamole*
2 tablespoons of your favorite salsa from this book

Spread spinach on plate, sprinkle ground flax seed and arrange hard boiled egg slices on top. Add shrimp and top with Mexican Guacamole* and your choice of salsa.

Yield: 1 serving

Fennel, Orange and Arugula Salad

1/2 cup shallots, minced
3 tablespoons extra virgin olive oil
1 1/2 tablespoons fresh lemon juice
Spike seasoning to taste
Tamari to taste
Black pepper to taste
2 large oranges, peeled and sliced
7 cups arugula (about 10 bunches), trimmed
1 large fennel bulb, cored, quartered and thinly sliced
1 small red onion, thinly sliced

Whisk minced shallots, olive oil and lemon juice in medium bowl to blend. Season to taste with Spike or tamari and pepper. Combine arugula, fennel and onion in large bowl. Toss with enough dressing to coat. Add orange slices; toss to combine.

Yield: 6 servings

Hawaiian Chicken Salad

1 pound mesclun lettuce mix or other chopped salad greens
1 pound grilled chicken breasts, sliced into thin strips
8 ounces red bell peppers, sliced into thin strips
8 ounces yellow bell peppers, sliced into thin strips
8 ounces fresh green beans, blanched, cut into 3" pieces
8 ounces cucumber slices
4 ounces red onion, cut into small pieces
8 ounces fresh papaya, cut into small pieces
1 teaspoon tamari
1/4 teaspoon ground black pepper (optional)
3/4 cup vinaigrette salad dressing
1/2 cup raw macadamia nuts, chopped
1/2 cup carrots, peeled, sliced into 1" thin strips
2-3 green onions, sliced into 1" thin strips

Place lettuce/salad mix, chicken, bell peppers, green beans, cucumber, red onion and papaya into a large mixing bowl. Season the ingredients with tamari and pepper. Drizzle the vinaigrette dressing over the salad ingredients and gently toss together.

Sprinkle the macadamia nuts over each salad serving. Garnish with sliced carrots and green onions.

Yield: 4 servings

Leftover Fish Salad

1 pound leftover fish and/or other seafood, already cooked
2 medium tomatoes, coarsely chopped
1 cup celery, sliced into 1/2 inch slices
1/2 cup red onions, thinly sliced
1/4 cup fresh cilantro, chopped
1/2 cup fresh parsley, chopped
1/4 teaspoons Spike or Mrs. Dash seasoning
1/4 teaspoons black pepper

Break fish/seafood into small chunks. In a large serving bowl add all vegetable ingredients. Toss with Lemon Mint Dressing.* Add fish/seafood and toss in the salad.

Yield: 4 servings

Mediterranean Salad

2 medium cucumbers, peeled and diced
3/4 cup tomatoes, chopped fine
3/4 cup celery, diced
1 cup Jerusalem artichokes (sun chokes), chopped fine
2 cups curly parsley, chopped
2 cups flat leaf Italian parsley, chopped
1 cup fresh mint leaves, chopped
1 tablespoon pine nuts
3 tablespoons fresh lemon juice
3 tablespoons extra virgin olive oil
1 teaspoon Morton Salt Substitute or 1/2 teaspoon regular salt
1/4 teaspoon freshly ground black pepper (optional)

Combine all chopped vegetables in large bowl. Mix lemon juice, olive oil, salt and pepper together. Pour over vegetables and toss thoroughly.

Yield: 4 servings

Raw Veggie Delight

1 zucchini, shredded
1 carrot, shredded
3-4 lettuce leaves, shredded
Handful of alfalfa sprouts or bean sprouts
Handful of cauliflower, chopped into small bite-sized pieces
1/2 red bell pepper, diced
Handful of red cabbage, chopped

Shred zucchini and carrots in food processor. Put all of above ingredients in a large salad bowl and mix together. Top with Veggie Topping (below) or choose one of our Sauces and Dressings recipes.

Veggie Topping
2 tomatoes
1 stalk celery
2 small-medium carrots
Juice of one lemon
1/2 cup soaked seeds, nuts or avocado, depending on desired thickness and consistency

Blend the above 5 ingredients in a blender. Pour mixture over salad and mix thoroughly.

Yield: 1 serving

Salade Niçoise

1/2 pound green beans
2 eggs, hard boiled
6 cups assorted lettuces or other greens
2 cans tuna (substitute fresh grilled if you have it)
3 tomatoes, cut into wedges
6 anchovies (optional)
1 teaspoon capers (optional)
3/4 cup olives, pitted
2 tablespoons red wine vinegar
1/2 cup extra virgin olive oil
Morton Salt Substitute or regular salt (optional)
Black pepper (optional)
1 shallot, minced
1 teaspoon Dijon mustard

Steam green beans for 4 minutes. Drain, dump into ice water to set color.
Refrigerate until time to use. Boil eggs, cool and refrigerate until ready to use.

Arrange greens on a platter. Top with tuna, green beans, eggs, tomatoes, anchovies, capers and olives. Mix in small bowl or blender the red wine vinegar, olive oil, shallot, Dijon mustard, and salt and pepper to taste. Drizzle over salad.

Note:
A number of these ingredients can be prepared in advance and stored in the refrigerator until you are ready to assemble the salad. Improvise with the ingredients if you don't have certain things on hand.

Yield: 4 - 5 servings

Salmon Salad

4 cups romaine lettuce leaves, torn into bite-size pieces
1 cup Jerusalem artichokes, peeled and cut into matchsticks
3/4 cup jicama, peeled and cut into matchsticks
8 ounces sunflower sprouts (or any other sprouts you have)
1/2 avocado, cubed
2 teaspoons capers (optional)
4-6 ounces leftover baked or poached wild salmon, chunked
8-10 black or green olives, pitted
Lemon wedges
3 tablespoons Omega 3 Mayonnaise*
1 green onion, minced fine
1 teaspoon fresh parsley, chopped
1 teaspoon Dijon mustard
1 teaspoon fresh lemon juice

Arrange Romaine lettuce on serving platter. Arrange vegetables on top of lettuce.
Top with salmon chunks and garnish with olives and lemon wedges.

Mix mayonnaise, green onion, parsley, mustard and lemon juice together.
Serve as topping on salad.

Yield: 1-2 servings

Shoestring Carrot Salad

3 - 4 large carrots, cut into shoestrings
1/2 medium onion, chopped fine
1/2 green bell pepper, chopped fine
1/2 teaspoon celery seed or 1-2 tablespoons chopped fresh celery
1/2 teaspoon dried parsley flakes or 1/2 tablespoon fresh parsley
1/2 teaspoon Salt-Free All-Purpose Seasoning*
Black pepper to taste
2 tablespoons extra virgin olive oil
1/4 cup lemon juice

Place carrots, onion, and green pepper in steamer for 3-4 minutes only. Remove and place in bowl. Add celery seed and parsley. Combine the seasoning, pepper, olive oil and lemon juice. Pour over vegetables and blend entire mixture well.

Yield: 4 servings.

Spinach and Pink Grapefruit Salad

8 cups spinach (about 1/2 pound), washed, stemmed, chopped or torn into bite-size pieces
2 pink grapefruit, sectioned
Grapefruit Vinaigrette*

Place spinach in salad bowl with grapefruit sections and dressing. Toss well.

Yield: 4 servings

Spinach Salad

2 bunches fresh spinach, washed and stemmed
1 bunch scallions, chopped
2 tablespoons lemon juice
2 teaspoons tamari
1 tablespoon extra virgin olive oil
Black pepper to taste (optional)

Drain spinach, pat dry and chop. Add scallions, lemon juice, tamari, olive oil and pepper.

Yield: 2 servings

Variation:
For some added heartiness, add either 1/4 cup chopped walnuts or 1 sliced hard boiled egg

Turkey and Broiled Eggplant Salad

1 pound eggplant
1-2 teaspoons tamari
1-2 teaspoons Salt-Free All-Purpose Seasoning*
2 large heads of lettuce (leafy)
2 cucumbers, shredded
1 cup cooked turkey, chunked
1 tablespoon capers (optional)
1/2 cup Olive Lemon Dressing*

Preheat broiler. Slice eggplant into slices about 1/4 inch thick and sprinkle with tamari and Salt-Free All-Purpose Seasoning.* Broil eggplant until brown (about 3 - 4 minutes on each side). While eggplant is broiling, tear washed lettuce into bite-size pieces and shred cucumbers. Plate the salads. Remove eggplant from broiler.

Cut turkey into chunks and divide over salads. Slice cooled eggplant and arrange over salads. Garnish with capers and drizzle with Olive Lemon Dressing.*

Yield: 4 servings

Turkey Citrus Salad

2 cups turkey, cooked and chopped
1/2 cups celery, chopped fine
1/4 teaspoon Salt-Free All-Purpose Seasoning*
1/4 teaspoon curry powder
1 orange
1/2 cup seedless grapes
2 tablespoons Omega mayonnaise*

Combine turkey, celery, and seasonings in a bowl. Peel and chop the orange.
Add orange, grapes and mayonnaise. Toss gently to mix.

Yield: 4 servings

Warm Beef and Walnut Salad

Assorted lettuce leaves, torn into pieces
8 ounces lean beef strips (or buy a thick piece of fillet or rib eye steak and slice thinly)
1/4 cup red pepper (any kind), cut into thin strips
1 small onion, cut into wedges
2 teaspoons extra virgin olive oil
1 tablespoon walnut pieces
Walnut dressing (see below)
1 tablespoon fresh chives, chopped

Walnut Dressing:
2-3 teaspoons walnut oil or extra virgin olive oil
2 teaspoons white wine vinegar
1 teaspoon Dijon mustard
Black pepper (optional)

Tear lettuce leaves into bite-size pieces. Arrange on two dinner plates.

Trim fat from meat. Slice finely into strips if necessary. Remove seeds and inner membranes from pepper and cut into thin strips. Peel and slice onion. Have ready near the stove.

Heat wok or deep 10 inch nonstick skillet. Moisten wok or bottom of pan with 2 teaspoons water and then add 2 teaspoons oil and stir-fry the pepper and onion for 1-2 minutes over high heat to soften. Push contents to the sides of the wok to clear a space in the middle and add sliced meat. Continue to stir-fry for another 1-2 minutes until meat just turns brown at the edges.

Add walnuts and 1 tablespoon of the dressing. Stir to combine and heat through. Serve on top of lettuce leaves. Pour remaining dressing on top. Sprinkle chives and serve.

Yield: 2 servings

Warm Nut and Cress Salad

1 tablespoon extra virgin olive oil
1 large garlic clove
2 tablespoons pine nuts
2 tablespoons hazelnuts, finely chopped
1/2 teaspoon tamari
1/4 teaspoon black pepper (optional)
1 pound watercress, washed and finely chopped

In a heavy 12" skillet, heat olive oil on low heat. Cut garlic clove in half lengthwise and add to oil. Cook for 2 minutes, stirring constantly. Remove garlic and discard.

Add all nuts and cook for 5 minutes or until they are slightly browned. Add tamari and pepper. Cook 2 to 3 more minutes.

Working fast, toss watercress into nut and seasoning mixture, making sure it is well coated and barely heated through. If left too long it loses some of its crispiness. Serve immediately.

Yield: 2 servings

Wild Greens Salad

6 cups mixed wild greens (whatever is available in your area)
4 teaspoons fresh lemon juice
4 teaspoons walnut oil
1 teaspoon tamari
1-2 teaspoons capers (optional)

Pour lemon juice into small bowl. Gradually whisk in oil. Season with tamari or any other flavors to your liking. Pour over greens and toss until evenly dressed. Garnish with capers. Serve at once.

Yield: 4 servings

Note:
Wild greens in your area might include: chickweed leaves, Miner's Lettuce, lamb's lettuce, dandelion greens, wild mustard, purslane, lamb's quarters or sorrel. If no wild greens are available to you, look for unusual greens that are locally available in some supermarkets, health food stores, ethnic markets or local farmer's markets.

13.2.7 Vegetables

Recipes in This Section

Apples 'n Onions
Baked Cabbage with Dill
Braised Onions, Shallots and Leeks
Broccoli with Garlic and Lemon
Cabbage Roll Ups
Cauliflower with Mushrooms
Celery Slaw
Cole Slaw
Cooked Cabbage
Leeky Carrots
Mashed Cauliflower
Mustard Greens with Vinaigrette
Ratatouille
Roasted Vegetables No. 1
Roasted Vegetables No. 2
Roasted Yellow Peppers
Sautéed Broccoli Italian Style
Spicy Wilted Greens
Steamed Asparagus
Stir-Fried Bok Choy
Stuffed Mushrooms
Tomato Cups
Tomatoes Dijon
Vegetables and Dip
Vegetables in Ginger Sauce
Walnut Watercress Stir Fry
Zucchini Sauté

Apples 'n Onions

2 tablespoons olive oil
4 large Spanish onions, sliced
3 large cooking apples, sliced
1/2 cup water or free-range chicken stock
2 teaspoons tamari
Dash of nutmeg

Preheat non-stick skillet. Moisten bottom of skillet with a little water, then add oil. Add onion slices and cook until nearly soft. Add sliced apples and 1/2 cup water or chicken stock. Cover and cook 15 minutes or until apples are tender but not mushy. Sprinkle with nutmeg and serve.

Yield: 4 servings

Baked Cabbage with Dill

1/4 cup water
6 cups finely sliced cabbage
1 tablespoon finely chopped dulse (seaweed)
2 teaspoons dried dill or 2 tablespoons fresh dill, chopped fine
3 tablespoons olive oil

Preheat oven to 350° F. Put water in bottom of baking dish. Add sliced cabbage. Sprinkle cabbage with chopped dulse and dill; drizzle with olive oil. Cover tightly with foil and bake for 35 minutes or until cabbage is tender.

Yield: 2 - 4 servings

Braised Onions, Shallots and Leeks

1 teaspoon extra virgin olive oil
3 red onions, cut into thick wedges
3 Vidalia (or yellow) onions, cut into thick wedges
4 or 5 shallots, halved
3 leeks, cut lengthwise, rinsed well and sliced into 2" lengths
Fresh basil, minced, or dried basil
Juice of 1 lime

Heat deep skillet over low heat. Moisten bottom of skillet with 1 teaspoon water and then add oil. Add onions and cook until they begin to soften (about 10 minutes), stirring occasionally. Add shallots, stir and cook, 4 - 5 minutes. Stir in leeks and continue cooking until they are bright green and tender (about 5 minutes). Add a little more water and a sprinkling of basil. Cover and simmer until any remaining liquid has been absorbed. Remove from heat and stir in lime juice.

Yield: 4 servings

Broccoli with Garlic and Lemon

1 bunch broccoli, about 1 pound
1/4 cup extra virgin olive oil
3 cloves garlic, cut into thin slivers
1/8 teaspoon pepper
3 tablespoons fresh lemon juice

Cook broccoli in a large saucepan of boiling water 5-6 minutes, or until tender-crisp. Drain in a colander. Arrange on a serving dish and cover to keep warm.

In a small frying pan, warm olive oil over low heat. Stir in garlic and cook slowly until golden brown, being careful not to burn the garlic (about 1-2 minutes). Add pepper and lemon juice. Pour sauce mixture over broccoli.

Yield: 2 servings

Cabbage Roll Ups

Have on hand any (or all) of these ingredients:
Chopped shrimp
Avocado, sliced into thin strips (small to moderate amount)
Cucumber, sliced into thin strips
Roasted red pepper, sliced into thin strips
Roasted zucchini, sliced into thin strips
Chopped cilantro or parsley
Sesame seeds (small amount)
Leftover vegetables
Steamed, cold green beans
Roasted or raw onion, chopped
Green onion sliced into thin strips
Minced garlic
Chopped fresh tomato

Use several leaves of green cabbage. Steam them for a couple of minutes just to soften. Remove from steamer and allow to cool. Fill with any combination of the above ingredients.

Suggested Serving: 2 - 4 rolls

Cauliflower with Mushrooms

1 large head of cauliflower
1 teaspoon extra virgin olive oil
1/4 pound fresh mushrooms, thinly sliced
1/3 cup green onions (with tops), thinly sliced
1 cup chicken broth

In a saucepan containing 1 inch of water, steam whole cauliflower until tender (about 20 minutes). Meanwhile, in a skillet, steam-sauté mushrooms and onions in oil on medium heat until mushrooms are tender. Add chicken broth. Bring to a boil over medium heat, stirring constantly. Cook and stir for 2 minutes. Place cauliflower in a large bowl; pour mushroom mixture over it and serve immediately.

Yield: 3-4 servings

Celery Slaw

1 large bunch of celery, chopped fine
2 red bell peppers, chopped fine
3 or 4 tomatoes
4 ounces fresh walnuts

Put chopped celery and peppers in a bowl and set aside. Put tomatoes and walnuts in a blender, cover and blend until smooth. Pour over celery and peppers.

Yield: 2 servings

Cole Slaw

1 head of cabbage, sliced very thin
1 small-medium carrot, shredded
1/2 yellow, white or red onion, thinly sliced
1 small, tart green apple, shredded (optional)
1 teaspoon Spike seasoning
1/2 teaspoon freshly ground black pepper
1/4 cup rice vinegar
1/4 cup cider vinegar
3 tablespoons extra virgin olive oil

Place cabbage, carrot, onion and apple in a bowl. Mix the seasonings, vinegars and oil together and pour over vegetables. Toss very well. Cover and refrigerate for at least 1 hour before serving.

Note:
You can use all green cabbage with this recipe, use half red cabbage, or use a mix of green, red, Napa, curly, or Chinese cabbages. The total quantity of cabbage should be the equivalent 1 full head of cabbage, or roughly 2 - 3 pounds.

Variations:
Eliminate rice vinegar and increase cider vinegar to 1/2 cup. Mix vinegar with 1/2 teaspoon Dijon mustard. Sprinkle 1 tablespoon whole caraway seed into slaw.

Eliminate apple and sprinkle slaw with 3 tablespoons chopped fresh dill or 2 tablespoons dried dill.

Replace carrot with jicama.

Eliminate rice vinegar in the dressing and replace with 2 tablespoons of Omega 3 Mayonnaise* and 1 clove of pressed garlic mixed well with the cider vinegar. Pour over salad and toss well.

Yield: 2 - 4 servings

Cooked Cabbage

1 small head of cabbage
1 tablespoon extra virgin olive oil
1/2 teaspoon fresh rosemary (or 1/4 teaspoon dried)
1/2 teaspoon fresh oregano (or 1/4 teaspoon dried)
1/2 teaspoon fresh thyme (or 1/4 teaspoon dried)

Wash and finely chop cabbage. Moisten bottom of frying pan or Dutch oven with 1 tablespoon water, then add 1 tablespoon olive oil and heat on medium low. Add cabbage and stir, adding fresh rosemary, oregano and thyme.

Turn heat to low, cover and stir every few minutes to prevent burning. Cook 7-10 minutes.

Variation:
Use ginger and garlic as flavoring rather than the spices listed above. Add about 5 minutes into the cooking if using fresh ginger and fresh garlic.

Yield: 2 servings

Leeky Carrots

1 tablespoon extra virgin olive oil
4 tablespoons free range chicken stock
3 medium leeks, white and palest green parts only, rinsed and chopped
4 large carrots, peeled and sliced
Pinch of nutmeg (optional)
Salt Free All Purpose Seasoning (to taste)

Heat the oil and chicken stock in a wide skillet. Add the leeks and carrots, cover, and cook over medium-low heat, for about 8 to 10 minutes, or until tender-crisp. Uncover and sauté, stirring frequently until the leeks and carrots begin to turn golden. Stir in the nutmeg, if desired. Add seasoning and serve.

Yield: 4 - 6 servings

Mashed Cauliflower

1 tablespoons butter
2 tablespoons olive oil
1/4 cup water
1 clove garlic (optional)
6 cups cauliflower, chopped fine
2 tablespoons tamari
Onion powder to taste

In a large pot, slow cooker, or electric skillet (on the lowest temperature) add butter, olive oil, water, garlic and cauliflower; stir and toss until coated. Cook over low heat until cauliflower is very soft. Season with tamari and onion powder.

With hand blender or beaters, whip mixture until cauliflower is creamy and fluffy.

Try with Mushroom Gravy.*

Yield: 3 - 4 servings

Mustard Greens with Vinaigrette

2 cups water
1/4 teaspoon tamari
1 pound mustard greens, washed, stemmed, cut into 1/4 inch strips
Balsamic Vinaigrette* dressing

Using a large skillet with a lid, add water and tamari and bring to a boil. Add prepared greens, cover, and cook over high heat, stirring occasionally until tender, about 5 minutes. Drain in a colander, using a cooking spoon to push greens against side to squeeze out excess moisture. Drizzle with dressing, stir quickly, and serve hot.

Yield: 2 - 3 servings

Ratatouille

2 large onions, thinly sliced
2 large eggplant, sliced 1/2" thick
4 ripe tomatoes, stemmed and sliced thickly
4 red or yellow bell peppers, stemmed, seeded and sliced into 3-4 pieces
10 cloves garlic, peeled
1 teaspoon fresh rosemary or thyme
1 tablespoon tamari
Black pepper to taste (optional)
1/2 cup extra-virgin olive oil
2 tablespoons fresh parsley or basil, minced

Preheat oven to 350° F.

In a covered casserole dish, make a layer of onion, then eggplant, tomatoes, peppers, garlic, herbs, tamari and pepper. Repeat layers as necessary. Drizzle with olive oil, cover and place in oven.

Bake about one hour. If mixture is too liquid, uncover and bake another 15 minutes. If too dry, add a little water or chicken stock and bake another 15 minutes. Garnish with parsley or basil and serve.

Yield: 8 servings

Roasted Vegetables No. 1

4 yellow summer squash
5 zucchini
2 red, yellow or orange peppers
15 - 20 small button mushrooms
1 red onion
3 tablespoons extra virgin olive oil
3 cloves garlic
2 teaspoons tamari
Dried cilantro or basil, chopped

Trim ends from summer squash. Cut into round about 1/4" thick. Trim ends of zucchini. Cut in half, then into 3 or 4 pieces. Cut peppers into strips. Cut onion in half, then into wedges, leaving root end in place so onion will stay together during roasting.

Preheat oven to 400° F.

Combine oil, garlic and tamari. Toss vegetables in that mixture. Spread out on large pan. Roast for about 15 minutes. Remove from oven and sprinkle with basil or cilantro.

Note:
Roasted vegetables are handy to make once a week and keep in the refrigerator for use as a snack or meal component.

Yield: 4 - 6 servings

Roasted Vegetables No. 2

4 medium carrots
1 eggplant, sliced about 1" thick
2-4 zucchini or summer squash, halved
2-3 small onions, cut in quarters
1/4 cup extra virgin olive oil
3 tablespoons fresh lemon juice

Preheat oven to 350° F.

Rub vegetables with olive oil and lemon juice. Bake carrots and onions for 35 minutes. Add eggplant and zucchini, and bake for an additional 20 minutes, turning if they become too brown.

Yield: 4 - 6 servings

Roasted Yellow Peppers

4 large yellow bell peppers, about 2 pounds
3 tablespoons extra virgin olive oil
2 tablespoons shredded fresh basil, or
1 1/2 tablespoons chopped fresh parsley combined with 1 teaspoon dried basil
Pepper to taste

Preheat oven to 475° F. Set peppers on a baking sheet. Brush with 1 tablespoon oil to lightly coat peppers. Bake for 20 minutes or until skins begin to blister (turn once or twice). Place peppers in a brown bag or plastic bag to steam for 10 minutes. Pull skins from peppers. Remove stems, seeds, and membranes. Tear peppers into 4 to 6 pieces each. Lay roasted peppers flat on a serving plate. Sprinkle with basil, parsley and fresh ground pepper.

Yield: 4 servings

Sautéed Broccoli Italian Style

1 head broccoli, cut into small flowerets, stems thinly sliced
1 teaspoon extra virgin olive oil
2 or 3 cloves garlic, minced
1 onion, diced
4 or 5 button mushrooms, brushed clean and thinly sliced
1 or 2 tomatoes, diced

Bring a large pot of water to boil over high heat. Add broccoli and cook until bright green but not completely tender, about 3 minutes. Plunge into cold water to stop the cooking process and to preserve the bright color.

Heat skillet over medium heat. Moisten bottom of skillet with 1 teaspoon water, then add oil. Add garlic, onion and mushrooms. Cook and stir for 2-3 minutes. Add tomatoes and stir well. Cover and simmer 10-15 minutes. Remove cover and stir in broccoli. Simmer, uncovered, 2-3 minutes. Serve hot.

Yield: 4 servings

Spicy Wilted Greens

4 teaspoons extra virgin olive oil
2 tablespoons shallots, minced
1 tablespoon ginger, grated
2 teaspoons ground cumin
2 teaspoons turmeric
1 teaspoon coriander
1 jalapeno pepper, cored, seeded, and finely minced
1/2 teaspoon tamari
1 1/4 - 1 1/2 pounds collards or Swiss chard (about 2 bunches), thinly sliced
1 bunch scallions, trimmed and chopped

In a large skillet, warm the oil over low heat. Add the shallots, ginger, and cumin and sauté for 3 minutes. Stir often; do not allow ingredients to burn.

Add turmeric, coriander, jalapeno, and tamari. Sauté for 3 minutes longer. Add greens and scallions and mix with oil and spice mixture. Cover and allow greens to wilt, stirring occasionally. Collards take about 10-12 minutes; chard takes about 8 minutes. If there is too much liquid, remove cover, turn heat to high, and cook off moisture while stirring greens. Serve immediately.

Note:
This recipe can be made fiery or simply highly flavored by varying the amount of jalapeno.

Yield: 2-4 servings

Steamed Asparagus

1 bunch fresh asparagus (green or white)
1 teaspoon lemon juice
1 teaspoon fresh parsley, minced

Bring 1 inch of water to a boil in covered stock pot with steamer inserted. Wash asparagus and snap off tough ends. Put into steamer; steam until crunchy-tender. Serve with lemon juice and minced parsley.

Yield: 2 servings

Stir-Fried Bok Choy

2 tablespoons extra virgin olive oil
1 large onion, quartered and thinly sliced
1 medium-large bok choy (10-12 ounces), chopped crosswise in medium-large chunks
1 teaspoon grated fresh ginger, more or less to taste
2 teaspoon tamari (optional)

Moisten bottom of stir-fry pan or wide skillet with a little water, then add oil and heat. Add onion and sauté over medium heat until golden. Add bok choy (both stalks and leaves) and ginger. Stir-fry briefly, just until leaves are wilted. Season with tamari.

Yield: 4 servings

Stuffed Mushrooms

1/3 cup pine nuts
3 cloves garlic, minced
1/3 cup fresh cilantro, packed leaves, chopped
1/3 cup fresh basil, packed leaves, chopped
1 tablespoon lemon juice
2 tablespoons tamari to taste
1 tablespoon extra virgin olive oil
1 cup tomato, chopped
8-10 large button mushrooms, stems gently removed

Put all ingredients except mushrooms and tomatoes into a food processor and pulse chop several times. Stop to scrape down the sides and repeat. Add tomatoes and continue to pulse chop until just blended. Keep mixture at a coarse texture, more like a pesto than a puree. Spoon into mushroom caps and drizzle with olive oil. Bake for 10-15 minutes at 350° F.

Yield: 2 servings.

Tomato Cups

6 medium tomatoes
1/2 small cucumber, chopped fine
2 sticks celery, minced
2 -3 green onions, chopped fine
1/2 cup fresh parsley, minced
1 tablespoon fresh mint, minced
1 clove garlic, minced
1/2 cup pine nuts
1 tablespoon lemon juice
1 tablespoon olive oil (optional)
Tamari to taste (optional)

With a very sharp knife, cut tomatoes in half and scoop out the center pulp. Add pulp to other ingredients (saving a little parsley for garnish) and mix well. Fill tomato halves.

Yield: 12 tomato cups

Tomatoes Dijon

4 cloves garlic, mashed
1 tablespoon Dijon mustard
1/2 teaspoon dry mustard
Salt-Free All-Purpose Seasoning*, Spike or Mrs. Dash (to taste)
2 tablespoons extra virgin olive oil
4 small tomatoes, cut in half

In bowl, combine garlic, Dijon mustard, dry mustard and seasonings to taste. Add oil, a little at a time, whisking until smooth. Place tomatoes in oiled baking dish and spread with mustard mixture. Broil tomatoes 3 inches from heat for 1 minute or till tops are bubbly and golden.

Yield: 2 servings

Vegetables and Dip

1 medium kohlrabi
1 small jicama
1 red pepper, seeded
2 small yellow squash
4 medium stalks of celery
2 cups broccoli flowerets
2 cups cauliflower flowerets
1 cup snow or sugar snap peas
1 cup Mock Sour Cream*

Wash all vegetables. Cut the kohlrabi, jicama, pepper, squash and celery into sticks. Break the broccoli and cauliflower into small flowerets. String the snow peas if necessary. Arrange on tray with a dish of Mock Sour Cream in the center for dipping.

Yield: 10-15 servings

Vegetables in Ginger Sauce

1 1/2 tablespoons olive oil
3 cups broccoli, chopped in quarter sized heads
1 head fennel, washed and sliced into small pieces
2 carrots, sliced
1 cups fresh spinach, chopped
3 cloves of garlic, minced
1 tablespoon ginger, minced
3 scallions
1/3 cup fresh basil, chopped
1 teaspoon tamari
1 teaspoon red pepper chili flakes (less if you want the dish less spicy)
1/2 cup free-range chicken stock

Chop all ingredients. Heat non stick skillet to medium high, and when hot, add 2 tablespoons water to moisten bottom of pan and add olive oil. Then add garlic, ginger, scallions, basil, tamari and chili flakes. Sauté for one minute, stirring well. Add carrots and fennel and stir for another minute. Add broccoli and chicken stock. Cover for 30 seconds. Remove from heat and garnish with scallions.

Yield: 2-4 servings

Walnut Watercress Stir Fry

2 teaspoons extra virgin olive oil
1 teaspoon fresh ginger, peeled and minced
Leaves from 2 bunches watercress, coarsely chopped
1/4 teaspoon red pepper flakes
1 tablespoon tamari
1/2 cup chopped walnuts
1 teaspoon walnut oil (optional)

Moisten bottom of large skillet or wok with small amount of water. Add olive oil. When oil is hot, add the ginger and cook until fragrant, about 30 seconds. Add watercress, red pepper flakes, tamari and walnuts. Stir-fry until wilted but not overcooked, about 3 minutes. Serve hot, drizzled with the walnut oil, if desired.

Yield: 2 servings

Zucchini Sauté

2 tablespoons water
1 large red onion, sliced thin
2 small zucchini, sliced into 1/4 inch rounds
2 small yellow summer squash, sliced into 1/4 inch rounds
1 large ripe tomato, chunked
1 handful of fresh basil, chopped

Heat pan on medium heat. Add 2 tablespoons water, followed by onion. Sauté for about 5 minutes. Add zucchini and summer squash. Stir occasionally only for about 5 minutes. Add tomato and basil. Cover and cook for another 5 minutes or until everything has blended together well.

Yield: 4 servings

13.2.8 Soups

Recipes in This Section

Chicken Vegetable Soup
Cilantro Chicken Broth
Curried Squash Soup
Gazpacho
Italian Beef Soup
Louisiana Gumbo
Minestrone
Scallion Soup
Steak and Vegetable Soup

Chicken Vegetable Soup

2 cloves garlic
1 medium onion
1 tablespoon extra virgin olive oil
2 quarts low-salt chicken broth
2 chicken breasts, bone and skin removed
6 tomatoes (or 24 ounces canned tomatoes if fresh not available)
2 zucchini, chopped
8 Brussels sprouts or other vegetables, chopped
1/2 cup fresh parsley
1/2 tablespoon turmeric
Pinch of pepper (optional)

Sauté garlic and onion in a little olive oil in a soup pot. Add broth and bring to a boil. Add chicken. Simmer 30 minutes. Remove chicken, cool and dice. Add vegetables and spices. Simmer another 15 - 20 minutes. Return chicken to pot and serve when chicken is reheated.

Variation:
Substitute a turkey breast for the chicken.

Note:
Use leftover soup for breakfast, lunch or dinner over the next few days.

Yield: 5 servings

Cilantro Chicken Broth

32 ounces free-range organic chicken broth
2 bunches of cilantro (leaves only), chopped fine
1 small minced onion (optional)
1/4 cup parsley, chopped
1 tablespoon tamari

Wash cilantro and parsley. Finely chop only the leaves of both. If using onion, chop it fine as well. Add all chopped ingredients and tamari to chicken broth. Heat slowly until broth is hot and onion is soft.

Yield: 4 servings

Curried Squash Soup

1/4 cup diced onion
1 tablespoon extra virgin olive oil
1 cup thinly sliced carrots
1 cup zucchini, thinly sliced
1 cup yellow summer or patty pan squash, thinly sliced
2 teaspoons chopped fresh parsley
1 teaspoons tamari
1/8 teaspoon pepper
1-2 teaspoons curry powder (to taste)
2 cups organic chicken broth

In a 1 1/2 quart saucepan, cook onion in oil until translucent. Add all other ingredients except broth. Cover and cook over low heat until vegetables are tender, stirring occasionally. Add broth and bring to a boil. (If you wish a thinner soup, add more broth or some water.) Reduce heat to medium and cook until vegetables are soft (about 20 minutes). Remove from heat and let cool slightly. Remove 2/3 of soup from pan and reserve; pour remaining soup into blender and process at low speed until smooth. Combine pureed and reserved mixtures in saucepan and reheat on low temperature, stirring constantly until hot.

Yield: 2 servings.

Gazpacho

1 cup fresh tomato juice (see below)
4 ripe tomatoes, quartered
1 small onion, coarsely chopped
1 clove garlic, peeled
2 tablespoons lemon juice
1 - 2 tablespoons Spike or Mrs. Dash No Salt Seasoning
pepper to taste
1/2 teaspoon cayenne pepper or hot chilies if you prefer
1 sprig fresh parsley
3 scallions, chopped fine
2 cucumbers, peeled and coarsely chopped

Make fresh tomato juice by adding several chunks of tomato to 1 cup water in blender and blend at high speed.

Blend all ingredients in blender or food processor, until vegetables are well chopped but NOT pureed. Serve cold.

Yield: 2 servings

Italian Beef Soup

1 pound organic lean ground beef
1 tablespoon olive oil
1 small onion, chopped
1 cup chopped celery
1 cup chopped carrot
1 clove garlic, minced
1/8 teaspoon freshly ground pepper
5 medium tomatoes, diced
2 medium tomatoes, pureed
28 ounces vegetable broth
1/2 cup fresh loosely chopped basil leaves
1 tablespoon chopped fresh thyme
1/2 (8-ounce) container sliced fresh mushrooms

Cook ground beef in a large Dutch oven about 5 minutes or until brown; drain and set aside. Heat same Dutch oven over medium heat. Add 2 tablespoons water and then the oil, onion, celery, carrot, and garlic. Sauté about 5 minutes or until vegetables are tender. Add pepper. Stir in tomatoes, broth, basil and thyme. Let simmer uncovered over medium-low heat for 20 minutes, stirring occasionally. Add mushrooms and beef and simmer 10 more minutes.

Yield: 6 - 8 servings.

Note:
This recipe is very adaptable. You can add the vegetables you like and take out the ones you don't!

Louisiana Gumbo

3 tablespoon extra virgin olive oil
2 cups onion, chopped
1 cup celery, chopped
2 large tomatoes, chopped
8 cups organic chicken stock
8 cups pure water
4 cloves garlic, minced
Tamari, black pepper and red pepper to taste
1/2 - 1 pound fish (any fish), in chunks
2 pounds shrimp, peeled and deveined
1 cup frozen clams
1 tablespoon parsley, finely chopped
1/2 teaspoon "gumbo file" (dried, ground sassafras leaves)

Moisten bottom of large soup kettle with 2 tablespoons of water, then add oil and heat with medium heat until hot. Add onions and celery. Cook until onions are wilted and then add tomatoes, chicken stock, water and garlic. Cook over medium heat for 1/2 hour and season to taste with tamari, black pepper and red pepper. Add fish, shrimp, clams and parsley. Cook another 10 minutes. Sprinkle a dash of gumbo file on each served dish of gumbo.

Yield: 6 servings

Minestrone

1 tablespoon extra virgin olive oil
4 cloves garlic, crushed
1 medium onion, chopped
3 stalks celery, sliced
1 medium carrot, chopped
1 zucchini, chunked
1 tablespoon Italian seasoning
1 teaspoon Spike
1/2 teaspoon ground black pepper
2 tomatoes, seeded and chopped
1 quart vegetable or free-range chicken stock
1 cup cabbage, shredded
1/2 cup Italian Basil Pesto*

Moisten bottom of soup pot or Dutch oven with a bit of water, then add olive oil and heat. Add garlic and onions and cook over medium heat until onion is soft. Add chopped celery, carrot and zucchini. Continue cooking for about 5 minutes, stirring frequently. Add seasonings, tomatoes and stock and bring to a boil. Reduce heat and simmer 10 minutes. Add cabbage; taste and adjust the seasonings.

Ladle into bowls and serve with 1 tablespoon of Italian Basil Pesto* on top of each serving.

Note:
The longer this soup simmers, the better it gets.

Yield: 4 servings

Scallion Soup

3 teaspoons extra virgin olive oil
1 cup zucchini, shredded
1/2 cup white onion, chopped
1 clove garlic, minced
1 cup scallions, chopped
1/2 cup chives, chopped
2 1/2 cups chicken broth
2 teaspoons tamari

In saucepan, cook zucchini, onion and garlic in oil over low heat. Cook about 5 minutes, stirring occasionally. Add scallions and all but 2 tablespoons chives. Cook and stir until scallions are soft (about 2 minutes). Stir in broth and tamari and simmer for another 2 minutes or so. Cool slightly.

Place mixture in blender and process on low speed until pureed. Reheat and adjust seasonings as needed. Serve topped with remaining chives.

Yield: 2 servings

Steak and Vegetable Soup

1 pound organic round steak
1 teaspoon dried basil or 2 teaspoons fresh basil, chopped
1/2 teaspoon Salt-Free All-Purpose Seasoning*
1/4 teaspoon pepper
2 cloves garlic, crushed
1 tablespoon extra virgin olive oil
32 ounces organic beef stock
2 cups homemade Tomato Chili Salsa*
1 cup cabbage, chopped
1 cup zucchini, chopped
1/2 cup onion, chopped
1 cup celery, chopped
1 cup mushrooms, sliced
1/4 cup carrots, chopped
1 cup fresh spinach, torn into small pieces
1 cup fresh Swiss chard or other greens, torn into small pieces
1/2 cup fresh basil, cilantro or parsley (or all three), for garnish

Cut beef into 1/4 inch thick strips; cut each strip into 1 inch pieces. In medium bowl, combine beef, basil, seasoning, pepper, garlic and oil; toss to coat.

Heat Dutch oven or large saucepan over medium-high heat until hot. Add 2 tablespoons water and then add beef mixture. Cook and stir 4-5 minutes or until browned. Stir in beef stock, salsa and vegetables except spinach and chard. Bring to a boil over medium-high heat. Reduce heat to low; simmer 10 minutes. Stir in spinach and chard. Garnish each serving of soup with fresh basil, parsley or cilantro.

Note:
This soup freezes well. Cool completely and put into plastic bags or freezer containers.

Yield: 10 servings

13.2.9 Juices and Smoothies

Recipes in This Section

Aloha Smoothie
Apricot Apple Flaxseed Smoothie
Berry Nut Shake
Cucumber Mint Smoothie
Garden Tonic
Raspberry Coconut Slush

~

Aloha Smoothie

2 tablespoons flax seeds
2 tablespoons raw macadamia nuts
2 tablespoons raw almonds
2 tablespoons pecans
2 slices organic ginger root
1 papaya
About 2 cups pure water
Stevia to taste

Soak nuts and seeds overnight, rinse. Add seeds, nuts, ginger, papaya and a little water to blender. Fit lid and blend on high until smooth. Add remaining water a little at a time and continue blending until all water is added. Add stevia to taste.

Yield: 2 servings

Apricot Apple Flaxseed Smoothie

3 fresh apricots, pitted
1/2 medium apple, chunked
2 tablespoons flax seeds
1/8 cup lemon juice
1 cup pure water
Dash of cinnamon
Stevia to taste

Soak flax seeds overnight before using this recipe. Drain seeds. Put all ingredients in blender or food processor and process until smooth, adding more water if necessary.

Yield: 1 serving

Berry Nut Shake

3 cups pure water
2 tablespoons almonds
2 tablespoons pine nuts
1 tablespoons flax seeds
2/3 cup blueberries and/or strawberries (fresh or frozen)
1/2 teaspoon vanilla
1/4 teaspoon nutmeg
Stevia

Soak flax seeds overnight before using this recipe. Process nuts on high in food processor or blender until ground. Add water slowly and process. Add berries, vanilla, and nutmeg. Add stevia to sweeten to taste. Blend well.

Notes:
If you wish a colder shake, substitute ice for some of the water. You may vary this recipe by using any nuts or seeds you desire.

Yield: 2 servings

Cucumber Mint Smoothie

2 medium cucumbers, peeled
2 tablespoons fresh basil
1 tablespoon fresh mint
1 apple
Pure water as needed

Put all ingredients in blender and blend until smooth.

Garden Tonic

Big handful of spinach
1 medium carrot
3 stalks of celery
2 stalks of asparagus
1 large tomato
Water as needed

If you use a juicer, juice spinach, carrot and celery together, followed by asparagus and tomato. Pour all into one glass and enjoy.

If you do not have a juicer, you can use a blender. Cut celery and asparagus crosswise in 1-2 inch pieces. Put all ingredients into blender. Cover and blend at high speed until well blended, adding water if necessary. Garnish with cherry tomato or lemon wedge.

Raspberry Coconut Slush

3 tablespoons shredded unsweetened coconut
1/2 cup almonds (soaked overnight)
2 tablespoons flax seeds (soaked overnight)
1 tablespoon psyllium seed (optional)
1/2 teaspoon ground cardamom (or other spice you prefer)
2 cups herb tea (brewed)
1 cup pure water
1/2 cup raspberries, fresh or frozen

Place coconut, almonds, flax, psyllium and cardamom in food processor or blender and enough brewed tea to process. Blend until smooth. Add remaining tea, water and raspberries and continue processing until thick and smooth. Serve in bowls. Or thin it with more water and drink it. Substitute ice for some of the water if you prefer a thicker, colder result.

Yield: 2 servings

13.2.10 Snacks and Handhelds

Recipes in This Section

Dried Veggie Chips
Flax Crackers
Lettuce Roll Ups
Sprout and Jicama Snack
Vegetable Leather
Vegetable Wraps

~

Dried Veggie Chips

1 medium eggplant, cut into thin slices
1 teaspoon sea salt
1 tablespoon extra virgin olive oil
2 teaspoons tamari
2 zucchini, cut diagonally into thin slices
2 medium kohlrabi, peeled, halved and cut into thin slices
1 medium jicama, peeled and cut into thin slices
1 red bell pepper, cut into thin strips

Cut eggplant and toss with 1 teaspoon sea salt and allow to set for about 30 minutes; this will remove any bitterness. Rinse and drain.

Meanwhile, mix olive oil and tamari in a large bowl. Add vegetables and toss to coat. Place coated slices on dehydrator screens or on lightly greased cookie sheet. Dehydrate at 110° F for 4-8 hours. If using an oven, adjust oven to lowest possible setting and cook for 3-4 hours until vegetables are dry and leathery. Thicker slices and wetter vegetables (like zucchini) may take longer.

Flax Crackers

4 cups whole flax seeds, soaked 4-6 hours
1/3 cup low-salt tamari
Juice of 2-3 lemons

Soak flax seeds for 4 to 6 hours in purified water. Pour off excess water. You will then have a gelatinous mixture. Add Braggs and lemon juice to taste and mix well. Keep moist and loose for spreading.

Spread mixture thinly on your dehydrator trays with a teflex sheet on top. Keep your hands wet as this will help on spreading the flax seeds (or use a spatula). Dehydrate at 105° F for 5-6 hours and then flip the mixture, removing the teflex sheet.
Continue dehydrating until the mixture completely dry (approximately 5-6 hours).

Variation:
Add garlic, onions, carrot juice, taco seasoning, Italian seasoning, chili powder or cumin in any combination. Be creative and make up your own recipe.

Lettuce Roll Ups

Use 2 large leaves of leafy or Romaine lettuce, washed and patted dry for each roll up.
Fill with any the following combinations. Roll leaves and secure with toothpick.
Wrap in wax paper, parchment or plastic wrap and store in refrigerator.

Mixture #1
1 avocado
1 orange
1/2 grapefruit
Sprinkle of rice vinegar

Mixture #2
Water packed canned salmon or tuna
1/2 cucumber, finely chopped
1/4 red onion, finely chopped

Mixture #3
1/2 cup ground walnuts
1/2 cup apple, finely chopped
Sprinkle of lemon juice

Mixture #4
1 red bell pepper, chopped fine
1 carrot, shredded
1 cup cabbage, finely shredded
1 stalk celery, minced

Mixture #5
4 tablespoons pine nuts, chopped
1/2 cup chopped wild mushrooms
1/8 teaspoon flaked seaweed
1 carrot, shredded

Notes:
Create your own recipe for roll ups. You can also use steamed cabbage leaves instead of
lettuce leaves if you wish.

To add different tastes or mouthfeel, you may wish to use one of the sauces or dips from the
Sauces and Dressings section of our recipes.

Yield: 1-3 servings per roll up

Sprout and Jicama Snack

2 cups mung bean sprouts
1 cup sunflower seed sprouts
1 cup lentil sprouts
1/8 cup radish sprouts
1/3 cup onion sprouts
1 cup additional mixed sprouts of your choice
1/2 cup grated jicama
1 tablespoon Salt-Free All-Purpose Seasoning*
1 teaspoon extra virgin olive oil
1 teaspoon Spike or Mrs. Dash seasoning

Mix sprouts and jicama together in large bowl. Drizzle olive oil over sprouts and toss well.
Sprinkle with seasonings.

Note:
Try different kinds and proportions of sprouts. Experiment with different seasonings.

Vegetable Leather

4 cups vegetables, your choice of any on Recommended list, or
4 cups thick, vegetable soup
1 teaspoon tamari
1 teaspoon lemon juice

Steam vegetables. Blend well in blender or food processor; and season with tamari and
lemon juice. Spread pureed vegetable mixture on Teflon tray in food dehydrator and
dehydrate at 135° F for about 6 hours or until no longer sticky. Remove and cool. Cut into
eighths, roll each one up and wrap tightly. Store in a dry place.

If using an oven, lightly grease a cookie sheet and spread puree onto sheet. Cook on lowest
possible oven setting until dry and leathery.

Yield: 8 roll ups

Vegetable Wraps

2 cups flax seeds, ground
1 1/2 cups water
1 teaspoon Spike
3 cloves garlic, peeled
1 cup fresh basil, chopped
1/2 cup fresh parsley, chopped
1/4 medium onion, chopped
1 cup sun-dried tomatoes
2 red bell peppers, chopped
1/4 teaspoon cayenne pepper
1 teaspoons marjoram
2 teaspoons lime juice

In a spice or coffee grinder, grind flax seed to a fine meal. Place all remaining ingredients except water and seed meal into blender or food processor and blend well. Add water and seed meal, then stir well and set aside for at least 30 minutes or until mixture has thickened. Drop by spoonful onto non-stick dehydrator sheets, spreading each wrap into a thin circular shape. Dehydrate at 105° F for 6 hours or until easily removable. Remove to mesh sheets and dry for another few hours until leathery.

Note:
Use as you would a tortilla. Store in plastic bags in the refrigerator for up to 30 days.

Yield: 8 wraps

13.2.11 Sauces and Dressings

Recipes in This Section

Asian Dressing
Balsamic Vinaigrette Dressing
BBQ Sauce
Dijon Vinaigrette
Fines Herbs
Ginger Dressing
Grapefruit Vinaigrette
Green Salsa
Herb Dressing
Herbs de Provence Spice Mix
Italian Basil Pesto
Latin Salsa
Lemon Mint Dressing
Lemon Vinaigrette
Lime, Oil and Garlic Dressing
Mango Salsa
Meat Marinade No. 1
Meat Marinade No. 2
Mexican Guacamole
Mock Sour Cream
Mushroom Gravy
Nut Pâté
Olive Oil-Lemon Dressing
Omega 3 Mayonnaise
Pork Loin Marinade
Salt-Free All-Purpose Seasoning
Spicy Salad Dressing
Tapenade
Tartar Sauce
Tomato Chili Salsa

Asian Dressing

1 cup raw hulled (white) sesame seeds
1 cup brewed black tea
1 tablespoon rice vinegar
1/2 teaspoon chili flakes (optional)
2 cloves garlic, chopped
2 tablespoons tamari
2 tablespoons fresh ginger, minced

Grind sesame seeds in coffee bean grinder or food processor into a fine meal. Place all ingredients in a blender and blend until smooth, adding a little water if necessary to get desired consistency. Refrigerate in tightly covered container. Use as dip or thin down and use as salad dressing.

Yield: 2 cups

Balsamic Vinaigrette Dressing

1 tablespoon extra virgin oil
1/4 teaspoon tamari
1 teaspoon balsamic vinegar
Fresh ground pepper to taste
1 teaspoon Dijon mustard
2 teaspoons freshly squeezed lemon juice
Dash of hot sauce

Blend all ingredients. Store in airtight container in refrigerator. Use on any salad.

Yield: 1 serving

BBQ Sauce

1 cup walnut or hemp oil
2 cups cider vinegar
2 tablespoons poultry seasoning
3 tablespoons Spike seasoning
1/2 teaspoon black pepper (optional)
1 egg

In heavy pan, combine oil, vinegar and seasonings. Bring to a boil, reduce heat and simmer for 5 minutes. Remove from heat. Whisk in the beaten egg and allow to cool. Store in container with lid in refrigerator. Keeps for up to 60 days.

Yield: 3 cups

Dijon Vinaigrette

1/2 cup extra virgin olive oil
2 tablespoons red or white wine vinegar
1 teaspoon Dijon mustard
1 small shallot, minced (optional)
A little salt and pepper

Blend all ingredients together in blender or shaker with lid. Keep refrigerated in covered container. Recipe can be doubled.

Yield: approximately 1/2 cup

Fines Herbs

1 tablespoon dried thyme
1 tablespoon dried savory
1 tablespoon dried marjoram
1 tablespoon dried sage
1 tablespoon dried basil
1 tablespoon dried grated lemon peel

Fine Herbs is a mixture of chopped aromatic herbs in varying proportions. The above list is just an example. You could also use such herbs as parsley, chervil, tarragon and chives. The mixture could be used to flavor sauces, meat, poultry, fish, sautéed vegetables, soups and omelets.

Mix herbs and lemon peel. Store in airtight container. Keep in cool, dry place.

Yield: 1/3 cup

Ginger Dressing

1 teaspoon grated ginger root
2 tablespoons walnut oil
2 shallots, finely chopped
1 teaspoon tamari
3 tablespoons rice vinegar

Combine all ingredients in jar. Cap and shake well.

Grapefruit Vinaigrette

1/4 cup freshly squeezed grapefruit juice
3/4 cup extra virgin olive oil
1 teaspoon Mrs. Dash, Spike, or Salt Free All Purpose Seasoning*

Blend and bottle. Keep refrigerated. Recipe can be doubled.

Yield: 1 cup

Green Salsa

4-7 jalapeno or Serrano chilies
1 clove garlic
1 pound tomatillos (husked)
1 ripe avocado
1/2 cup chopped cilantro
1 lime
Morton Salt Substitute or regular salt

Roast chilies and tomatillos on the grill. Blend garlic first with a little water in blender or mash with a garlic press. Combine garlic with roasted chilies and tomatillos and blend at low speed.

Mash or cut finely the avocado. Combine avocado, cilantro and contents of blender in a bowl. Squeeze lime into salsa and add salt or salt substitute to taste.

Yield: Approximately 2 cups

Herb Dressing

2 stalks celery and leaves, chopped fine
2 small green onions, chopped fine
4 sprigs parsley, chopped fine
1 teaspoon paprika
1/4 teaspoon dried basil
1/8 teaspoon marjoram or rosemary
1 cup olive oil
2/3 cup lemon juice

Combine all ingredients in blender and blend well. Allow to stand in refrigerator overnight or until flavors are blended.

Yield: Approximately 2 cups

Herbs de Provence Spice Mix

3 tablespoons dried marjoram
3 tablespoons dried thyme
3 tablespoons dried savory
1 teaspoon dried basil
1 teaspoon dried rosemary
1/2 teaspoon dried sage
1/2 teaspoon fennel seeds

Combine all ingredients. Mix well and spoon into small jars. Use to season chicken, vegetables or meat.

Yield: 3/4 cup

Italian Basil Pesto

2 cups fresh basil leaves, stemmed and packed
3/4 cup fresh parsley, chopped
1/2 cup raw walnuts or pine nuts
2 cloves garlic, peeled (use more if you wish)
1/2 teaspoon grated lemon rind
1/2 cup extra virgin olive oil
1 1/2 teaspoons Morton Salt Substitute or Spike

In blender or food processor, combine all ingredients and process until fairly smooth. Store in refrigerator. Will keep up to 3 weeks.

Yield: About 24 servings

Latin Salsa

6-8 cloves garlic, peeled
3-5 Serrano chilies or jalapeno peppers, seeds removed
1 cup cilantro
Juice of 1 lime
3-4 tomatillos, outer husks removed (or use 2 more tomatoes instead)
3-4 medium tomatoes
1 teaspoon ground cumin
1 medium-large red onion, chopped into 1/4 pieces

Best tool for salsa making is a blender. In order to achieve a chunky texture, add ingredients to blender in the order specified below and don't over-blend in the last step. Blend enough to break up the last few tomatoes but not so much as to pulverize them.

Place garlic, chiles, cilantro and lime juice into blender. Pulse blender repeatedly, until garlic is a paste and chiles and cilantro leaves are finely chopped. Scrape down the sides of blender if necessary.

If mixture is too dry to process well, add a couple of tomatillos, or a tomato. Add remaining tomatillos and pulse to break them up. Then add tomatoes and cumin and pulse just enough to break up tomatoes. Pour salsa into a bowl.

Stir onion into salsa by hand. Let salsa stand for one hour at as the flavors combine. Then refrigerate in sealed container.

Yield: 2 cups

Lemon Mint Dressing

5 tablespoons extra virgin olive oil
3 tablespoons lemon or lime juice
2 tablespoons white vinegar
1 clove garlic, minced
1/2 teaspoon dried mint (or 1 teaspoons fresh mint, minced)
1/2 teaspoon dried basil (or 2 teaspoons fresh basil, minced)

Put all ingredients in jar or blender and shake or blend. Makes 2/3 cup of dressing.

Lemon Vinaigrette

1/4 cup freshly squeezed lemon or lime juice
3/4 cup extra virgin olive oil
A dash of Mrs. Dash seasoning
1 teaspoon parsley (fresh or dried), or any fresh herbs you like (rosemary, savory, thyme, dill, sage, etc.)

Blend and store in bottle. Keep refrigerated. Recipe can be doubled.

Yield: 1 cup

Lime, Oil and Garlic Dressing

1-2 teaspoons tamari
1 teaspoon garlic, peeled and finely chopped
2 tablespoons shallots, finely chopped
1/3 cup lime (or lemon) juice, plus extra if needed
1 cup extra-virgin olive oil, plus extra if needed
Freshly ground black pepper

In a small bowl, whisk tamari, garlic, and shallots with lime juice. Slowly whisk in the oil until emulsified. Taste and adjust seasonings, adding more lime juice if needed. Store in airtight container overnight or until flavors are well blended.

Yield: 1.3 cups

Mango Salsa

1 ripe mango, diced
1 papaya, diced
1/2 medium red onion, chopped
1 Serrano or jalapeño chili pepper (or use milder Anaheim), minced (optional)
1 small cucumber diced
2 tablespoons fresh cilantro leaves, chopped
3 tablespoons fresh lime juice
Pepper to taste

Put all ingredients into bowl and mix. Let salsa stand for one hour at room temperature to let flavors combine. Refrigerate in sealed container.

Yield: 2-3 cups

Meat Marinade No. 1

1 tablespoon honey
1/3 - 1/2 cup olive oil
4 cloves garlic, crushed
1/4 cup tamari
2 teaspoons rice vinegar

Put all ingredients in small bowl and whisk until well blended.

Put meat or poultry into zip lock bag. Pour in marinade. Refrigerate and leave overnight, if you have time. Otherwise, let it marinade for 1 - 4 hours.

Remove meat and set out to cook or barbeque. Baste some of the marinade on top of meat before cooking. When you turn the meat, baste other side. If barbequing, baste meat frequently to keep it moist.

_____

Meat Marinade No. 2

1 tablespoon honey
1/3 - 1/2 cup olive oil
3 tablespoons lime juice
2 teaspoons fresh ginger root, finely grated
1/4 cup tamari

Same instructions as above.

Mexican Guacamole

2 avocados
1 onion, chopped fine
1 tomato, chopped fine
1-2 limes or 1 lemon, juiced (to taste)
2 cloves garlic, minced
1 tablespoon cilantro, minced
1 jalapeno or Serrano pepper, finely chopped (optional)

Cut avocados in half, pop out the pit, scoop out the flesh with a spoon   Ingredients can be chopped by hand or put into food processor or blender, depending upon whether you like your guacamole smooth or chunky. Place all ingredients, except lemon or lime juice, into bowl and mix. Add lemon or lime juice to taste and mix again.

Store in sealed container in refrigerator.

Variation: Take Mexican Guacamole and mix some of it with any salsa dish for a different taste and texture.

Yield: 1 - 2 cups

Mock Sour Cream

1 cup Brazil nuts, soaked overnight
1/4 cup lemon juice
1/2 teaspoon tamari

Add 1/3 cup water to food processor or blender. Combine nuts, lemon juice, and tamari until light and creamy, about 3 or 4 minutes. Add more water as necessary.

Variation:
Replace lemon juice with lime juice and add chili powder and cumin to taste. Use a different nut or seed if you wish.

Yield: 1 1/4 cups

Mushroom Gravy

1/2 cup soaked almonds
1/2 cup organic beef broth (use more if needed)
2 cups shitake mushrooms (use another mushroom if shitake not available)
1/4 teaspoon garlic granules or 1 clove garlic
2 teaspoons tamari
Additional seasonings if you wish

Blend almonds and beef broth until smooth; set aside. Blend mushrooms with just enough beef broth to get desired gravy consistency. Add almond mixture, garlic, tamari and seasonings. Blend again until smooth, adding more broth if necessary. Heat and serve.

Yield: Approximately 2 cups

Nut Pâté

1 cup walnuts
1/2 cup almonds
1/2 cup macadamia nuts
1/4 cup sesame seeds
1 red bell pepper, finely chopped
3 stalks celery, finely chopped
1 small leek (white part only), finely chopped
2 tablespoons lemon juice
1-2 teaspoons powdered kelp
1-2 tablespoons tamari

Soak all nuts and seeds 12-24 hours in pure water, then rinse. Using a food processor, process all nuts and seeds until reduced to a meal. Add red bell pepper, celery, leek, lemon juice, kelp, tamari and mix well.

Yield: 2 - 3 cups

Olive Oil-Lemon Dressing

3 tablespoons fresh-squeezed lemon juice
1/2 cup olive oil (may also use flax, walnut or hemp)
1 clove garlic, peeled and crushed (optional)
Herb seasoning for taste

Herb seasoning ideas:
Oregano - for a more Italian flavor
Thyme - for a mild herbal flavor
Basil - for a strong herbal flavor
Cayenne - for people who like spicy food

Shake all ingredients in a container with a tight-fitting lid. Keep refrigerated. If olive oil solidifies, remove from refrigerator one hour before using. Use on salads or vegetable dishes.

Yield: about 2/3 cup

Omega 3 Mayonnaise

1 tablespoon lemon juice
1 whole egg
1/4 teaspoon dry mustard
1/3 cup olive oil
1/3 cup flaxseed oil
1/3 cup walnut oil

Put lemon juice, egg and mustard into blender. Blend 3 to 5 seconds. Continue blending and slowly add oils in a thin stream while blender is on low. Blend until mayonnaise is thick. Store in sealed plastic container. Use within 5-7 days.

Note:
If you don't have both flaxseed oil and walnut oil, use 2/3 cup of the one that you do have.

Yield: 1 cup

Pork Loin Marinade

1/4 pineapple
1 orange
2-3 tablespoons olive oil
1/3 - 1/2 cup tamari
1 teaspoon ground ginger
1 small onion, chopped
2 cloves garlic, minced

Slice away outer skin of pineapple and peel orange. In a blender or food processor, puree pineapple and orange. In a jar with a tight fitting lid, combine all ingredients. Shake well. Pour over meat. In refrigerator, marinate, turning occasionally, for several hours or overnight before cooking.

Salt-Free All-Purpose Seasoning

1/4 cup dried minced onion
4 teaspoon dried vegetable flakes
1 tablespoon garlic powder
1 tablespoon dried orange peel
1 teaspoon dried lemon peel
1-2 teaspoons coarse ground black pepper (optional)
1 teaspoon dried parsley
1/2 teaspoon dried basil
1/2 teaspoon dried marjoram
1/2 teaspoon dried oregano
1/2 teaspoon dried savory
1/2 teaspoon dried thyme
1/2 teaspoon cayenne pepper (optional)
1/2 teaspoon cumin
1/2 teaspoon coriander
1/2 teaspoon dried mustard
1/4 teaspoon celery seed
2 teaspoon dried Nori flakes (or other dried seaweed flakes)
Dash of dried rosemary

Combine all of the ingredients in a grinder and grind to powder. Store the spice blend in a covered container or a sealed shaker bottle.

Yield: Approximately 2/3 of a cup.

Spicy Salad Dressing

6 tablespoons extra virgin olive oil
2 tablespoons lemon juice
1 teaspoon dry oregano
1 teaspoon dried parsley
1/2 teaspoon curry powder
1 clove garlic, peeled and minced
Dash of Salt-Free All-Purpose Seasoning*
Dash of freshly ground black pepper

Mix all ingredients and let them to rest for at least 10 minutes. Add to any salad. Top with avocado, onion and tomato.

Yield: 2 servings

Tapenade

6 tablespoons walnuts or pine nuts
2 cloves garlic, peeled and pressed
1 green onion (white part only)
1/2 cup Italian parsley, stemmed and chopped
1 cup fresh spinach, stemmed and chopped
1/4 fresh thyme
1/2 teaspoon grated lemon peel
1/2 teaspoon Morton Salt Substitute or 1/8 teaspoon regular salt
3/4 cup black olives, pitted
3 tablespoons extra virgin olive oil

Put nuts and garlic in food processor and process until nuts are ground. Add onion, parsley, spinach and thyme and process well. Add lemon peel, salt, olives and olive oil and blend until smooth. Transfer to covered container and store in refrigerator.

Yield: 1 1/2 cups

Tartar Sauce

1 cup Omega 3 mayonnaise*
2 tablespoon red onion, finely chopped
1/2 tablespoon lime or lemon juice
1/2 teaspoon dried dill
1/4 teaspoon paprika
1/2 tablespoon Dijon mustard
1 tablespoon drained capers
1 tablespoon cucumber, peeled and finely chopped

Put Omega 3 mayonnaise* into bowl. Add all ingredients and whisk until mixed. Serve immediately or refrigerate in sealed container for 2-3 days.

Yield: 1 cup

Tomato Chili Salsa

1 clove garlic, peeled and minced
1 pound tomatoes, chopped small
1/2 cup bell, Anaheim or Serrano peppers, chopped
1/2 small red onion, finely chopped
1/4 cup fresh cilantro, finely chopped
1/4 cup fresh parsley, finely chopped
1 tablespoon lime juice
1 teaspoon white vinegar
1/2 teaspoon Spike seasoning

Mix garlic, tomatoes, peppers, onion, cilantro, parsley, lime juice, vinegar and seasonings. Cover with plastic food wrap and let stand at room temperature for 1 hour. Keeps in the refrigerator up to 10 days.

Yield: 2-1/3 cups.

Variation:
RED HOT SALSA: Increase the garlic to 2 cloves, the lime juice to 1 1/2 tablespoons and add 1 tablespoon chopped jalapeno pepper, plus 1/4 teaspoon red pepper sauce. Proceed as directed above.

Part 3

Additional Steps To Take

Section 14

Other Things You Can Do

3

14.1 Exercise

Physical activity is an essential key to managing PCOS, increasing fertility and a healthy life.

Our bodies were made to move. For thousands of years, human beings were nomadic, following or seeking out the food supply. Once we learned how to *create* our food supply, we were able to stay in one place. As time passed, we began to enjoy the benefits of advancing technologies, which provided us with more leisure time. We used our minds more and more, while using our bodies less and less. Today we find ourselves in a modern life that actually demands very little of us physically. Although our bodies are still hard-wired for movement, most of us no longer honor the very real need of the "natural self" to get up and move about.

Appreciating your body — for its miraculous ability to carry out millions of intricate functions without conscious direction, for its continual pursuit of equilibrium, for its complex adaptive ability — is the first step on the road to total fitness. Lay aside your judgments, fears, expectations and disappointments in favor of a positive framework that sets the stage for a lasting and consistent exercise program.

Benefits of Exercise

Unlike drugs or fad diets, there are no downsides to regular exercise. Here are a few ways you will benefit from exercise.

- Increased endurance and fatigue resistance
- Increased strength and flexibility
- Better balance
- Improved coordination
- Improved posture
- Higher self esteem
- Tension release
- Better sleep
- More energy
- Mood improvement
- Decreased insulin resistance
- Leaner body
- Tendency to normalize hormones
- Improved general health

Why Women with PCOS Should Exercise

A number of studies have demonstrated that women with PCOS or insulin resistance can greatly benefit from regular exercise.

For example, a study conducted at the University of Adelaide in Australia showed that a six month program of diet and exercise helped 18 overweight PCOS women normalize their hormones.[240] They experienced an 11% reduction in central fat, 71% improvement in insulin sensitivity, 33% fall in insulin levels, and a 39% reduction in LH (luteinizing hormone) levels. The women in this study achieved surprising results with a combination of diet and exercise in just six months. This study is relevant because insulin resistance and chronically high insulin and LH are reasons why PCOS women don't ovulate and why they have a number of other troubling symptoms.

Exercise Necessary for Loss of Belly Fat
Exercise is necessary for the loss of belly fat in diabetic women according to a new study from Syracuse University.[241] Thirty-three women were divided into "diet only" and "diet plus exercise" groups. Since diabetic women have metabolic problems similar to PCOS women, the study results are relevant.

Either diet alone, or diet plus exercise, caused an average weight loss of 9.9 lbs in three months. However, only the diet plus exercise group had a loss of visceral fat, which is the belly fat that surrounds internal organs.

This study suggests that you can lose weight with diet alone. But if you also want to significantly lose abdominal fat, you'll want to add regular exercise to your diet program.

Reduction of Homocysteine
Women with PCOS tend to have elevated homocysteine, especially those who are taking metformin (Glucophage). Homocysteine is an amino acid in the blood. A normal amount is okay — but an elevated level means that your metabolic processes are not working properly. Elevated homocysteine is associated with coronary artery disease, heart attack, chronic fatigue, fibromyalgia, cognitive impairment and cervical cancer.

A recent study at the University of Warwick in England has provided the first evidence that regular exercise significantly lowers homocysteine in the blood of young overweight women with PCOS.[242] In this study, a group of women who exercised for six months had a significant drop in their homocysteine levels. They also reduced their waist-to-hip ratio, meaning that their bellies got smaller. In contrast, there was no change in the non-exercising group.

Insulin Resistance and Exercise
Insulin resistance is a primary cause of PCOS and infertility. Does exercise reduce insulin resistance?

A very interesting study from Otago University in New Zealand may provide the answer.[243] Two groups of men and women were put on one of two dietary and exercise programs for four months.

The "modest" group was given a diet commonly recommended by health authorities. They were required to cut their cholesterol intake and increase their fiber intake. Their diet consisted of low-glycemic foods, fish, nuts, seeds, grains, pasta, rice, fruit, vegetables, legumes and low-fat dairy products. This is the type of diet your doctor might recommend. The participants were also required to exercise for 30 minutes five times a week. No instructions were given on how hard to exercise.

The "intense" group was given a diet similar to the "modest" group, although their fiber intake was somewhat higher and the total fat intake was somewhat lower. In addition, the exercise requirement was different. The "intense" group was asked to exercise for at least 20 minutes five times a week at 80-90% of the maximum heart rate for their age. In other words, they were requested to exercise quite hard for 20 minutes.

After 4 months, only the "intense" group had a significant reduction in their insulin resistance (a 23% drop vs. a 9% drop for the "modest" group). Also, their aerobic fitness increased 11% vs. a 1% increase for the "modest" group.

This study demonstrated that healthier diet recommendations combined with a greater intensity of exercise are effective in reducing insulin resistance. This study is especially relevant for lean PCOS women who have insulin resistance. It's well known that insulin resistance can be reduced by losing a lot of weight. But if you're not overweight and have insulin resistance — what can you do? This study suggests that a better diet and regular exercise at 80-90% of your maximum heart rate will improve your sensitivity to insulin and thus reduce your PCOS symptoms.

Can You Get Better by Exercise Alone?

Even if you don't follow our healthy PCOS diet at all, you can still get some benefit from regular exercise. (Of course, we strongly recommend that you do *both!*).

A small study conducted at the University of Florida showed that non-dieting sedentary adults who got a few hours of exercise each week and did not lose weight still were able to significantly improve their glucose and fat metabolism.[244]

And, according to a new study of premenopausal women by researchers at Queen's University in Ontario, Canada, moderate exercise without dieting caused a reduction in total body fat, belly fat and insulin resistance.[245] However, these women did not lose any weight. So, with moderate exercise alone, you may not lose much weight, but you will improve your body fat percentage and reduce insulin resistance.

Regular exercise provides numerous health benefits, including improvement in some PCOS symptoms such as insulin resistance. We also know that a healthy diet provides additional numerous benefits. If you combine a healthy diet with a regular exercise program, you will accelerate your progress towards managing PCOS, improving fertility and being more vital and healthy.

What Is an "Exercise Program"?

An exercise program is a commitment to move your body in a variety of ways beyond your normal day to day activity. Some people are put off by the term "workout" or "program" because it conjures up images of gymnasiums or hard-body clubs where everyone sweats and grunts their way toward fitness. If you're turned off by clanging barbells, mirrored walls and loud, overhead music, then simply create our own workout routine wherever and however you choose…and call it whatever you like.

You can start with small things like:
- Parking a little further away from your destination and walking
- Taking stairs instead of elevators
- Pacing rather than sitting while talking on the phone
- Getting up and stretching whenever possible

Your program can utilize a variety of exercise activities, at varying degrees of intensity. You can join a health club or spa, go to the pool and swim or do water aerobics. Or find a park or hiking trail near your home where you can go for a brisk walk. There's no end to what you can do to be more active. Ultimately, you'll find a safe and steadily challenging program that works for you.

Most find that they get maximum benefit by including several different types of exercise during their daily routine, including flexibility, strengthening, balancing and aerobic activity.

Exercises and physical activity can be divided up into 10-15 minute periods or done all at once for a much longer period of time. Most people need to exercise at least 30 minutes a day, although some individuals with insulin resistance may need to do considerably more. If you're not physically fit, or quite overweight, or don't have the energy to exercise for 30 minutes or more, just do what you can, even if it is only 5 minutes at a time.

Here are some exercise options that can be done at varying levels of intensity and duration:
- Stretching
- Yoga
- Pilates or Gyrotonic
- Resistance Training (free weights, machines, bands, pushups, sit-ups, etc)
- Water Exercise (water walking, water aerobics, swimming, surfing)
- Organized Sports (basketball, badminton, softball, soccer golf)
- Individual Sports (biking, roller blading, ice skating, skiing, snowboarding)
- Dancing

- Aerobic classes or Jazzercise
- Walking, jogging or running
- Martial arts (karate, tai-chi)

Some exercise works best if it is structured, like stretching, resistance training and some aerobic activities. Other exercise, like walking, biking, gardening or housecleaning can simply be worked into your day however you can do it.

If you're just beginning an exercise program, it's smart to consult with a health care professional and/or a personal trainer before you begin. Both can help you figure out what routines would be best for your health limitations, fitness level, body type and lifestyle.

How Much Should You Exercise?

There are three aspects to the question of how much you should exercise: frequency, duration, and intensity.

Frequency:
Ideally, you would do some kind of exercise every day, especially if you have troublesome PCOS symptoms. There's no need to do the same type or amount of exercise every day.

Duration:
The duration of your exercise will depend on your physical limitations, the type of exercise and its intensity. If you're walking, you may be able to continue for an hour or more. If you're doing any high-intensity exercise, you may be able to last only 20 minutes or possibly much less.

Intensity:
The intensity of your exercise could range up to 80% of the maximum heart rate for your age. But you may want to start out quite a bit lower, perhaps at 60-70% of maximum. Wherever you start, be absolutely certain to consult with your physician before starting any high intensity exercise, especially one that is putting stress on your heart. To find out the maximum heart rate for your age, consult with your doctor, personal trainer, or get a heart rate chart from the Internet.

As we said earlier in this chapter, high-intensity exercise may be especially helpful for reducing insulin resistance. It has also been shown to be more effective in reducing body fat percentage in women.[246] And, according to one study of women, those who did high-intensity aerobic dance lost more weight than women who did low-intensity walking.[247]

There will be some combination of frequency, duration and intensity that will work for you. The most important thing is that you enjoy what you are doing. The second most important thing is to try to gradually increase the frequency, duration and/or intensity of your exercise program.

In general, the more exercise, the better. Most of us don't exercise nearly enough on a consistent basis.

How Hard Should You Exercise After You've Lost Weight?

If you eat a healthy PCOS diet and exercise on a regular basis, what happens when you reach your target weight? To avoid possible re-gain of your weight, you will want to continue with your exercise program.[248]

A study at the University of Chicago suggested that women require 35 minutes of vigorous exercise or 80 minutes of moderate exercise to minimize future weight gain after initially losing weight and reaching their target weight.[249]   In this study, 32 women (average age 38) had lost at least 26 pounds and reached their target weight. One year later, the physically active women had gained back an average of 5.5 pounds, moderately active women gained 21.8 lbs. and sedentary women gained 15.4 pounds. There appears to be an activity threshold above which you can maintain your weight loss. But if you fall below the threshold and are only mildly active, you may regain much of your lost weight.

Walking

Walking is a wonderful, natural form of exercise. It's easy to do and almost anyone can do it, regardless of fitness level. Not only does walking contribute to fitness, it relieves stress and lifts your spirits.

Brisk walking an hour a day reduces your risk of obesity by 24% and diabetes by 34%, according to a study from researchers at Harvard University.[250] Even standing or walking around the house reduced obesity risk by 9% and diabetes by 12%. In contrast, watching television for 2 hours a day increases obesity risk by 5% and diabetes by 7%. So, turn off your TV for one hour and take a walk instead. What could be easier? If it's not easy, just grit your teeth and do it anyway.

If you can't walk for an hour, walk around the block or down to the mailbox on the corner. Look for every opportunity to take a walk, whether it is short or long.

If you can stay with walking for a long time, you will see results. For example, some men and women started a one-year walking program (with no dieting) after they had heart attacks.[251] Their daily walks increased from 20 minutes to 43 minutes over 3 months, and then were maintained at that level for an additional 9 months. By year's end, the women had lost 7% of their total body weight, their body fat percentage dropped 3.2% and their triglycerides dropped.

We recommend that you buy and use a pedometer. People who use pedometers tend to walk and be more active than people who don't use one.

Be Physically Active

We also recommend that you be as physically active as you possibly can. Take the stairs instead of the escalator or elevator. When shopping, park farther away from the store door. Develop active recreational activities such as gardening. If you have a desk job, get up every hour or two and briskly walk around the office building.

"No-assist" days can help you become fit. A "no-assist" day means that you don't use any powered mechanical contrivance, such as a car, elevator or escalator to help you move about. You use your two legs or a bicycle. You are completely under your own power. Try to have at least one "no assist" day per week.

Tips for a More Satisfying Workout

There are many resources available that offer suggestions for exercise regimes of varying intensities. Consult with your physician and/or professional trainer to design a workout that you can live with on a daily basis. Here are a few tips that can make any workout more satisfying:

- Exercise offers you a way to cultivate health and well-being by discovering who you are and what you're made of. It gives you the chance to "fall in love" with, and cooperate with, your true and spontaneous nature. Think about this before a workout so you will approach the session with an attitude of cooperation rather than resistance.

- Put aside rigidity and practice being fluid. Recognize that when you are breaking new ground physically or emotionally, the little hobgoblins of resistance, reluctance, discouragement, fatigue or failure begin to show up. Respect the information they're giving you about your condition. Recognize that with perseverance, these little hobgoblins will quiet down and take their place on the bench. What replaces them ultimately is a remarkable sense of well-being, satisfaction and self-esteem.

- Find a balance point between healthy exertion and injury and *stay conscious of that point* as you strive to improve the quality and duration of your workout.

- Precede each workout with 5-10 minutes of deep breathing to focus your energy. As you breathe, quiet your mind and begin to gently stretch and warm up. This tells your body that you're about to do something wonderful with and for it. It sets your intent. Intent + focus + attention = success.

- Focus your attention on your body when working out. Rather than let your mind wander, practice "being present" with your muscles as they stretch and contract. This amplifies your workout because your attention is inside your body rather than on outside distractions.

- Cultivate the habit of breathing deeply through your nostrils to bring oxygen into your entire body.

- Be attuned to your body's natural cycles, its ebbs and peaks. Your energy fluctuates during the day, just as it does during the week, month and year. There are just some days that your body is tired. There are some times of the day when you're perkier than other times. Try to understand and cooperate with these fluctuations rather than stressing yourself by working against them.

- Visualize success. In your mind's eye, see your body in top form, moving freely and easily. As you work out, form clear and vivid images of your muscles becoming strong and flexible, your body shedding what no longer serves your well-being, your cells absorbing plenty of oxygen, and your entire being becoming strong and healthy.

- Use affirmations to create a positive thought pattern. "I love to work out," is a good one to start with. Other affirmations might be, "I love feeling fit," or "My body loves to move!" or simply, "I can." You can make up your own affirmations if you want to. The only rule is to keep them simple and positive. The word affirmation means to "make firm." Affirmations are direct and repeated efforts toward changing negative patterns.

- Let go of perfectionism. It's a seduction. Replace it with a *process of excellence* — doing your personal best and feeling complete about it. This way, results become a byproduct of a healthy internal process rather than an external obsession. Keep an exercise journal of what activities you do and how you feel about yourself when you do them. It's a good way to keep track of the process and will tell you a lot about who you are.

- Exercise is transformational if you flow with it. When you focus on your body and muscle group(s) being worked, and when you pay attention to what you're doing and how you're doing it, you're less likely to exhaust yourself and you'll be more energized afterwards.

- See your workout as a dance between you and your body, a joyful process of natural movement that can lead to great satisfaction.

- Stay conscious of your physical state. Accept what you cannot change and change what you can. As you get more fit, you will want to expand your workout. Recognize that each time you expand, it's important that you commit to 'going the distance' to the new level. Remember that fitness is a process, not a destination.

- Make exercising a priority and a habit. A good way to do that is to choose a time of day, e.g., first thing in the morning, before work, over lunchtime, after work or in the evening. Sometimes people stay on track with an exercise program more easily if they exercise with a friend. But if you choose to do it that way, don't let your friend's schedules or attitudes interfere with your resolve to get and stay fit.

- Goals create a relationship between what you dream and what you do. They direct your energy to what's most important. Set exercise goals for yourself and strive to reach them. Research from the University of Minnesota has shown that people with high physical activity goals have more long-term weight loss than those who had less ambitious goals.[252] And when you reach your goal, celebrate!

Be patient. It takes time to develop endurance, strength, willingness, perseverance and a healthy body. Every time you exercise, you're proving that you're worth the time and energy it takes to become healthy and happy.

14.2 Stress Management

Understanding and managing stress is a crucial component of your plan to control PCOS and improve your fertility odds.[253]

Stress is any stimulation to the body that challenges its sense of balance and triggers a significant set of biological responses. These responses include a release of stress hormones, an increase in blood sugar, tightening of muscles, shallowness of breath, rising blood pressure and rapid heart rate.

This stress response is a kind of a "biochemical insurance" that enables you to fight, flee or fortify. Some stress actually keeps us alert and motivated. Without it, we wouldn't want to get out of bed in the morning, let alone respond to life's challenges. But at some point, the physical effects of stress cease to work for us and begin working against us.

Even though stress is most readily observed in our emotions and behaviors, the stress response is mostly an internal biochemical process. A stress response is like stepping on the gas pedal while your car is in neutral…the engine revs way up. As soon as you take your foot off the pedal, the engine slows down. But if you keep your foot pressed on the gas pedal all the time, the engine stays revved up way too high, resulting in engine damage. So it is with chronic stress and your body: cell and organ damage are the inevitable result.

Modern life frequently presents unrelenting stressful situations over which we may have little control. These chronic stressors may include work pressures, long-term relationship problems, loneliness, abuse and persistent worry.

Continual or frequent stress reactions eventually cause your body to become exhausted and no longer able to adequately respond to stress. You want to avoid this end point because it represents a very serious threat to your health.

External and Internal Stressors

You can experience both external and internal stressors.

External stressors include things like pain, hot or cold temperatures, a constant sense of danger, abuse, adverse working conditions, persistent noise and other physical stimulations that are intolerable or beyond your control. External stressors can also be invisible and insidious. Environmental chemical pollution is one example of a pervasive stressor that you can't see, taste or smell.

Internal stressors can be physical, such as infections, inflammations and diseases, or toxins stored in your cells. Internal stressors can also be your thoughts and feelings — persistent worry, loss, unexpected change, a sense of helplessness, abandonment, or any deep emotional event that requires you to go into overdrive.

Consequences of Stress

The first thing to understand about any stressful event is that its effect on your body is **universal.** There is no organ or gland or tissue that is unaffected, either directly or indirectly.

Your hypothalamus (master gland in the brain), pituitary, ovaries, thyroid, adrenals, pancreas, liver, and GI tract are all affected in some way.[254] [255] [256]   So is your immune system.[257]   So are your brain chemicals ("neurotransmitters"). Most of your hormones and other signaling molecules are altered.

Your mind and body is an enormously complex web of interrelated parts that are in a state of homeostasis, or balance. The balance is maintained by constant communication among your millions of cells.

When a stressful event occurs, your body is thrown out of balance. Your cells start to send out "alarm" messages (such as hormones) to other cells and very quickly your entire body is alerted to the new situation. Your body then does everything in its power to restore its balance.

For example, if you eat some spoiled food, you will probably vomit or have diarrhea to get rid of it. This is your body's reaction to a "spoiled food" stressor, which has thrown it out of balance. After you have gotten rid of the bad food, your body is back into a state of balance. However, your balance after the bad food is not quite the same as before the food. Your GI tract, your immune system, and many organs and glands had to do a lot of communicating and expend a lot of energy to get rid of that bad food. After the episode, your body will be somewhat depleted, in a slightly less desirable state of balance.

An isolated, infrequent stressor is not a problem. But what if you ate some bad food every day? This is an example of chronic stress. Your body will find a new place of balance, which is a continual state of alarm. In other words, you would always be in a state of stress and alarm as your body unsuccessfully tries to reclaim its equilibrium — because there is always another stressor coming along. The new homeostasis is a continual state of alarm rather than a state of ordered calm and natural balance.

As all of your organs, hormones, central nervous system and every part of your body are recruited to deal with multiple chronic stressors, your body as a whole becomes somewhat disordered.

Manifestations of this disordered state include:
- Elevated blood pressure
- Loss of muscle mass
- Low energy
- Cold and hot sensitivity
- Depression

- Increased abdominal fat accumulation
- Muscle pain
- Inability to concentrate
- Depressed thyroid function
- Altered thyroid hormone metabolism
- Elevated C-reactive protein and other inflammatory proteins
- Impaired fertility
- Impaired pulsation of hormones
- "Resistance" to hormones beside insulin
- Lack of, or disordered, menstruation
- Increased miscarriage
- Insulin resistance
- Prone to infections
- Amplified startle reflex
- Impaired digestion
- Decreased sex drive
- Increased oxidative stress (free radical molecules that damage cells)
- High cortisol and stress hormone levels
- Altered sex steroid hormone levels (estrogen, progesterone, testosterone)
- Altered neurotransmitters (serotonin and catecholamines)

As you can see, the consequences of uncontrolled chronic stress are profound and far-reaching. Here are a few more comments about stress consequences:

Psychological Effects
A continual state of stress depresses serotonin, which increases anxiety, increases appetite and is a trigger for depression.

Stress also diminishes quality of life by robbing you of your sense of pleasure, security, accomplishment and empowerment. Alienation from enjoyment and a sense of well-being interrupts your ability to truly thrive.

Weight Gain
Stress-induced cortisol, insulin resistance and numerous other factors predispose you to gain weight, especially around the middle. Abdominal fat gain is a predictor of diabetes and cardiovascular problems.

Stress Hormone and Belly Fat
Women with central obesity (belly fat), whether obese or not, produce more of the stress hormone cortisol under repeated stress than women without belly fat.[258] This is one example of the many vicious cycles caused by chronic stress. Elevated levels of the stress hormone cortisol contribute to belly fat and increased belly fat increases the responsiveness of cortisol to stress.

Stress Stimulates Eating
High cortisol reactivity in response to stress may lead to eating after stress. One study showed that women with a high level of cortisol reactivity consumed more calories on the stressful day compared to those without high cortisol levels.[259] They also ate significantly more sweet food (refined carbohydrates).

Eating Disorders
Anorexia and bulimia are very complex eating disorders. Both conditions are associated with stressful emotional issues. If you think that you suffer from anorexia or bulimia, seek professional help right away. These conditions are quite serious. You deserve so much more than to be victimized by an eating disorder. Nothing on this earth is more important than your health and nothing is worth its ruin.

Sexual Function
Stress tends to diminish your sexual desire and responsiveness.

Fertility and Reproductive Hormones
Some women who don't menstruate have higher cortisol levels than menstruating women.[260] Cortisol (a stress hormone) also interferes with progesterone. Since cortisol and progesterone compete for common receptors in the cells, cortisol impairs progesterone activity, setting the stage for estrogen dominance and subsequent menstrual cycle irregularities. Progesterone insufficiency and estrogen dominance are characteristics of PCOS women and contribute to infertility.

The cumulative effects of long-term, "real life" stress on reproductive capacity aren't well known. However, a study recently published by the University of Michigan sheds some light on this issue.[261] Twenty four Guatemalan women were assessed for one year. The researchers discovered that increased cortisol from stress disturbed the timing of reproductive hormones during the menstrual cycle. One of the disturbances caused by high cortisol was diminished production of progesterone after ovulation, thus making it more difficult for the egg to implant into the uterus.

Effects on Pregnancy
Stress during pregnancy has been linked to a higher risk for miscarriage, premature births and lower birth weights.[262] [263] High stress in expectant mothers can influence the baby's brain and nervous system and how they react to stress.[264] Stress has a constricting effect on arteries that can interfere with normal blood flow to the placenta.

Stress also produces an inflammatory state that appears to reduce success with in-vitro fertilization (IVF).[265]

Ovarian Cysts
Stress may contribute to ovarian cysts. Experiments on rats showed that stress created ovarian cysts.[266]

PCOS and Infertility Is a Stressor

Polycystic ovarian syndrome is itself a major stressor. Most women have some version of "female perfection" that influences their self-perceptions. Most want to see themselves as healthy, attractive, fertile and "juicy." But women with PCOS report feeling abnormal, even freakish.[267] Excess hair growth, hair loss, overweight, acne, absent periods and infertility all diminish self esteem.

You may feel betrayed by your body and become stressed over feeling stigmatized and robbed of your womanhood.

But the truth is you're not a failure or freak. You are a vibrant and lovely expression of humanity and you can do much to correct PCOS with your understanding and commitment. Befriending your body, whether it meets your expectations or not, is the first step toward being successful because when you love who you are, you understand your worth and value. You become friends with yourself and can more easily lay your judgments aside. And that single embrace will relieve you of an enormous amount of stress and free up energy to persevere and succeed.

Stress Management

Control of stress is a lifelong process that contributes to better health and a greater ability to succeed with your own agenda. A good philosophy for reducing stress is Reinhold Niebuhr's elegant passage: "Grant me the serenity to accept the things I cannot change, the courage to change the things I can, and the wisdom to know the difference."

Professional Help for Stress
Some stress symptoms such as tension headaches are mild and can be managed by rest, herbal supplements or over the counter medications. However, a medical practitioner should be consulted for physical symptoms that are out of the ordinary, that increase in severity or awaken you at night. A health professional should be consulted for unmanageable stress or for serious anxiety or depression. Often, short-term therapy can resolve stress-related emotional problems.

Stress Reduction Strategy
In choosing specific strategies for dealing with stress, consider these factors:
- A combination of approaches is usually more effective than a single method.
- What works for one person does not necessarily work for another.
- Stress can be positive as well as negative. Appropriate and controllable stress provides interest and excitement. Mild stress can motivate you to greater achievement. A lack of stress invites boredom and depression.
- Chronic stress makes you vulnerable to illness. Get professional help if you have chronic or worsening physical or emotional symptoms.

Obstacles to Success

You may encounter these or other obstacles as you make efforts to manage stress.

People often succeed in reducing stress temporarily, but fall back into habitual ways of stressful thinking and behaving. Learn how to change your habits and sustain new habits that relieve stress. There are lots of books on this subject, or you might consult with a counselor or ask someone in your support group.

Another obstacle is the stress of a specific situation. The very idea of relaxation can feel threatening because it is perceived as letting down one's guard. For example, an over-demanding boss may force a subordinate into a "siege mentality" where there is no safe opportunity to fight back or express anger. The only solution is to internalize the feelings and always be "on guard." Stress builds up, but the worker has the illusion, even subconsciously, that being hyper-vigilant and always on guard is a necessary protective measure and thus does nothing to correct the problem.

Some are afraid of being perceived as selfish if they engage in stress-reducing activities that benefit only themselves. This is particularly true for women who, in most cultures, are trained to put everyone else's interests before their own. However, self-sacrifice is probably inappropriate if it makes you unhealthy, unhappy, resentful, angry or unsafe.

Some believe that certain emotional responses to stress, such as anger, are innate and unchangeable features of personality. But fortunately, you can learn to change your emotional reactions to stressful events with various therapeutic techniques.

Be aware of obstacles and finds ways to get around them. Take time to relax and clear your mind so that you can come up with some creative solutions to any obstacle.

Stress Reduction Methods

Healthy Lifestyle
Stress can be significantly reduced with a healthy lifestyle, consisting of regular exercise, healthy diet, and avoidance of excessive alcohol, caffeine and tobacco.

Create a healthy lifestyle plan. As you implement your plan, you'll develop feelings of mastery and control. Be patient with yourself and start modestly.

Cognitive-Behavioral Techniques
Cognitive-behavioral methods are an effective way to reduce chronic stress. They include identifying sources of stress, restructuring priorities, changing your response to stress, and finding methods for managing and reducing stress.

Identify Sources of Stress

Identify what is stressing you out so that you can deal with the situation. One method is to keep an informal diary of daily events that you experience as stressful and your responses to them. A few words will suffice.

Question the Sources of Stress

After you've identified the sources of your stress, ask yourself:
- Do these stressful activities meet my own goals or someone else's?
- Have I taken on tasks that I can reasonably accomplish?
- Which tasks are within my control and which ones aren't?

Restructure Priorities

Shift the balance from stress-producing to stress-reducing activities. It may not be possible to eliminate a particular source of stress. However, you can add activities that reduce your experience of stress.

Treat yourself to pleasant activities and remember that the benefits of small, daily decisions for improvement will accumulate. Ultimately they will help you turn a stressed existence into a pleasant and productive one.

Consider as many relief options as possible. A few examples:
- Take long weekends or vacations.
- If the source of stress is at home, plan times away, even if it's only an hour or two a week.
- Replace unnecessary time-consuming chores with pleasurable or interesting activities.
- Delegate some chores to others.
- Take long, aromatherapy baths by candlelight.
- On beautiful mornings, take your morning tea out in the sunshine.
- Sit quietly or meditate, close your eyes and maybe listen to your favorite music.
- Buy yourself little non-food treats, such as a beautiful scarf or flowers.
- Take yourself to a movie.
- Get regular massages.
- Enroll in a yoga, tai chi or self defense class.
- Deep breathe. Deep breaths center you, oxygenate your body and calm you.
- Make time for joy and recreation, i.e., "re-create" yourself.

Discuss Feelings

Feelings of anger or frustration that are not expressed in an acceptable way lead to hostility, helplessness and depression.

Expressing feelings does not mean venting frustration on waiters and subordinates, boring friends with emotional minutia or wallowing in self-pity. A better approach is to just talk rather than "vent" your anger. Explain and assert your needs to a trusted individual in as positive a way as possible. Direct communication may not even be necessary. Writing in a journal, writing a poem or writing a letter that is never mailed may be enough to reduce your stress considerably.

Of course expressing your feelings is only half of the communication process. Learn to listen, empathize and respond to others with understanding. Communication cannot be effective until you become a good listener.

Keep Perspective and Look for the Positive
Reversing negative ideas and focusing on positive outcomes reduces tension and helps you achieve your goals. These steps may be useful:
* Identify possible outcomes...the good, the bad and the ugly.
* Rate the likelihood of these outcomes happening.
* Envision a favorable result.
* Develop a specific plan to achieve the positive outcome.
* Recall previous situations that ended with a positive outcome.

Use Humor
Maintaining a sense of humor during difficult situations is very effective for coping with stress. Laughter releases the tension of pent-up feelings, helps keep perspective, relaxes your body and reduces stress hormones.

Reduce Job Stress
While paying lip service to stress reduction, many employers put intense pressure on individuals to behave in stress-provoking ways. Here are some ways you can deal with stress in your job:
* Seek out someone in the Human Resources department or a sympathetic manager and communicate your concerns about job stress. Work with them to improve working conditions, letting them know that productivity can be improved if some of the pressure is off.
* Establish or reinforce a network of friends at work and at home.
* Restructure priorities and eliminate unnecessary tasks.
* Focus on positive outcomes.
* If the job is unendurable, plan and execute a career change.
* Schedule daily pleasant activities and physical exercise during free time.

Establish or Strengthen a Support Network
Most people who remain happy and healthy despite life stresses have good networks of social support. Having a pet also reduces stress.

Relaxation Techniques
Relaxation reduces blood pressure, respiration, pulse rates, muscle tension and emotional strains. Relaxation techniques include yoga, massage and progressive muscle relaxation.

Deep-Breathing Exercises
During stress, breathing becomes shallow and rapid. A deep breath is an automatic and effective technique for winding down.

Inhale through your nose slowly and deeply to the count of ten. Make sure that your stomach and abdomen expand but your chest does not rise up. Exhale through your nose, slowly and completely, also to the count of ten. To help quiet your mind, concentrate fully on breathing and counting through each cycle. Repeat five to ten times and make a habit of doing the exercise several times each day, even when you're not feeling stressed.

Muscle Relaxation
Muscle relaxation techniques, often combined with deep breathing, are easy to learn and very useful for getting to sleep. In the beginning have a friend or partner check for tension by lifting an arm and dropping it; the arm should fall freely. Practice makes this procedure more effective.

After lying down in a comfortable position without crossing the limbs, concentrate on each part of your body. Maintain a slow, deep breathing pattern throughout this exercise. Tense each muscle as tightly as possible for a count of five to ten and then release it completely. Experience the muscle as totally relaxed and heavy. Begin with the top of your head and progress downward, focusing on all the major muscle groups in your body.

Meditation
The goal of meditation is to quiet the mind (essentially, to relax thought). Meditation reduces stress hormone levels, heart rate and blood pressure.

Some recommend meditating for up to 20 minutes in the morning after awakening and then again in early evening before dinner. Even once a day is helpful.

It can be difficult to quiet the mind so don't be discouraged by lack of immediate results.

Mindfulness Meditation
Mindfulness focuses on breathing. Sit upright with the spine straight, either cross-legged or sitting on a firm chair with both feet on the floor, uncrossed. With eyes closed or gently looking a few feet ahead, observe the exhalation of the breath. If the mind wanders, simply note it as a fact and return to the out breath. It may be helpful to imagine your thoughts as clouds gently drifting away.

Transcendental Meditation
TM uses a mantra (a specific chanting sound). The meditator repeats the word silently, letting thoughts come and go.

Mini-Meditation
This involves heightening awareness of the immediate surrounding environment. Choose a routine activity when you are alone and really concentrate on doing the activity. For example: while washing dishes concentrate on the feel of the water and dishes. Allow your mind to wander to any immediate sensory experience (sounds outside the window, smells from the stove, colors in the room). If your mind begins to think about the past or future, abstractions or worries, redirect it gently back. This redirection of brain activity from your thoughts and worries to your senses disrupts the stress response and prompts relaxation.

Biofeedback

Here's how biofeedback works. Electric leads are taped to your head. You are encouraged to relax. Brain waves are measured and an audible signal is emitted when alpha waves are detected, a frequency that indicates a state of deep relaxation. By repeating the process, you begin to associate the sound with the relaxed state and learn to achieve relaxation by yourself.

Massage Therapy

Massage therapy slows down the heart and relaxes the body. Most massage involves the manipulation of muscles, such as Swedish massage. Shiatsu is a different form of massage that applies intense pressure to parts of your body. It can be painful but people report deep relaxation afterward. Reflexology manipulates acupuncture points in your hands and feet to promote relaxation.

Recite Poetry

Hearing the rhythmic sounds of poetry appears to have a calming influence and reduce your heart rate, according to one study.[268] Any kind of enjoyable reading reduces stress.

14.3 Emotional Factors

PCOS can be an emotional drain, wearing away at your self confidence and body image. Women report feeling unworthy, unwomanly, inferior, defective, abnormal, depressed, scared, confused and embarrassed. Perhaps most difficult is feeling out of control, because in spite of everything you do and how hard you try, your PCOS and infertility problems stay with you.

Judgments and the attitudes of others (real or imagined) are an additional burden. Some cannot understand why you can't lose weight or can't become pregnant. And it can be heartbreaking to see your friends have babies when you can't. Others may not find you feminine and attractive because of thin scalp hair, excess facial hair, acne or body size.

The challenge is that you want to be normal like everyone else, but you're not able to. Over time, discouragement, resentment or self-anger can set in.

So let's begin with making one thing clear — the emotions that arise from self disapproval are toxic and *don't serve you in any way*. Does this mean we're going to tell you that you have to learn to like, even love, yourself? Well...yes, it does. And you're probably thinking, "They've got to be kidding!" We're not. The first step toward dealing with polycystic ovary syndrome is to unconditionally accept yourself as you are right now. Self-acceptance is the foundation for constructing a new perspective on your life and taking action to gain a measure of control over PCOS.

Let's explore some of the emotional factors of PCOS and discuss how you can move yourself to a place where you clearly see possibilities for improving the outcome of your health challenge.

Infertility

For some women, infertility is not a major issue. For others, it's crisis. If you fall into the latter group, we recommend you consult with a counselor if you're:
- plagued with feelings of sadness or guilt
- experiencing severe mood swings, high anxiety or depression.
- isolating yourself socially and are losing interest in everyday activities
- having trouble sleeping
- obsessed with your infertility
- turning to drugs or alcohol
- experiencing increased problems in your significant relationships
- having thoughts of suicide

A good counselor can work with you to help you realize your worth and reclaim your self confidence. Support groups are also a healthy option because they help you see that you're not alone.

Body Image and Cultural Expectations

Body image is how you see your physical self and how you feel about how you look. It is part of your self-esteem. There are many cultural expectations about how a woman should look and behave. How you should dress, act, look and wear your hair is dictated (with varying degrees of success) by trends, fashion, culture, religion or the community you live in.

Some of these cultural values may suggest that being overweight, having a hairy body or not having a head of full, lustrous hair is unacceptable.

When you're unable to conform to the pressures of others' expectations, fear of rejection, failure or abandonment can creep in. Under these circumstances, self confidence diminishes. Self confidence, after all, is tied to success, and we may be feeling quite unsuccessful.

What to Do?

Take a look at your expectations of yourself. There are some things you can do and some things you can't. Everyone has limitations and no one is perfect, regardless of how it may appear. Accepting who you are, including strengths and faults, is the beginning of emotional health.

When you value yourself you're better able to give priority to your own happiness and needs. And you're better able to forgive your body its idiosyncrasies and move forward with increased self respect.

You care about and value who you are. You care about your health and happiness and act accordingly. You recognizes both illness and health as part of life and don't buckle under the judgments of others. Improved self esteem reduces anxiety about being unlovable, unacceptable or unworthy. You no longer see yourself through the lens of external opinion.

How to improve self esteem and self confidence:
- Improve your knowledge
- Upgrade negative beliefs to positive beliefs
- Replace failure-oriented behaviors with success-oriented behaviors
- Let go of the concepts that don't serve your overall well-being
- Release perfectionism and accept "what is"
- Practice forgiveness of self and others

Negativity

Negativity of any kind drains your personal power and creates self-limiting beliefs. Here are a few ways to determine whether you're caught in a web of negativity:

- You allow someone else to define who you are rather than creating your own definitions and sticking to them.
- You allow people around you to disrespect you or to treat you badly (whether they intend this or not). You let them dump their disappointment or guilt on you. (Instead, show them how to become supportive of you.).
- Nothing appeals to you. Your passion for life appears dead.
- The words you use to describe yourself are downbeat, pejorative and harmful.

Remember that you're at the center of your own life…the star in your own movie. Ultimately you're responsible for shaping it, creating it and producing it so that it is satisfactory to you. And although PCOS presents real and serious challenges, you can still create a masterpiece.

Emotional Eating

There's a big difference between emotional eating and eating in response to physical hunger, but people often have trouble making the distinction.

There are a number of emotions that generate eating behaviors in the absence of true hunger. Stress and the emotions of sadness, depression, loneliness, anger, boredom, frustration, nervousness, anxiety, hopelessness, exhaustion and feeling out of control are all known activators of non-physical hunger.

If you think you may be an emotional eater, it's well worth the effort to keep a daily journal of stressors, emotional reactions and eating behaviors. Over time, you'll have a good awareness of what causes you to eat and you can take steps to deal with those causes.

Emotional vs. Physical Hunger

Emotional hunger often begins in the mind, with cravings or obsessive thoughts about certain specific foods or tastes, e.g., bread, pasta, rice, salt, chocolate or sweets. It often comes on suddenly and may be associated with an upsetting emotion. Emotional hunger demands to be satisfied immediately and has an almost automatic pattern to it, as if someone else is in charge. Emotional eating doesn't stop with fullness because it's not about hunger — it's about becoming anesthetized to the emotion that is so uncomfortable. Emotional eating often concludes with regret, remorse and self judgment.

Physical hunger, on the other hand, begins with an empty feeling or rumbling in the stomach that comes on gradually several hours after your last meal. It asks to be satisfied before making you lightheaded or dropping your energy level, but does not demand that you let go of everything right now and go get pizza. In fact, real physical hunger is satisfied when you consume healthy food because it stems from the body's desire to have proper fuel and nourishment. Healthy satiation of natural, physical hunger does not bring on guilt but rather it creates a feeling of satisfaction and well-being.

How to Deal with Emotional Hunger

Recognition.
The first step is to recognize what's going on. Use a daily journal or other tools to help you identify the dynamics of your eating patterns.

Education.
Next, gather as much information about healthy eating behavior and healthy foods as you can. Seek to understand the nature of emotional hunger, as well as understanding how hormonal imbalances can increase appetite. Once you have sufficient information and understanding, you can lay out your action plan for dealing with your hunger and appetite.

Action.
Then take action. Carry out your plan.

If you're looking for ideas to help you avoid emotional eating when you're not actually hungry, consider these:
- Call someone
- Take a walk
- Exercise
- Stretch
- Do Yoga or Tai Chi
- Meditate
- Clean
- Read
- Write in your journal
- Walk the dog
- Run an errand
- Take an aromatherapy bath
- Dance
- Do something nice for yourself
- Do something nice for someone else

The list is endless. Make up your own. Write down all the things you love to do or could do and keep it where you can see it. The next time you feel hungry, become conscious of your hunger and give yourself a 10 minute "time out" to focus on your body so that you can tune in to why you want to eat and whether or not this hunger is physical. This is a supreme act of self respect. Once you've determined whether the hunger is emotional or physical, you can then act appropriately.

Evaluation.
Finally, evaluate and adjust your actions in a compassionate way.

Remember that Rome wasn't built in a day. You developed eating habits as a child, long before you had any conscious control over your life. Retraining takes time, patience and understanding. Everyone's process is individual so don't compare yourself to others or to some external timeline. There is also no need to undermine your progress with any blame, self-hatred, impatience or hopelessness. What you need most is your own approval, even in the face of setbacks. And don't forget to celebrate your successes!

Believe in Yourself

Control of emotional hunger is not an issue of willpower; it is an issue of understanding and self acceptance. You are learning to recognize *real* hunger from *false* hunger…and that is no small task, particularly if you've lived your life not knowing the difference. But now you know. Keep in mind that inside each of us is a person trying to do the best possible thing. If you remain positive as you befriend yourself, the rewards will be rich and many.

14.4 Liver Health

The liver is possibly the most overlooked and under-appreciated organ in the body. You'll often hear about the ovaries, thyroid, adrenals or hypothalamus. Rarely do you hear anyone talk about your liver.

A healthy liver is essential to recovering your hormonal balance, maintaining blood sugar control, improving your fertility and performing other work that will keep your PCOS symptoms under control.

The liver performs several hundred different functions. Below are a few of its primary functions.

Detoxification

The liver is the primary organ responsible for detoxifying hormones such as estrogen, environmental chemicals, drugs and any other toxic substance. The liver takes these fat-soluble substances and makes them water-soluble so that the kidneys can excrete them in the urine.

Normalization of Blood Fats

The liver is responsible for the synthesis of cholesterol and triglycerides. Since the liver can create cholesterol, elevated serum cholesterol may occur as a result of liver malfunction, regardless of the amount of cholesterol in the diet. Abnormalities in the ability of the liver to normalize blood fats can lead to increased cardiovascular disease.

Synthesis and Normalization of Serum Protein

The liver is responsible for metabolizing protein fragments and amino acids (the building blocks of proteins) that are absorbed from the intestines. It takes various amino acids and creates proteins out of them, according to the needs of the body.

The liver produces albumin, which circulates in the blood and provides an amino acid pool source from which other tissues of the body can ultimately get the amino acids essential for their function and protein metabolism.

The liver can break down protein so that pieces of it can be burned as fuel, as needed.

The liver also has an internal mechanism called the "Cori cycle" that normalizes blood sugar.

Manufacture of Bile

The liver manufactures bile, using cholesterol as raw material. Bile is used for the emulsification of dietary fats and oils for their proper absorption and assimilation. Bile is also necessary for the absorption of the fat-soluble vitamins A, D, E, and K.

Elevated serum cholesterol may reflect a reduced ability of the liver to convert cholesterol into bile salts. Since bile is stored in the gallbladder, low liver production of bile means the gallbladder will have less bile to help with fat digestion. The result is reduced absorption of essential fats and fat-soluble vitamins.

Synthesis and Storage of Glycogen

Glycogen is the storage form of glucose (blood sugar). Glycogen is stored in the liver in order to stabilize blood sugar levels. The glycogen stored after eating is released as glucose into the bloodstream as needed between meals or when you are exercising. Remember that the preferred fuel for your brain is glucose. Your brain is very active and requires a large amount of fuel. It may use up as much as 25% of your entire glucose supply. So the liver is a good fuel reserve for your brain.

People with liver glycogen storage problems may experience insulin fluctuations or hypoglycemia (low blood sugar).

The liver creates and stores chromium in a form known as "glucose tolerance factor" or GTF. GTF is secreted into the bloodstream to sensitize cells to insulin after a meal rich in carbohydrates (sugars and starches). This feature of the liver is important for those of you who may have insulin resistance or hyperinsulinism.

Your Liver Senses Types of Fat

There is a very intricate and not fully understood relationship between your liver and the type of fats you eat.

A diet that provides 2-5% of calories as highly unsaturated omega-6 or omega-3 fats appears to inhibit fat production by the liver and stimulate the liver to burn fat. This process results in a reduction of triglycerides (fats in the blood).

The liver appears to use unsaturated fatty acid levels as a sensor to determine whether fats are to be stored or oxidized (burned).[269] In this way highly unsaturated fats may function to reduce the risk of developing fatty liver degeneration and insulin resistance, according to a study at Louisiana State University.

Liver Lab Tests

It's hard to tell if your liver is operating sub-optimally. Many symptoms of liver malfunction are non-specific, meaning that the liver cannot be positively identified as the source of the symptom.

One easy way to determine if you have a liver problem is with a common blood chemistry test. Most blood chemistries will include measurements of two liver enzymes, "ALT" and "AST." When liver cells die, they release these enzymes into the bloodstream. So, if you have lots of liver cells dying, these enzymes will be higher than normal on your blood test. Elevated liver enzymes suggest some kind of liver pathology.

On the other hand, it's possible that your liver enzymes may be at the low end of normal, or even below the normal range. In this case, you may have an overly sluggish liver.

Fatty Liver Degeneration

You may have a liver that is sluggish because, for a variety of reasons, cholesterol and triglycerides are accumulating in the liver and getting in the way of proper liver function.

Fatty liver degeneration can occur if you have high levels of cholesterol and triglycerides, if you eat a high-fat diet, and if you are overweight.

One example of fatty liver impairment is the liver's reduced ability to remove insulin from the bloodstream. When the insulin is not removed, it remains high in the blood and may contribute to insulin resistance and the other insulin-related disorders you are experiencing such as infertility. Remember that insulin will keep you in "fat storage" mode so that you will continue to store calories as fat in your liver, in your belly and throughout your body. Of course, this is a vicious cycle, because the high insulin leads to further fatty liver degeneration.

PCOS diet designed to ease the fat load on your liver by providing healthy fats in moderation and by providing nutrients that the liver needs to do its work. The PCOS diet also is free of toxins and unhealthy foods that cause the liver to work overtime.

14.5 Your Health Care Team

To deal effectively with PCOS and infertility, you may need to assemble a team of health professionals to help you develop a treatment plan that will yield good results.

There are several reasons why you may need to work with more than one health practitioner:
- PCOS is not well understood by many physicians.
- PCOS and infertility are often quite difficult to treat.
- Medical knowledge has expanded so fast that no one individual "knows it all." The general practitioner is ill-equipped to effectively deal with PCOS and infertility.
- Modern health care is divided into compartments called "specialties." Specialists tend to look at a health problem only from the perspective of his or her specialty.

Your health care team may consist of one or more of the following:
- Medical doctor - family doctor
- Endocrinologist
- Gynecologist
- Licensed naturopathic physician
- Oriental medical doctor
- Acupuncturist
- Psychologist
- Personal fitness trainer

Components of a Diagnostic Workup

You should start with a thorough diagnostic workup by an experienced physician so that the nature and causes of your unique health problems can be discovered. The workup would include:
- Your complete medical history, including a review of past and present treatments
- Medical history of your family
- Physical exam and functional assessment of body systems
- Laboratory tests as indicated by the interview, medical history, and exam findings

Taking Time to Listen

During the initial interview, the physician must take the time to listen to everything you have to say and answer the questions you ask.

If the physician will not listen or take time to address your concerns, it is unlikely that a truly effective treatment program can be developed. This is because it takes time to elicit from you all of the important and relevant information that is required to accurately identify what the problems and issues are. The information that is obtained from this interview is the foundation for an effective treatment plan.

Secondly, the doctor must answer your questions and listen to your concerns. This is necessary in order to build a strong bond of trust and understanding. Without this bond, there is little to support the implementation of the proposed treatment plan.

Lab Tests

Laboratory testing may be fairly extensive, depending on your medical history, current health status and previous blood tests.

A good basic screening for PCOS or infertility would include:
- Multi-channel blood chemistry panel, including lipid profile and complete blood count
- 2-hour glucose tolerance test including insulin levels
- LH (luteinizing hormone) - FSH (follicle stimulating hormone) ratio
- Testosterone
- DHEA (dehydroepiandrosterone)
- SHBG (sex hormone binding globulin)
- Androstenedione
- Prolactin
- Thyroid panel

In addition, there is an extensive array of more in-depth testing that can be done as needed. What is tested will depend on what your specific needs are and your health care budget.

Your Treatment Plan

After a careful review of your lab test results and other findings, your doctor should recommend a well-thought-out and comprehensive plan for successfully managing PCOS and increasing your fertility. The doctor should take the time to review and explain your lab test findings.

Your treatment plan should include recommendations for medications, diet, exercise, stress management, emotional support and other natural therapies such as acupuncture or naturopathic medicine. Any potential side effects of medications should be explained.

The treatment plan should focus on your entire body and health, not just on how to make your ovaries behave differently.

PCOS is a systemic disorder. It is not very amenable to a piecemeal approach. For example, simply prescribing birth control pills does not always yield lasting, satisfactory results. We believe that a more comprehensive approach is appropriate.

14.6 Check for Food Allergies

An allergic reaction is an inappropriate immune reaction to an otherwise harmless substance. Allergens can be environmental, chemical, or food-based. Common allergens include dust mites, pollen, animal dander and certain foods. Allergens can be absorbed into the body through the skin, respiratory or gastrointestinal tract.

Allergens are proteins, protein fragments or other very small substances that the body identifies as antigenic or "foreign" and marks for elimination by your immune system. The immune system reaction against an antigenic substance is known as a hypersensitive or allergic reaction. These allergic reactions may produce symptoms ranging from almost unnoticeable to life threatening.

In this book, we're concerned about food allergies, although an allergy to anything can be a factor that worsens PCOS symptoms. Allergenic substances lead to inflammation. Chronic inflammation creates substantial oxidative stress, the production of unstable free radical molecules that damage cells. Chronic inflammation also releases a variety of alarm messengers that spread throughout your body and disturb your hormonal balance and organ function.

Compared to normal women, those with PCOS already have a higher level of inflammation. Exposure to allergenic substances only adds fuel to the inflammatory fires. You want to reduce inflammation, not increase it. So avoidance of any allergens is highly desirable, including foods to which you are allergic.

Types of Food Allergies

There are four types of allergic reactions. The two types you are most likely to encounter are Type I and Type IV.

Type I reactions are immediate, resulting in anaphylactic reactions within minutes of exposure to an antigen. If you have a Type I allergy, you will certainly know it. For example, you might break out in hives when you eat strawberries. Or your throat will swell and cut off your air supply if you eat shrimp. People with a Type I food allergy know what they are allergic to and they avoid those foods.

A Type IV allergy is much different. Type IV reactions, known as delayed hypersensitivity reactions, appear 24 to 72 hours after exposure to an antigenic substance. For example, if you have a Type IV allergy to milk, you could have a glass of milk on Monday and not have any symptoms appear until Wednesday. You may think the cause of your allergic symptoms is something you ate on Wednesday when actually it was the milk you drank on Monday. Therefore, a Type IV food allergy is difficult to detect.

Diagnosis of Food Allergies

Most doctors are not familiar with diagnosing Type IV allergies and therefore they are under-recognized and overlooked. It is thought by some researchers that Type IV food allergies are more common than we think. We agree with this assessment.

When doctors suspect an allergy, they will typically order a "scratch test" or intradermal test. These tests involve exposing your skin to specific allergens. If an inflammatory response is noted on your skin, you are deemed allergic to the substance that was applied to that area of your skin. The limitation of these tests is that they are only useful for identifying Type I allergies, not Type IV.

The only way to identify a Type IV allergen is with a blood test. The recommended test is called an ELISA (Enzyme Linked Immunosorbent Assay). It measures your reactions to various panels of foods, usually 50 or 100 of the most common foods.

After allergic foods are identified, the best treatment is to avoid the offending foods. After a period of perhaps six months, you might be able to reintroduce them into your diet. However, there may be some foods that you will always be allergic to and those foods should be avoided indefinitely.

We suggest you get an allergy test done so that any offending foods can be removed from your diet. Anything that you can do to reduce inflammatory stress in your body is a step in the right direction.

14.7 Measure Your Progress

It is well documented that what we hold to be true, our 'world view' and our relationship to that worldview, provides the fertile ground for developing our sense of what is possible. Although old habits die hard, it is certainly within your power to change your self concept, your perennial attitudes, your habits and your future vision even if you've held them for a long time.

Again, this is not a question of will power. Change relies heavily on the process of self-reflection, a process that enables us to view ourselves more clearly. When we are self reflective, we can evaluate what works and what doesn't; what limits us and what moves us closer to our desired outcome. We can ascertain if what we've 'always' done, or believed to be true, does, in actual fact, work; whether it is congruent with what we want as a desired outcome.

The information we gather through self-reflection acts as a rudder. It enables us to improve by eliminating what doesn't work, setting and achieving goals and measuring our progress toward those goals. The result is a greater sense of self control and stronger self esteem.

How does one become self-reflective? The best way we know is journal writing. The reason is that we can think in multiple channels simultaneously, but we can only write and record in one. Writing helps us focus. Recording what is *actually* happening gets us out of the lofty realm of wishes, fantasies and ideas and places us squarely 'on the ground,' with a real map that we can look at and see where we've been and where we'll end up if we keep going in the same direction.

Keep a Food Journal

A food journal is a great way to become aware of what you're eating and how much. If you're like us, you may tend to eat more than you think, especially if you are busy, distracted or under stress.

An awareness of exactly what you are eating and drinking is a powerful tool to help you improve your diet and thus reduce PCOS-related problems.

We suggest you keep a log of everything you put into your mouth for one week. It's not as hard as it may sound. Just keep a small notebook in your bag or your pocket and write down everything you eat as you go about your busy day. After a week, review what you've eaten and compare it to the recommendations in this book. Without judging or criticizing yourself, carefully review where you can make positive changes to improve the quality of your diet.

You may discover that you --
- are eating more food than you thought
- are eating foods that are not very healthy
- have erratic eating patterns (skipping meals)
- snack unconsciously or excessively
- are eating unbalanced meals (not enough vegetables and fruit)
- are eating more refined or convenience foods that pack more calories than you realized

A food journal provides you with an honest reality check that can guide you to make smart, small changes over time. By increasing your awareness of what you eat and drink, you provide yourself with a basis for changing dietary habits that don't work for your body. Once you change and improve your habits, you will be healthier.

A Word about Change

Don't try to change too many things at once. Start with one or two elements that capture your interest. Consistently stick with the new habit for at least 21 days because it takes that long to change a habit. After the new habit is ingrained, you can move on to changing another food or behavior habit. Over a year's time, you will have made significant changes.

Reward Yourself

There are many ways to reward yourself. And rewarding yourself positively (with non-edible delights) serves to reinforce your efforts. Look at it as an act of self love. Taking a vacation, going on retreat, buying yourself something special like a spa membership or a new pair of shoes...all are harmless ways of celebrating a goal well won and a job well done. Rewards needn't be expensive. They should simply bring you joy.

Keep Track of Your Physical Changes

It's also important to keep track of your physical changes so that you know where you are improving and where you many need more help.

Until regular exercise is an ingrained habit, we recommend you keep track of how often and for how long you exercise. If you are overweight, an exercise journal can be especially helpful — see if you can incrementally increase the frequency, duration and intensity of your exercise.

In addition to exercise, you should keep track of how your body shape is changing as you gain muscle and shed extra fat. Measure and record these items once a week:
- Neck
- Bust at the nipple line

- Upper arm, 3 inches away from your armpit
- Waist
- Hips
- Thigh, 6 inches away from your crotch (3 or 4 inches if you are less than 5'4" tall; the place doesn't matter, just measure the same place each time)

Notice that we are not focusing solely on keeping track of your weight. That's because many women have a strong aversion to seeing that number on the scale because of the negative judgments of others about how much you weigh. It's hard to understand how you can feel so good, be so fit and still weigh something more than the magical 118 to 125 pounds!

The number on the scale and our relation to it is complicated by a great deal of inaccurate mythology and emotional distress. Tracking your physical dimensions will give you all the information you need to monitor your progress as you make healthy changes in your diet and exercise.

You do not have to weigh yourself unless or until you are peacefully curious about what that number is. We hope you will track your weight only when you understand what it means — and doesn't mean — about your health as well as your value as a person.

Some women have found that weighing at the same time every day, first thing in the morning, is a useful learning tool. Weight will fluctuate by 1 to 3 pounds overnight, for a variety of reasons — hormonal cycles, salt and water intake, exercise intensity, and amount and composition of food recently consumed. If you are paying close attention to your food choices and exercise habits, you can watch these fluctuations and learn what works for you in what way.

If you use a specific program of eating and journal your choices, you can have a valuable learning experience instead of outrage and despair when you see unexpected weight gain. "Aha," you might think, "I know exactly what I ate and drank yesterday, the same sort of choice that has led to steady weight loss up till now — so this gain is related to something other than my food, drink and exercise." Or, you might have the occasion to think "Wow! So that's what happens when I have a piece of birthday cake and 2 glasses of wine! Carbohydrates call up insulin, which encourages water retention and by golly, there it is right on my scale!" And back you go to your regular program and watching the scale cha-cha up occasionally and eventually ever-downward, as you maintain your new healthy habits over time.

After you have settled at the weight and dimensions you are happy with, daily weighing can help you stay there. A recent study followed 291 people (80% of whom were women) who had lost an average of 44 pounds for 18 months afterward. 68% of the participants who did not weigh themselves regained five or more pounds in that time. Only 39% of those who did weigh themselves daily regained five pounds or more in the following year and a half. Staying alert to small weight increases allows you to use your enhanced self-knowledge to adjust any behaviors that may be causing you to regain.

Keep Track of Your Lab Data

Whenever you get a blood test, always get a copy for your personal records, even if you don't understand everything the report says. Your doctor will tell you which findings are "abnormal."

On a common blood chemistry tests that are taken from time to time, you can watch for long-term trends in fasting glucose and triglycerides. These two blood markers may be high in women with PCOS, especially if overweight. With the passing of time, these two markers should be declining or at least be stable.

If you see a blood test value you don't understand, ask your doctor, or get the answer on the Web.

Section 15

Nutritional Supplements

15.1 Why You Need Nutritional Supplements

If you think you don't need dietary supplements, read this chapter. It may have implications for your future health.

Finally, after more than 50 years, leading medical journals now recommend all adults take multivitamins. Both the *New England Journal of Medicine*[270] and the *Journal of the American Medical Association*[271] [272] have concluded that:

- "Most people do not consume an optimal amount of all vitamins by diet alone."
- "Inadequate intake of several vitamins has been linked to chronic diseases, including coronary heart disease, cancer and osteoporosis."
- "Suboptimal folic acid levels, along with suboptimal levels of vitamins B6 and B12, are a risk factor for cardiovascular disease, neural tube defects, and colon and breast cancer; low levels of vitamin D contribute to osteoporosis and bone fracture; and low levels of the antioxidant vitamins (vitamins A, E and C) may increase risk for several chronic diseases."
- "It appears prudent for all adults to take vitamin supplements."

A large body of research has demonstrated that the nutrients found in dietary supplements reduce your risk of chronic disease, improve quality of life, and increase longevity.

Why You Can't Depend on Food Alone for Essential Nutrition

Listed below are 22 reasons why you cannot depend on food alone to provide you with all of the nutrition you need to stay healthy.

Reason #1. Overfed and undernourished. The average American is overfed and undernourished. It's no secret. Just look around you. Most people are gaining weight. Even kids are overweight these days. You or someone you know has a chronic disorder of some kind.

If you're like most Americans, you're consuming fabricated convenience foods high in calories but low in food value (nutrition). This type of diet leads to "subclinical" or marginal deficiencies that lead to vague health complaints such as nervousness, listlessness, recurring minor infections, general aches and pains, difficulty concentrating, irritability, depression, muscle weakness, fatigue, insomnia, and just not feeling right.

A large body of research has demonstrated that most Americans are not getting what they need from their diet. For example, in one recent U.S. Dept. of Agriculture survey of 20,000 people, not a single person was consuming adequate levels of all the vitamins and minerals. In this study, the percentage of Americans were found to be deficient as follows: 90% in vitamin B6, 75% in magnesium, 68% in calcium, 57% in iron, 50% in vitamin A, 45% in vitamin B1, 41% in vitamin C, 34% in vitamin B2, 34% in vitamin B12....and the list goes on.

There are literally hundreds of medical studies to suggest it's a virtual certainty that you and every member of your family are deficient in one or more essential nutrients.

Reason #2: Soil depletion. Modern mass-production agriculture depletes nutrients from the soil without replenishing them. The application of synthetic fertilizers stimulates the growth of beautiful-looking plants. However, the nutrient content is missing.

So when you bite into that healthy salad or slice of whole-wheat bread, you're getting less nutrition today than from the identical foods grown in the same soil fifty years ago.

Reason #3: Commercial food processing. Much of the food you eat is processed in one way or another. When foods are processed, they are exposed to heat, light, oxygen, or drastic change in temperature or humidity. This exposure causes the destruction of vital but fragile nutrients. Examples of processing include baking, extruding, milling, grinding, boiling, cooking, recombining, spray-drying, etc.

Reason #4: Food storage and transportation. All foods deteriorate as they age. This is a problem for the food industry because many foods are shipped over great distances. Therefore chemicals are added to preserve foods and give them a longer "shelf life." Unfortunately, in spite of chemicals, the nutrient content of foods decline over time, even though they may look the same.

Even fresh fruits or vegetables may be sprayed, gassed or fumigated in order to make them look "ripe" and "fresh." So what looks healthy isn't necessarily as healthy as you may think.

Reason #5: Preparation and cooking of foods. Many people eat out or bring something home from the market that is already cooked. Even if you prepare your meals at home, most of your food is probably cooked, not raw. Here's the problem: the more you cook a food, the less its nutrient value.

Of course, there are some foods, such as grains and dried legumes that you have to cook because they're inedible when raw. You're obviously not going to eat a bowl of raw rice. However, if you overcook rice, you lose nutrients.

Reason #6: Home storage of food. Have you looked in your refrigerator lately? How long has that head of lettuce been in there? What about those leftovers from three days ago? Refrigeration does slow down the deterioration of food, but it certainly does not stop it. As every day goes by, whatever is in your refrigerator is losing its nutritional value.

Some people will eat something out of the refrigerator that is three weeks old, or something from the pantry that is a year old. By this time, some vital nutrients have been completely lost.

Reason #7: Food irradiation. Exposing foods to gamma rays, x-rays or other radiation extends their shelf life by destruction of microorganisms, inhibition of sprouting and delay of ripening. Some meats, chicken, and vegetables are irradiated. Foods served in restaurants or schools may be irradiated. The problem with irradiation is that vital nutrients, especially antioxidants and fat-soluble vitamins, are destroyed. There's no label to tell you if a food has been irradiated.

Reason #8: Pesticides in foods. A pesticide is a poison. A little bit of pesticide will kill a bug. A lot of pesticide will kill you. Most foods contain pesticides. Even organic produce contains pesticides, although a lot less than regular produce. Pesticides may be applied to the soil, to the growing plant, or to the food while in storage or shipment.

Keep in mind that you can't see, smell or taste these pesticides. So you have no way of knowing if what you're eating contains pest poisons. But your body knows. Some pesticides can accumulate in the body and cause problems. Your body has to deal with the problem by expending valuable vitamins and minerals to detoxify and try to eliminate these poisons.

Reason #9: Genetically modified foods. Millions of acres of genetically modified corn, cotton and potatoes have been planted in the U.S. (Cotton is mentioned here because cottonseed oil is found in many processed foods, and cottonseed meal is fed to cattle.) These foods, which are now in our food supply, have been engineered to produce a naturally occurring pesticide that is supposedly toxic only to insects.

There are no long-term human studies to indicate that genetically modified foods are safe. However, rats fed genetically modified potatoes had increased intestinal infections, reduced immunity, and reduced weight of intestine, pancreas, kidneys, liver, lungs and brain. Since you may be unknowingly consuming genetically modified or irradiated foods, you would need dietary supplementation to offset the invisible but potentially negative effects of such foods.

Reason #10: Environmental pollution. We dump nearly six billion pounds of chemicals into our environment every year. While some of it ends up in our food, much of it is in our air and water. If you breathe air and drink water, you are ingesting chemical pollution. Medical research has clearly established that environmental chemicals contribute to degenerative diseases.

You have no choice but to eat food, drink water, and breathe air. Therefore, you will need dietary supplements to help you process and detoxify the pollution entering your body every day.

Reason #11: Bioaccumulation of pollution in animal foods. There are certain "persistent" pollutants that tend to accumulate in any living thing, whether animal or plant. The higher up the food chain, the greater the accumulation. Take swordfish for example. Swordfish is known to have high levels of mercury, a toxic metal.

The problem starts when small bait fish eat organic material that contains mercury. They metabolize the organic material but retain the mercury. Small predatory fish then eat the bait fish, thus inheriting their accumulated mercury. The more bait fish they eat, the more mercury they accumulate. Finally a swordfish comes along and eats a bunch of small predatory fish and picks up a load of mercury. So a big swordfish can gather a lot of mercury over time. But the swordfish is not the end of the chain. You are! You eat the swordfish and now all that accumulated mercury is stored in *your* body.

Swordfish is only one example out of hundreds. The point is, you're at the top of the entire food chain on earth. Therefore, you unknowingly accumulate heavy metals and chemical pollutants which are proven to be detrimental to your health. If you consume animal foods, you need dietary supplements to help you handle the pollutants they contain.

Reason #12: "Energy" pollution. Energy pollution invisibly burdens your body. The form of energy pollution you're familiar with is radioactive fallout, like that from nuclear testing in Nevada which caused an increase in cancers downwind from the test site. Another, less well known form of energy pollution is altered magnetic fields from electrical motors and circuits and all kinds of energy transmissions (microwave, radar, cell phone, etc.). Not only can energy pollution destroy or damage cells directly, but also it causes a stress reaction in the body which leads to hormonal imbalances. For example, energy pollution reduces your levels of melatonin, an essential hormone. Once again, dietary supplements are a method to assist your body to compensate for another type of pollution from which there is no escape.

Reason #13: Genetic weaknesses. Each of us is genetically and biochemically unique. But none of us is perfect. We all have some kind of genetic weakness. For example, you might have a genetic abnormality in methionine metabolism called homocystinuria (methionine is an amino acid required to make your body function). In this case, taking large doses of vitamin B6 is a way to compensate for this weakness. There are hundreds if not thousands of possible genetic abnormalities. Many of them can be minimized with dietary supplementation.

Reason #14: Chronic Stress. "Stress" occurs when your body has a "fight or flight" response to any situation. Most of the time, you're not aware of it. Stress can come from anywhere at any time. It could be a barking dog, a disagreeable boss, a car that needs repair, an unpaid bill, a relationship that isn't working, or living alone. Anything at all. You become so accustomed to stress that you consciously tune it out — but your body doesn't.

When stress is repeated over and over, it is called chronic stress, which seriously depletes your body of energy and vital reserves. Chronic stress produces hormones that have a long-term weakening effect on your body that accelerates the aging process and leads to chronic degenerative disease. Supplements reduce the detrimental effects of chronic stress.

Reason #15: Your lifestyle. How you behave may increase your need for supplementation. For example, smoking or drinking alcohol to excess dramatically saps your reserves of vital nutrients. In both cases, dietary supplementation is not an option -- it's a requirement.

On the other hand, if you're an avid mountain climber or high-performance athlete, you use up nutrients faster than the average person. The same is true if you work in a physically demanding occupation. Your performance will be improved with dietary supplementation.

Reason #16: GI problems. Any kind of digestive or gastrointestinal problem will diminish your absorption of vitamins, minerals, protein, essential fats, and plant substances required to maintain a healthy body. Irritable bowel syndrome, colitis, Crohn's disease, or chronic diarrhea hurt your ability to absorb nutrients. Ditto for bacterial, viral, yeast or parasitic infections. Food allergies are notorious for causing GI problems. In short, any inflammation in your GI tract means trouble. Therefore, you will need supplements to help you deal with the inflammation, as well as to increase the amount of essential nutrients you are consuming and absorbing.

Reason #17: Weak digestion. Heartburn, bloat after eating, burping, or gas may suggest you have an impaired ability to digest your food. If you can't digest your food, it can't be absorbed into your body. Supplementary digestive aids may be indicated.

Reason #18: Getting older. Medical studies have proven that you lose your digestive power as you get older. By the time you're "elderly," you have a serious problem that can only be corrected by supplementation.

In addition, studies have shown that many elderly people eat less well than they did in earlier years. In this case, dietary supplements can augment an otherwise inadequate diet.

Reason #19: Teenager. It's no secret that adolescents eat and drink things that are very unhealthy, i.e., "junk food." This is no way to nourish a maturing body. Most teenagers need dietary supplementation.

Reason #20: Chronic disease or disorder. It doesn't matter what the disorder is. It could be arthritis, macular degeneration, cancer, diabetes, high blood pressure, asthma, eczema, PMS or anything else. Specific dietary supplements can help almost any disorder.

Reason #21: Medications. Americans consume an astounding quantity of prescription and over-the-counter medications. However, nothing in your body operates in isolated compartments - everything interacts with everything else in some way. Many drugs interact with supplements, or cause an increased need for them. For example, women on birth control pills may have an increased need for vitamin B6. People on Glucophage need more calcium, B12 and folic acid. The list is endless. So if you're on medication, consult with one of our physicians to determine the specific supplements you need.

Reason #22: Pregnancy. Your requirement for nutrients undergoes a big shift when you become pregnant. It's to your and your baby's benefit to take supplementation to reduce your risk of a miscarriage or pregnancy complications and to have a healthier baby.

Bottom Line: Because of worldwide pollution and degradation in the quality of our food supply, it's hard to imagine anyone who will not need nutritional supplements for the rest of his or her life. In addition, many people have health problems, a lifestyle or special situations where supplements are advisable.

15.2 Nutritional Supplement Quality

The clinical experience of naturopathic physicians has shown that you'll get healthier if you buy the highest quality dietary supplements. There are no standards for quality, so buy wisely. Use the quality guidelines listed below.

The primary requirement for any supplement is that it actually works. In order to be clinically effective, it must be of the highest possible quality. However, quality varies widely because there are no quality standards in the industry. So you can't rely only on the label.

Take vitamin E, for example. A study of various vitamin E products by laboratory analysis showed that a large percentage of the supplements had less vitamin E than stated on the label. A few of the products had no vitamin E in them at all! In addition, there are various forms of vitamin E: alpha, beta, delta and gamma. Most supplements have only the alpha form because that is the least expensive. The alpha form is beneficial, but not nearly as beneficial as all the forms together. All the forms together are called "mixed tocopherols." They have more health benefits but are also more expensive. This example illustrates the difficulty in selecting supplements merely by looking at the label.

Independent Lab Assay Is a Key to Quality

Some supplement manufacturers hire independent laboratories to verify what their products contain. This is the only way to know for certain what is in a supplement.

Listed below are some of the benchmarks that we look for in a lab assessment of a dietary supplement:
- No microbial contamination - bacteria, yeast, or mold
- No heavy metals - lead, mercury, cadmium, arsenic or aluminum
- Free of chemical solvent residue, pesticides and herbicides
- No rancidity
- Truth in labeling - the product contains what the label claims
- Stability - the product maintains potency until the expiration date
- No dioxins, mercury or PCBs in fish oil products

Additional Quality Considerations

Product manufactured according to standards. A top-quality supplement is manufactured according to the strict standards of United States Pharmacopeia, and the proposed Food & Drug Administration's Current Good Manufacturing Practice Guidelines.

Non-allergenic. Supplements with food colorings such as tartrazine are a common source of allergy problems. Many "natural" supplements come from food sources such as corn, soy, yeast, dairy, or egg, which may cause allergy problems. We stock only the most allergy-free products available.

Highest purity. Some supplement manufacturers try to save money by adding cheap fillers, including lactose, sucrose, hydrated aluminum silicate, modified corn starch, sodium chloride or sand. Binders, lubricants, and disintegrators might include talc, soap, rancid oils, shellac, tree sap, polyethylene glycol, waxes or cornstarch. If a product does not have a lab analysis to prove its purity, we utilize our extensive knowledge of the supplement industry to determine whether these impurities may be present.

Correct potency. Labeling can be deceptive. For example, it is legal to say "100 mg of citrus bioflavonoid complex" when in fact the "complex" you are getting is 30 mg of bioflavonoid and 70 mg of lactose (milk sugar). In addition, some manufacturers cut costs by simply not including the full amount of the nutrient. This is why we ask our suppliers for authentication from an independent laboratory.

Standardized herb potency. The potency of herbs in a supplement can vary wildly, depending on what part of the plant is used, the time of year it was harvested, how long it was stored or how it was processed. By potency, we're referring to the components of the plant that are biologically active in your body. The most reputable supplement manufacturers used herbs with a "standardized" potency, so that you will know exactly how much of the biologically active part of the herb you are getting. All of the herbs available through our website are standardized.

Quality DOES Matter

When it comes to buying dietary supplements, you essentially have two choices: buy according to price or buy according to quality.

If you buy the cheapest supplement, you'll end up with an inferior product that may not improve your health. Therefore buying the cheapest is a waste of your money. In fact, the lowest-price products may contain impurities or additives that could actually make you worse.

Our clinical experience indicates that you're definitely better off buying the highest quality supplements. By doing so, you maximize the probability of improving your health and thus minimizing future medical expenses. So, not only will you be healthier by taking the highest quality supplements, you will also save money in the long run.

15.3 Supplements for PCOS, Infertility and Insulin Problems

There is a wide range of supplemental nutrients that may help you alleviate the symptoms of polycystic ovarian syndrome, reduce ovarian cysts, and improve your chances of becoming pregnant.

However, not all of them are appropriate or necessary for every woman. You'll also notice that we do not recommend dosage levels of supplements. We recommend that you consult with a licensed healthcare professional regarding the best supplements for you. The type, dosage and duration of nutritional supplementation depends on your unique health history, present health status and body size.

In this chapter, we'll briefly list the dietary supplements that may be recommended by a physician for PCOS or infertility. Please do not rush out and buy all the supplements on this list. That is *not* the way to use nutritional supplements for PCOS. It may even be counterproductive — and unnecessarily expensive — to take a whole bunch of nutritional supplements or to take all of them at extremely high dosages.

To illustrate what you're dealing with, consider the two following examples.

Example of a Condition You May Want to Treat

Suppose that you have insulin resistance or want to prevent insulin resistance. Which supplement should you take?

Available information suggests that a number of nutrients may improve insulin resistance.[273] Minerals, including magnesium, calcium, potassium, zinc, chromium and vanadium, appear to have associations with insulin resistance or its management. Amino acids, including L-carnitine, taurine, and L-arginine also might play a role in the reversal of insulin resistance. Additional nutrients such as glutathione, coenzyme Q10, and lipoic acid appear to have therapeutic potential. Research on herbal medicines for the treatment of insulin resistance is limited, although silymarin may be helpful in some situations.

So should you take all of these? Or just some of them? Which ones? And in what dosage? It all depends on your unique needs.

Example of Individual Supplement Complexity

Let's take vitamin D as another example. It is likely that you will benefit from taking extra vitamin D. Vitamin D is essential for absorption of calcium. Women with PCOS often have calcium insufficiencies or disturbances that can be alleviated by taking supplemental vitamin D. Supplemental vitamin D and calcium have helped PCOS women resume menstruation and become pregnant.[274]

Vitamin D and calcium may also help with weight loss and insulin resistance. And some studies have shown that individuals with insulin resistance have low levels of vitamin D, suggesting a need for supplementation.[275]

As you consider these issues, you could easily think you should be taking vitamin D.

But how much should you take? If you are a dark-skinned woman living in northern Europe, you will need more supplemental vitamin D than a fair-skinned woman in Florida who likes to spend time on the beach. You will need more vitamin D if you live at sea level than if you live in the mountains. You will need more vitamin D if you live in a cloudy climate than in a sunny climate. You will need more in the winter than in the summer.

You may have heard that vitamin D is toxic in high doses. But a toxic dose for one person is not a toxic dose for another. A person with impaired liver function will experience toxicity at a lower dose than a person with a healthy liver. So, to be safe, should you take generally recommended amount of 400 IU per day? You could do that, but 400 IU may not be nearly the amount that you need.

On the other hand, some physicians have given their patients as much as 50,000 IUs per day for specific health situations. You might surmise that your dose might fall somewhere between 400 IU and 50,000 IU. But where? Should your does be 800 IU? Or 5,000 IU? This is where a licensed naturopathic physician or other licensed professional with expertise in clinical nutrition and infertility can help you.

The best way to benefit from nutritional supplementation is to consult with a professional. (By the way, we are most definitely *not* recommending you take 50,000 IU of vitamin D. We are only illustrating a point. *Always* consult with your physician before taking a very high dose of any supplement or drug.)

The Case for High-Dose Vitamin Therapy

Now that we've cautioned you about taking supplements, let's consider the advantages of supplementation.

According to research at the University of California (Berkeley), "…about 50 human genetic diseases due to defective enzymes can be remedied or ameliorated by the administration of high doses of the vitamin component of the corresponding coenzyme, which at least partially restores enzymatic activity."[276]

In other words, the processes of the body depend on vitamins and minerals. If a vitamin or mineral is missing or too low, the body process that depends on it cannot occur, or will occur at a lower than optimal rate. In addition, some body processes are genetically inefficient in some individuals. These individuals require higher-than-normal amounts of certain vitamins or minerals for their body processes to work.

The University of California study referred to genetic diseases. Although we wouldn't describe PCOS as an entirely genetic disease, it clearly does have genetic components. Depending on your specific genetic pattern, you may need extra amounts of some vitamins or minerals in order to optimize your metabolic processes.

Interactions Between Drugs and Supplements

Nutritional supplements and some foods may interact with prescription medications and vice versa. Some supplements will have an "additive effect" with certain drugs. For example, if you are taking drugs to reduce insulin resistance or lower insulin, many of the supplements listed here may do the same thing. Therefore, if you take those supplements, you may need less medication and will need to have your medication adjusted.

On the other hand, some supplements may be antagonistic with some drugs. In this case, you may need to avoid the supplement, or increase the dosage of your medication.

If you are taking any prescription medications, we strongly recommend that you consult with the prescribing physician before embarking on a nutritional supplement program.

Supplements Are Not a Substitute for Healthy Diet

Nutritional supplements are "supplements" to your healthy diet, not a substitute for it. A healthy diet, as outlined in this book, is the basis for the successful management of PCOS. All the supplements in the world will not correct the deficiencies and metabolic imbalances created by a poor-quality diet. Don't delude yourself into thinking that taking supplements is a magic short cut to good health. A healthy, sensible diet is the absolute prerequisite for improvement of PCOS problems and better overall health.

List of Supplements for PCOS and Infertility

Below is a partial list of nutritional supplements to consider, based on common reference sources.[277] We are not necessarily recommending that you take these supplements. Some women have benefited from using some of the supplements on this list. We don't know what is "right" for your unique needs. Consult with a qualified health professional about this list.

Many of these supplements are intended to improve insulin function and reduce insulin resistance. We mention these supplements because insulin resistance and dysfunction plays a major role in PCOS and infertility.

Alpha-lipoic acid

Alpha-lipoic acid reduces insulin resistance and lowers blood sugar levels in some studies. It is also an excellent antioxidant. There are two forms of this supplement: alpha lipoic acid, and r-alpha-lipoic acid. The r-alpha lipoic acid has recently been shown to be the most beneficial form of this supplement.

Banaba

Banaba is a species of crepe myrtle, an ornamental shrub. Extracts of the banaba leaves are popular in the Philippines and Southeast Asia. Banaba extracts contain corosolic acid and ellagitannins that seem to have an insulin-like effect and also activate insulin receptors.

Bilberry

Bilberry, a close relative of blueberry, has a long history of medicinal use. Bilberry fruit and its extracts contain a number of biologically active components, including a class of compounds called anthocyanosides.

Bilberry has been used traditionally in the treatment of diabetes and animal research suggests that bilberry extract can lower blood sugar levels. There is also some evidence to suggest bilberry acts as an antioxidant and anti-inflammatory.

Biotin

Biotin is a member of the B-complex family of vitamins. It improves disordered glucose metabolism by stimulating insulin secretion in response to blood sugar and by improving the liver's ability to process glucose. Biotin appears to improve insulin resistance.

Biotin is crucial for proper hair and nail growth. In high doses, biotin can be effective in restoring head-hair growth, with no known side effects.

Bitter Melon

Bitter melon (momordica) looks like a light green, pointed cucumber. It is a popular Southeast Asian natural product used for diabetes. Bitter melon, like banaba, also seems to have an insulin-like effect. Bitter melon contains a protein known as "plant-insulin," or "polypeptide-P."

Calcium

Calcium appears to improve insulin sensitivity. In one study, people taking calcium supplements had reduced insulin levels and improved insulin sensitivity as compared to people who did not take the supplements.

Recent studies also show that extra calcium helps with weight loss. In animal studies, those given extra dietary calcium or calcium supplements lost more weight than animals with lower calcium intake.

Chasteberry
Chasteberry (vitex agnus-castus) is a well-known herb that has been used for centuries in Europe for hormonal imbalances in women. Chasteberry helps the hypothalamus gland in the brain to shift the ratio of estrogen to progesterone, in favor of progesterone. Since most women with PCOS and infertility have a deficiency in progesterone, chasteberry is specific aid for this problem.

Some studies have shown that chasteberry restores the menstrual cycle and fertility. It may also reduce prolactin, which is too high in some PCOS women and inhibits fertility. Chasteberry may also help to relieve PCOS-related acne.

Chinese Medicines
A variety of medicines from Traditional Chinese Medicine may help with PCOS, infertility, insulin resistance and weight management. A couple of examples are Yu's Tonifying Recipe and Tiangui Recipe.

If you wish to explore Chinese medicines, consult with an Oriental Medical Doctor (OMD) or licensed acupuncturist (LAc) with training in the use of traditional Asian medicines. These professionals can diagnose your energy patterns and prescribe the appropriate medicine. Do not go into an ethnic market and buy Chinese medicines off the shelf. There is no quality assurance, plus you may purchase the wrong medicine by mistake. Unless you are thoroughly familiar with Traditional Chinese Medicine, you should always consult with an OMD or LAc first.

Chromium
It appears that a deficiency in chromium can result in insulin resistance. Evidence suggests diet-induced insulin resistance can be improved by chromium.

A diet high in sugar and refined carbohydrates may lead to a loss of chromium. The chromium loss may be due to high insulin levels when consuming this type of diet.

There are different forms of chromium available as supplements. There is controversy about which is best. The different forms include: GTF chromium, Chromium complexed with nicotinic acid, chromium chloride and chromium picolinate. Studies are somewhat contradictory as to the effectiveness of each of these forms.

Chromium has been used for decades to treat people with blood sugar or diabetic problems.

Cinnamon

A recent study suggested that cinnamon could lower fasting blood glucose by 18%-30%. Constituents in cinnamon appear to increase insulin receptor sensitivity. Cinnamon is safe and very well tolerated. You might sprinkle 1/2 - 1-1/2 teaspoons onto your food each day. The type of cinnamon that works the best is Chinese cinnamon (Cassia cinnamon). Chinese cinnamon is available in markets — just read the label.

CLA (Conjugated Linoleic Acid)

CLA is a fatty acid primarily found in dairy products and beef. It is available as a supplement, partly for the purpose of losing weight. The evidence for the efficacy of CLA is somewhat contradictory. It's theorized that CLA might shrink adipose tissue by inducing programmed cell death of fat cells.

Coenzyme Q10

Coenzyme Q10 (CoQ10) has shown some indication of being helpful in reducing glucose and insulin levels. It also aids energy production.

D-Chiro Inositol

D-chiro-inositol is a variation of the B-vitamin inositol.

You may have heard about d-chiro-inositol because a recent study suggested it reduced testosterone levels and helped to induce ovulation in overweight women with polycystic ovary syndrome. It is thought that it does this by improving insulin sensitivity. However, d-chiro-inositol is not commercially available at this time.

The basic inositol molecule is an essential component of cell membranes. Inositol may be helpful for fat transport and metabolism, hair growth and sensitizing serotonin receptors, which could relieve depression and improve appetite balance.

Fenugreek

Fenugreek seeds are used as a spice and taste similar to maple syrup. Diabetics who mix 15 grams of ground fenugreek seeds apparently have reduced blood sugar levels compared to those not using fenugreek seeds. Fenugreek seems to enhance insulin release.

Fish Oils

The most common forms of fish oils are cod liver oil and concentrated EPA/DHA. If you do not eat substantial amounts of cold-water fish, fish oil may be an important dietary source of essential fatty acids (EFAs). The role of EFAs is reviewed elsewhere in this book. EFAs from fish perform a wide variety of essential functions.

Folic Acid (Folate)

Folate and folic acid are forms of the same B vitamin. Folate is found naturally in food and folic acid is usually found in vitamins. Folic acid is required for DNA synthesis and optimal neurological function. It works in tandem with vitamin B12. Folic acid may be helpful in reducing homocysteine, which is a metabolic byproduct that is too high in some PCOS women, especially if they are taking metformin (Glucophage).

Garcinia

Garcinia is a fruit that contains hydroxycitric acid, which is theorized to inhibit the body's production of fat. It may also aid in the burning of fat. There's not much compelling evidence either way.

Ginseng

Ginseng root has been used for centuries as a "tonic" for improving energy and vigor. There are two types of ginseng: Panax ginseng and American ginseng. Panax ginseng appears to reduce blood sugar levels. Both Panax ginseng and American ginseng contain ginsenosides, which are thought to decrease insulin resistance. Ginseng may relieve fatigue.

GLA (Gamma Linoleic Acid)

As a supplement, GLA is found in oils extracted from the seeds of the borage plant or evening primrose. These oils contain significant amounts of GLA (gamma linoleic acid). Among other things, GLA appears to inhibit 3-alpha-reductase and 5-alpha reductase, which are involved in converting testosterone into its more active metabolite, dihydro-testosterone (DHT). Therefore, borage oil may be useful in some cases for acne and hirsutism.

GLA may have anti-inflammatory effects and can help prevent blood vessel narrowing, thus improving circulation.

Green Tea

Extracts of green tea are available as a supplement. Green tea is a powerful antioxidant and helps to prevent cancer. Although not all studies agree, green tea may help you lose weight, lose inches, boost your metabolic rate and possibly inhibit appetite.

Green tea also contains a substance called PQQ (pyrroloquinoline quinine), which has been shown to improve fertility in lab animals. In addition, green tea appears to inhibit the action of androgens (male hormones) and increases SHGB (sex hormone binding globulin) and thus may contribute to reduction of hirsutism.

Gymnema
Gymnema is an Indian plant whose extract seems to work by increasing insulin production and lowering blood sugar. In studies it has allowed diabetics to cut back on their insulin medication.

Indole 3 Carbanol
Indole-3-carbanol comes from cruciferous vegetables like broccoli or Brussels sprouts. Indole-3-carbinol shifts metabolism of estradiol from 16-alpha-hydroxyestrone to 2-alpha-hydroxyestrone, which is a weaker and more benign form of estrogen. This has the effect of reducing the risk of breast cancer.

L-Arginine
Arginine is an amino acid with a potential therapeutic role in the management of insulin resistance. It also appears to stimulate glucagon secretion. Glucagon is a hormone that raises blood sugar when it is too low. Glucagon is an opposing hormone to insulin.

L-Carnitine
Carnitine is an amino acid that also has potential to improve insulin sensitivity. It also helps the body to metabolize fat.

L-Tryptophan or 5-Hydroxy-Tryptophan (5HTP)
Tryptophan, or its metabolite 5-hydroxy-tryptophan (5HTP), is an amino acid that is an aid to weight loss because tryptophan is a precursor to serotonin. Serotonin is one the hormones that helps to regulate your appetite and thus help you avoid eating more food than you need.

Caution: This is an example of a supplement that is *potentially dangerous* if taken along with a prescription drug. *A person taking one of the serotonin reuptake inhibitor medications for depression should not also use 5-HTP.* A condition known as Serotonin Syndrome can result if the body produces excessively high levels of serotonin or if the body cannot break down serotonin at a sufficient rate. Symptoms include confusion, fever, shivering, sweating, diarrhea, and muscle spasms. This syndrome does not occur when 5-HPT is taken alone. However the medical literature contains reports of some cases that developed when L-tryptophan was combined with prescription drugs that inhibit activity (MAO or monoamine oxidase) that breaks down molecules of serotonin. Do not take 5-HTP at the same time as any prescription anti-depressant, (including Prozac and Zoloft) unless supervised by a physician. You should stop taking an MAO-inhibitor for at least 4 weeks before beginning therapy with 5-HTP or any other serotonin-active substance. Of course, do not stop taking any prescription medication without the guidance of the prescribing practitioner.

Licorice Root

Licorice root (glycyrrhiza glabra) has been shown to substantially reduce serum testosterone levels and thus may be beneficial to PCOS women who have elevated testosterone, acne or hirsutism. A component of licorice called glycyrrhizic acid inhibits an enzyme require for the creation of testosterone. Licorice may also aid in loss of body fat.

Chronic consumption of large quantities of licorice (50 grams) may cause high blood pressure, edema, depletion of potassium in the blood and other complications. Do not consume licorice if you are pregnant.

Magnesium

Magnesium is involved in numerous metabolic actions.

Insulin stores magnesium. Conversely, magnesium is necessary for the action of insulin and the manufacture of insulin. If your cells become resistant to insulin, you can't store magnesium so you lose it through urination. Studies have shown an association between insulin resistance and magnesium deficiency. Magnesium deficiency is relatively common in diabetics.

Magnesium is required for all energy-producing reactions that take place in the cell. Since magnesium is necessary to relax muscles, a magnesium deficiency would cause blood vessel constriction, leading to higher blood pressure.

Milk Thistle

Milk thistle (silybum marianum) contains an antioxidant flavonoid component called silymarin. It appears to reduce insulin resistance, as well as insulin and glucose levels. Silymarin is also a good antioxidant that is very helpful in protecting the liver from damage.

A small number of studies suggest possible improvements of blood sugar control in cirrhotic patients with diabetes. However, there is not enough scientific evidence to recommend milk thistle for this use.

NAC (N-Acetyl Cysteine)

NAC is a derivative of the amino acid l-cysteine. NAC is a potent antioxidant and appears to reduce inflammation. In at least one study, NAC reduced insulin resistance in women with PCOS.

Potassium

A potassium-depleted diet was found to lead to insulin resistance. You should be able to get most of your potassium from the diet recommended in this book. However, some potassium supplementation may be indicated.

Progesterone

Progesterone is used for treating amenorrhea, abnormal uterine bleeding and severe PMS. Progesterone is also used in combination with estrogens as part of hormone replacement therapy to prevent irregular bleeding as well as the increased risk of endometrial cancer associated with estrogen therapy.

Topically, progesterone is used for treating or preventing hormone-mediated allergies, bloating, breast tenderness, decreased sex drive, depression, fatigue, fibrocystic breasts, headaches, hypoglycemia, increased blood clotting, infertility, irritability, memory loss, miscarriages, osteoporosis, premenopausal bone loss, symptoms of premenstrual syndrome, thyroid dysfunction, unclear thinking, uterine cancer, uterine fibroids, water retention, and weight gain.

Intravaginally, progesterone is used for cervical ripening, mastodynia, and to prevent or treat endometrial hyperplasia. Progesterone is also used intravaginally or intramuscularly for treating infertility in women, anovulatory bleeding and for treating PMS.

Progesterone is secreted by the corpus luteum. The hormone is not available from any natural source without extraction and synthesis. "Natural" or "bio-identical" progesterone are products that are identical to the progesterone you make in your body. However, they are synthesized in the laboratory from diosgenin, found in wild yam. In the lab, diosgenin is converted to pregnenolone and then to progesterone. The human body is not capable of synthesizing progesterone from diosgenin.

Pushkarmoola (Inula Racemosa)

Pushkarmoola is an herb used in Ayurvedic medicine. Inula racemosa has improved glucose metabolism in animals, probably by improving insulin sensitivity.

Pyruvate

Pyruvate may have some utility as a weight loss aid. Pyruvate is the end product of glucose metabolism and is shunted to the part of the cell that burns fuel for energy where it used in the energy-producing cycle. When pyruvate is substituted for refined dietary carbohydrate, loss of weight and body fat can occur. However, you would need to consume a large amount and it is expensive.

Quercetin

Quercetin is a flavonoid found in many plants. Quercetin has antioxidant and anti-inflammatory properties, and has been used in the treatment of diabetes and cardiovascular disorders.

Saw Palmetto

The extract of saw palmetto is from the fruit of the saw palmetto, a small palm native to the southeastern U.S. It is widely used for the treatment of enlarged prostate glands in men. It is thought that the prostate gland becomes enlarged primarily because of a metabolite of testosterone called dihydrotestosterone, or DHT. Women with PCOS also tend to have higher levels of testosterone and DHT than other women. No studies have been done, but it is thought that saw palmetto might benefit women in the same way it has benefited men who have excess DHT.

Stinging Nettles

Stingling nettles (urtica dioica) may lessen the effects of androgenic hormones such as testosterone. In addition, there is some evidence that stinging nettle can decrease blood sugar levels, which is desirable for those women who have a problem with excessively high blood sugar levels.

Taurine

Taurine is an amino acid. There is some preliminary evidence with animals that suggests taurine can improve insulin sensitivity, blood sugar levels and possibly abdominal fat.

Vanadium

Vanadium is a trace mineral thought to enhance the action of insulin by activating insulin receptors. Vanadium is also thought to help the liver do a better job of controlling sugars and fats. Diabetics who take vanadium in the form of vanadyl sulfate have improved insulin sensitivity and reduced blood glucose.

Vitamin B6 (Pyridoxine)

Vitamin B6 is involved in numerous metabolic processes, including blood sugar metabolism. Vitamin B6 affects receptors for estrogen, androgen and progesterone. Vitamin B6 is required for the synthesis of serotonin. Mild deficiency of vitamin B6 is common.

Vitamin B12

Vitamin B12 is an essential vitamin commonly found in a variety of foods such as fish, shellfish, meats, and dairy products. Vitamin B12 is necessary for DNA synthesis and neurological health. It works in conjunction with folic acid.

Vitamin B12 is bound to the protein in food. Hydrochloric acid in the stomach releases B12 from protein during digestion. Once released, B12 combines with a substance called intrinsic factor (IF) before it is absorbed into the bloodstream. However, this absorption process is often compromised in unhealthy individuals or the elderly. Metformin

(Glucophage) and other medications may make vitamin B12 absorption more difficult.

Strict vegetarians or vegans may not get enough dietary vitamin B12.

Vitamin D

Vitamin D is required by the pancreas for the production of insulin. There is some evidence to suggest vitamin D improves insulin sensitivity and the body's ability to handle blood sugar.

Recent studies have shown that vitamin D and calcium, when taken together, suppress spontaneous food intake and burn fat. Higher calcium intake is consistently associated with lower body weight. As vitamin D significantly increases calcium absorption, it seems likely that higher intakes of vitamin D would decrease body weight even if the vitamin itself had no direct effect on weight.

Vitamin D levels are lower in obese people than in thin people.

In one small study, vitamin D combined with calcium supplementation resulted in normalized menstrual cycles within 2 months for seven women. Two became pregnant and the others maintained normal menstrual cycles.

Vitamin E

Vitamin E is a well-known antioxidant. Studies on vitamin E for improving insulin sensitivity are inconsistent. Vitamin E adequacy should be maintained at least because of its important antioxidant functions.

Zinc

Preliminary evidence suggests a relationship between zinc deficiency and a poor response to insulin. Zinc plays an important role in many metabolic processes.

Note: The above is only a partial list of supplements that may be relevant to PCOS, weight problems or infertility. There are many other specialty nutrients that could be helpful. In addition, the descriptions of each supplement are not complete.

Please visit **www.ovarian-cysts-pcos.com/supplements** to get additional information about supplements that may be useful to you.

Section 16

More About Hormones, Weight and Inflammation

16.1 What Makes You Hungry?

As a woman who has polycystic ovary syndrome, you may have discovered that you have a hard time staying away from food, especially if you are overweight. In spite of tremendous willpower, you are driven to eat. Or, even if your willpower prevails and you don't overeat, you are usually hungry and cannot lose fat weight.

The reason that you are having these problems is that the hormones that govern your appetite and fat regulation are just not working properly. There are dozens of hormones and other signaling molecules that either stimulate or inhibit food intake. They form an exceedingly complex web of interrelationships.

You may have heard that if you could just get control of your insulin, you will not feel as hungry and your weight will melt away. While this is partially true, it's an oversimplification. In fact, you may have numerous hormones or signaling molecules that are out of balance — either overactive or underactive.

There is no single factor that governs your weight, your fat metabolism or your hunger. It is a bewildering combination of factors, all interacting or influencing one another. An imbalance or disturbance of one signaling molecule will affect others, which in turn will affect still others.

No one, including research scientists and doctors, fully understands the functions and relationships of all these various signaling molecules, particularly as they exist in each unique woman. And, there are probably additional signaling molecules that haven't yet been discovered.

However some basic information about this fascinating internal world is becoming clearer. In this chapter, we'll briefly review a few of these hormones so that you can better understand the complexity involved and why you are having problems.

How the Hunger Process Works

The amount of food you eat is determined mainly by the intrinsic desire for food called "hunger." Hunger means a craving for food and is associated with a number of sensations. For example, if you haven't eaten for many hours, your stomach undergoes intense rhythmic contractions called hunger pangs.

The type of food you preferentially seek is your appetite. Your appetite helps you choose the quality of food you eat.

Satiety is the opposite of hunger. It's a feeling of fulfillment in the quest for food.

The hypothalamus, a gland in the brain, is the main control center for hunger and satiety. It tells your body whether it is hungry or not. The hypothalamus is especially important because it produces a variety of hormones that influence or determine the hormone production of other endocrine glands, which in turn tell various cells what to do.

The hypothalamus is sensitive to hormonal and other feedback signals from the body. This feedback is used by the hypothalamus to decide what hormones to produce.

An important feedback mechanism is the level of glucose (blood sugar) in the blood. Much of the food you eat gets converted to glucose — some is used immediately for energy, some is stored as glycogen and some is converted by the liver into fat for later use. When the levels of glucose are low, the liver sends signals to the hypothalamus that levels are low. The hypothalamus in turn triggers whatever habits you have accumulated relating to food seeking and consumption.

The hypothalamus actually tells you more specifically what foods you need, and seems to be responsible for many of our "cravings."

There are also certain hormones that are released when food begins to move from the stomach to the intestines that signal the hypothalamus that it's time to stop eating. There is also a hormone released by the fat cells themselves called leptin that decreases appetite via the hypothalamus.

From here on, we'll briefly discuss three of the signaling factors that influence your appetite and your weight. There are dozens of factors that we could discuss but these may be the ones you have heard about or will hear about.

Ghrelin

Ghrelin is a "hunger hormone" that was discovered in 1999. A lot of research is being done on ghrelin so you may be hearing more about it.

It helps to regulate how much food you eat and how much weight you gain. In normal individuals, ghrelin levels go up before meals and down after meals.[278] Elevated ghrelin triggers strong feelings of hunger. In addition to regulating eating behavior, ghrelin may slow your metabolism and reduce your ability to burn fat.

Ghrelin is secreted primarily in the stomach and intestines. Very obese people who have a gastric bypass operation to lose weight subsequently produce relatively little ghrelin, since their stomach is smaller and presumably produces less ghrelin.[279] This may help explain why their appetites decrease markedly after the surgery.

In slim people, ghrelin typically levels peaks right before a meal but rapidly declines soon afterwards. That's not what happens with overweight people — their ghrelin remains steady before and after a meal.[280]   In other words, since their ghrelin does not decline after a meal, they were still hungry after eating.

Also, dieters who lose weight and then try to keep it off make more ghrelin than they did before dieting, which may help to explain why it's so difficult to stay on a diet for a long time and why so many do "yo-yo" dieting, where they go off the diet to binge for a while, then return to the diet, then binge again, etc.

Ghrelin and Diet

Since ghrelin is a recently discovered hormone, much research still needs to be done to conclusively determine how the composition of the diet would affect ghrelin levels.

However, there is one interesting study from the University of Naples, Italy.[281]   The researchers fed 14 non-obese healthy women meals that were either high-fat or a high-carbohydrate. Ghrelin dropped after both the high-fat and high-carb meals. However, it dropped further after the high-carb meals. In addition, the women reported that the high-carb meal did a better job in suppressing their feelings of hunger.

Another study, from the University of Washington in Seattle, showed that a low-fat diet helped individuals avoid increases in ghrelin and thus avoid hunger.[282] They also lost weight.

Other studies have shown that consumption of high-glucose meals suppressed plasma levels of ghrelin, whereas this response was less after high-fructose meals.[283] Glucose and fructose are simple sugars that are found in carbohydrates.

Glucose and fructose have identical chemical formulas but the structure of their molecules is slightly different. Therefore they behave differently in the body. Since fructose is much sweeter than glucose, and very cheap, it is found throughout our food supply. Introducing a lot of fructose into your body will do little to reduce your ghrelin "hunger" hormone, thus propelling you in the direction of eating more food.

We believe that eating the right type, quality and quality of carbohydrate is important for controlling the hormones that govern your hunger and the behavior of your fat cells.

Ghrelin and PCOS

Several studies suggest that women with PCOS have disordered ghrelin levels or have an impaired ability to regulate ghrelin.[284] [285] For example, one study conducted at the University of Adelaide in Australia showed that PCOS women were less satiated and hungrier after a meal than normal women.[286] The ghrelin levels of the PCOS women did not decline after a meal as much as the non-PCOS women. Interestingly, the composition of the test diets (high protein vs. standard protein) had no effect on ghrelin levels.

In a study of overweight PCOS women at the Center for Applied Biomedical Research in Bologna Italy, there was a negative correlation between ghrelin and insulin resistance; the worse the insulin resistance, the lower the ghrelin level.[287] However, in overweight non-PCOS women, there was no such correlation. It's not clear to us what this means, although it demonstrates that there is a relationship between ghrelin and insulin resistance.

There appears to be some interplay among caloric intake, glucose, insulin and ghrelin. It is not clear whether ghrelin stimulates or inhibits insulin secretion. The authors also reported a strong correlation between decreased ghrelin and increased androstenedione, which is a precursor to testosterone. Moreover, the ovaries have a high concentration of binding sites for ghrelin, suggesting that ghrelin may play some kind of role in the production of hormones from the ovaries.

There is much to be learned about ghrelin. What we know at this point is that ghrelin imbalances occur in PCOS. We don't know whether obesity causes the ghrelin disorder, or whether the ghrelin disorder causes the obesity.

The diet in this book is intended to reduce insulin resistance. Possibly, as insulin resistance diminishes and you lose some weight, you will also be more sensitive to ghrelin and it will start to normalize.

Cholecystokinin (CCK) and Satiety

Cholecystokinin (CCK) is a hormone secreted in the gastrointestinal tract when you eat a meal. It slows down the digestive process and functions as a short-term satiety signal to inhibit food intake and thus decrease meal size.

However, some women with PCOS have reduced CCK secretion after a meal and deranged appetite regulation. Impaired CCK secretion may play a role in the greater frequency of binge eating and overweight in women with PCOS.[288]

There may be a number of factors at play. A primary factor is that short-term CCK must work in concert with the long-term hormonal regulators of energy balance, such as insulin and leptin. (Insulin and leptin are reviewed in the next chapter). The size and composition of your meals will influence insulin and leptin. Since the caloric size of the meal is partly determined by CCK, CCK influences insulin and leptin. However, as long-term regulators of your body fat, insulin and leptin will also influence CCK.

In the next chapter, we discuss how insulin resistance and leptin resistance can have serious consequences for your weight and your health. You may need to normalize insulin and leptin in order to get CCK to normalize.

In addition, there is some evidence to suggest that impaired CCK output is associated with increased levels of testosterone.[289] Some of the excess testosterone may be due to high insulin and insulin resistance. Our diet should help to keep your insulin under control and thus reduce your propensity to produce testosterone. The high fiber content of our diet will also help to slow the breakdown of CCK and keep you feeling satisfied for longer.

Beta-Endorphin & Sweet Cravings

Another brain chemical is called "beta-endorphin." One or two of the popular diet books mention it, so let's review it very briefly.

You may have heard about a "runner's high," a euphoric feeling that occurs when exercise causes the release of endorphins. Beta-endorphin increases your tolerance for physical or emotional pain, decreases appetite and anxiety and may induce feelings of euphoria.

Some individuals apparently tend to have lower levels of beta-endorphin. To compensate, additional endorphin receptors are created and thus the cells can take better advantage of whatever beta-endorphins happen along.

When beta-endorphins are low, you may feel isolated, inadequate or helpless. Some may experience feelings of withdrawal, like a runner who is prevented from running, or a drug addict who does not have access to drugs.

Sugar and sweets are capable of increasing beta-endorphins. This may partially explain why some people get a "high" by eating sweets and refined carbohydrate products. These individuals are predisposed to be quite sensitive to endorphins, feeling well when they are high and feeling depressed when they are low.

There is some evidence to indicate the PCOS women have disturbed beta-endorphin function. At least one study has indicated that some PCOS women have a greater beta-endorphin response to dietary glucose than normal women.[290] If you are overweight, this could mean that you may tend towards sweets to keep your beta-endorphin levels up.

Other studies have shown a close association of excess weight with increased beta-endorphin levels in PCOS women.[291] Beta-endorphins play a regulatory role in the menstrual cycle, and they appear to influence insulin and luteinizing hormone (LH) levels.[292] [293]

Our diet avoids refined carbohydrates and sugars that might cause excessive jumps or swings in beta-endorphins.

As you can see just from our short discussion of ghrelin, cholecystokinin and beta-endorphin, PCOS women with appetite or overweight problems have multiple hormonal disorders.

A healthy diet, as outlined in this book, is a powerful tool you can use to start getting your hormones back into balance and to get them to do their job more efficiently.

Our diet helps you with hunger and energy balance in basic ways:
- Provides all of the co-factor nutrients you need to make hormones work more efficiently
- Is free of refined carbohydrates and sugars that cause hormones to overreact
- Contains plenty of plant fiber and healthy fats, which slow down the absorption of dietary starches and sugars into the bloodstream
- Is free of chemicals and additives that may interfere with hormonal signaling
- Contains essential fatty acids that support communication between cells and hormones

16.2 'Evil Twins': Insulin Resistance and Leptin Resistance

In this chapter, we'll talk about insulin and leptin, two hormones that do much to determine your hormone status, how your reproductive tract functions and how fat you are.

Leptin is a hormone produced in your fat cells. Insulin is produced by your pancreas gland. Although these two hormones and their receptors appear unrelated and structurally distinct, they exert overlapping effects on the hypothalamus gland in your brain. The hypothalamus is the "control center" for maintaining your energy balance, that is, how fat or lean you are. Insulin and leptin keep your hypothalamus informed about the status of the energy stores in your body. They also appear to be able to "cross-talk" with each other in the hypothalamus.

Defects in either insulin or leptin signaling in the central nervous system and brain result in overeating, disturbed blood sugar balance, reproductive dysfunction and weight gain.

It is common for women with PCOS or those who have fertility problems to have excessively high levels of insulin (insulin resistance), especially if they are overweight. What is not so well known is that there is another hormone, leptin, which is also disordered in many PCOS women.

If you are overweight and infertile, you may have both insulin resistance and leptin resistance. Let's review these two centrally important hormones.

Insulin

If you adhere to any of the diets that are popular today, please read this section carefully.

Popular diet writers have made insulin the "bad guy," the hormone that makes you fat. They say that if you cut out the carbs, your blood sugar will not rise as much when you eat a meal. Rising blood sugar triggers an increase in insulin, which causes excess energy (calories) to be stored into cells.

Insulin has been characterized as the "obesity" hormone because it causes fat cells to take in glucose (blood sugar), which is converted to fat, and it inhibits the cells from breaking down fat so that it can be burned as energy.

Actually, an increasing body of evidence indicates that insulin can also be thought of as an "anti-obesity" hormone, because it can suppress food intake and thus prevent weight gain and obesity.

It appears that popular diets are concerned with the short-term effects of insulin but ignore its long-term effects.

Insulin is a long-term regulator of food intake, energy balance and body fat.[294] Insulin secretion from the pancreas gland is stimulated when you eat and digest glucose from carbohydrate and amino acids from protein.

Both fasting insulin levels and insulin responses to meal ingestion correlate with body fat. Accordingly, over a 24-hour period, overall insulin secretion and the insulin levels in the circulation are proportional to both the amount of body fat as well as to recent carbohydrate and protein intake. In other words, the fatter you are, the more insulin you will have in circulation between meals. And, you will produce more insulin in response to a meal containing carbohydrate and protein than a lean person would produce.

Insulin receptors exist in a number of brain regions that regulate feeding behavior, including the hypothalamus. Insulin transport into the brain is not rapid, occurring over a period of hours after circulating insulin concentrations increase after a meal. The slow transport indicates that insulin plays a role in the long-term regulation of body fat rather than as a short-term satiety signal.

However, insulin does not act alone in the hypothalamus to reduce food intake. It works in conjunction with leptin and other hormones to produce a combined effect.

In addition to inhibiting food intake, insulin increases burning of calories. Thus, insulin can modulate energy balance by inhibiting energy intake and by increasing thermogenesis (the burning of calories to produce heat).

Some researchers think that insulin signaling in the brain limits food intake and that over the long term, insulin secretion functions as a negative feedback signal to control caloric intake and body fat.[295]

However, a misconception that insulin causes weight gain and obesity has evolved because insulin works in the tissues to increase fat synthesis and storage. The idea that insulin promotes obesity has led to popular diets that propose to induce weight loss by avoidance of foods that stimulate insulin secretion.

But we need to distinguish between insulin responses to meals in which circulating insulin concentrations rapidly rise and then return to baseline levels within a short period of time — and the chronic excessively high levels of insulin being produced by the pancreas because of insulin resistance.

In fact, increased insulin secretion in response to blood sugar is predictive of a smaller degree of subsequent weight gain, rather than a factor leading to greater weight gain and obesity. Insulin plays a critical long-term role in balancing your energy and weight.

Dietary Fat and Insulin

Insulin content in the hypothalamus gland in the brain is increased after high carbohydrate meals, but not after high fat meals. This is likely due to the much smaller circulating insulin responses when high fat meals are consumed. If insulin in the hypothalamus does not increase, the hypothalamus is less effective in controlling your food intake and the amount of fat you are carrying.

In dogs, chronic consumption of a high fat diet impairs insulin transport to the brain, and the impairment predicts weight gain in response to the high fat feeding.[296] If insulin cannot efficiently get to the hypothalamus, then the hypothalamus cannot do its fat-regulating job.

The effects of reduced insulin secretion and reduced insulin transport to the brain could contribute to the increased calorie intake and obesity observed in animals and humans consuming high fat diets.

The Insulin - CCK Connection

There may be a synergistic relationship between insulin as a long-term signal in regulating energy balance, and CCK (cholecystokinin) as a short-term satiety signal. (CCK was discussed in the previous chapter).

In experiments with baboons, administration of both insulin and CCK resulted in a 50% reduction in calorie intake.[297] Insulin's action in the brain appeared to enhance the meal-suppressive effect of CCK.

The Insulin - Serotonin Connection

Serotonin is a brain chemical with several important functions throughout the body, including mood and appetite regulation. Serotonin is made from tryptophan, an amino acid. When serotonin is low, you may feel depressed and be in the mood to eat something.

Insulin controls serotonin synthesis. It causes stored tryptophan to be released and transported into the brain where it is converted into serotonin.

When you eat carbohydrates or something sweet, insulin increases in order to control the blood sugar. The insulin increase also causes serotonin to increase and thus you feel better after having a carbohydrate. This mechanism explains why dieting women with low serotonin tend to develop uncontrollable carbohydrate cravings.

But suppose you're on a low carb (high protein, high fat) diet in order to lose weight and get your insulin under control — what happens then? Since the blood sugar derived from your diet is lower, your insulin is also lower and so is your serotonin. When your serotonin is low, you will not be in the best of moods. You may find yourself sneaking a few carbs even though they are not allowed in your diet.

Insulin Resistance

Insulin resistance is a condition where the body does not fully respond to insulin. When cells and tissues do not fully and efficiently respond to insulin, critical metabolic work cannot get done. For example, blood sugar (glucose) from food cannot be stored into cells.

Another problem is that the hypothalamus gland may be insulin resistant. In this case, insulin sent to the hypothalamus won't be "heard" by the hypothalamus; thus it cannot properly exercise its food intake control function or its energy-balancing function.

To compensate for the lack of body's response to insulin, the pancreas gland produces additional insulin. This creates a condition called "hyperinsulinemia," or chronically high levels of insulin in the blood.

Very high levels of any hormone, such as insulin, can be disturbing or even toxic to the cells. So, to protect themselves from too much insulin, the cells become more insulin resistant.

We now have a chicken-and-egg problem, where insulin resistance causes chronically high levels of insulin and chronically high levels of insulin create more insulin resistance.

The endless cycle of insulin resistance and hyperinsulinemia, by direct action on the tissues and indirectly via the hypothalamus, prevents the breakdown of fat deposits for energy and removes the brakes on eating more food.

There are many reasons for insulin resistance, including genetic factors. In this book, we are concerned only with the dietary factors that can reduce insulin resistance and thus allow you to burn more fat and better control your appetite.

Insulin Resistance and "Nutrient Toxicity"

Although there are some genetic causes for insulin resistance, the most common cause is an excess of nutrition called "nutrient toxicity."[298] Both excess glucose (blood sugar) and excess fat can cause insulin resistance in muscle and fat tissues. Excess fat can cause insulin resistance in the liver.

The goal of our diet is to break the cycle of insulin resistance by reducing refined carbohydrates that cause excessive blood sugar, and by reducing undesirable fats. Once insulin resistance has diminished, your hormones, weight and appetite will start to normalize.

Leptin

Leptin, a hormone produced by your fat cells, is involved in reproduction and long-term weight and appetite regulation. It signals the hypothalamus gland in your brain when fat cells are full. The hypothalamus uses this information to maintain energy homeostasis (balance) in your body.

Leptin levels should be in a balance, not too high and not too low.

Low levels can result in food cravings. People with leptin deficiency or defects in the leptin receptor overeat and are severely obese. Small doses of leptin reduce overeating and cause loss of fat weight in leptin-deficient people. However, administration of leptin to people with no leptin deficiency induces only a modest and variable weight loss. Leptin is not an "anti-obesity" hormone.

If low leptin stimulates eating, you would think that high leptin levels would inhibit eating. But this is not the case, especially with overweight individuals. Overweight women tend to have higher leptin levels than lean women, but that doesn't stop them from eating.

It's thought that seriously overweight people may become resistant to the effects of leptin and, despite higher circulating levels of the hormone, do not experience its beneficial effects. Leptin resistance could result from decreased leptin transport to the hypothalamus gland in the brain, or from impaired leptin receptors in cells.[299]

In addition to sending signals to the hypothalamus, leptin appears to reduce cravings for sweet foods by altering taste receptors on the tongue. Therefore, either a lack of leptin, or leptin resistance, may contribute to a "sweet tooth." In mice, it has been shown that a lack of leptin, or defects in the leptin receptors, causes their taste buds to prefer sweets; so they eat more sweets.[300] This leptin receptor defect might be described as "leptin resistance," where even a normal level of leptin is not enough to suppress the desire for sweets.

Leptin and Insulin Influence Each Other

Insulin responses to meals are the primary cause of changes of leptin levels. Insulin increases leptin production indirectly via its effects on fat cell metabolism.

Conversely, leptin has direct inhibiting effects on insulin and insulin secretion by inhibiting insulin gene activity and insulin secretion.

Insulin and Leptin use some of the same signaling pathways, suggesting they may have a combined effect on the hypothalamus gland.[301] [302] [303]

Leptin and CCK

An important interaction between leptin as a long-term regulator of energy balance and the short-term satiety signal CCK has recently been demonstrated.[304] The synergistic actions of leptin and CCK on food intake are an example of the integration of long-term and short-term signals regulating energy balance. CCK may work more effectively if leptin resistance can be reduced.

Leptin, PCOS and Fertility

Leptin also plays a role in fertility and reproduction.[305] Here is some of the relevant evidence we've gathered. It's pretty technical, but the gist of it is that a leptin imbalance contributes to weight and fertility problems.

Ovarian follicle cells have leptin receptors, so leptin may directly affect ovarian function. Also, leptin may stimulate gonadotropin-releasing hormone (GnRH) release from the hypothalamus as well as luteinizing hormone (LH) and follicle stimulating hormone (FSH) secretion from the pituitary. All of these hormones are involved in your ability to ovulate and become pregnant.

A synchronicity of LH and leptin pulses has been observed in healthy women, suggesting that leptin probably also regulates the episodic secretion of LH. Leptin levels and leptin pulses for PCOS women is similar to women with regular ovulatory cycles, although the synchronicity between LH and leptin pulses in PCOS women is weaker and somewhat out of phase with LH as compared to cycling women.[306]

Some researchers think that the inappropriate LH secretion pattern in PCOS women may be due to leptin resistance.[307] As you know, inappropriate LH secretion prevents ovulation.

There is some evidence that estrogen causes an increase in leptin levels while androgens (male hormones) and insulin resistance will suppress leptin levels.[308] [309]

Overweight women with PCOS have leptin levels similar to overweight women without PCOS. However, overweight and obese PCOS women with higher levels of insulin appeared to produce insufficient leptin for a given fat mass.[310] This issue is important because adequate leptin production and leptin sensitivity appears to be required for long-term weight loss, especially if you are on a low-fat weight-loss diet.[311]

Leptin is influenced by diet, genetics, gender, amount of fat weight and a substantial number of other hormones. Women seem to have higher incidence of leptin resistance than men, suggesting a possible interaction with estrogen. Women with PCOS and infertility often have multiple hormonal disorders, including excessively high levels of estrogen, insulin, insulin resistance and cortisol (a stress hormone). These hormone imbalances could contribute to leptin resistance, especially in overweight PCOS women.[312] [313] [314]

Leptin and Diet

Fats and sugars appear to affect leptin production.

Fat and Leptin

The amount and type of fat in the diet appears to make a difference in leptin production. Studies of rats have shown that fish oil or polyunsaturated oils allowed higher leptin production that did saturated animal fats.[315] Other studies have shown that rats on a long-term, high-fat diet developed some level of leptin resistance, regardless of whether the animals were lean or fat.[316]

A diet high in saturated fats may contribute to leptin resistance, as shown in a study of at the St. Louis University School of Medicine.[317] Leptin resistance appears to arise from impaired leptin transport across the blood-brain barrier, defects in leptin receptor signaling, and other metabolic blockades.

The researchers demonstrated that milk, for which fats are 98% triglycerides, immediately inhibited leptin transport across the blood-brain barrier. In contrast, fat-free milk was without effect. High levels of triglycerides may underlie the impairment in the blood-brain transport of leptin.

If you are overweight and have PCOS, there's a good probability you have elevated triglycerides. If so, the triglycerides may be causing you to be leptin-resistant.

Sugars and Leptin

The amount and type of carbohydrate also affects leptin. Since leptin production is dependent on insulin's metabolism of glucose in fat cells, meals high in carbohydrate, which induce larger after-meal insulin and glucose increase, tend to increase circulating leptin more than low-carbohydrate meals do.

A study conducted at the MRC Dunn Clinical Nutrition Centre in England compared the effects over 6 months of a low-fat, complex-carbohydrate diet, a low-fat, simple-carbohydrate diet, and a control diet in overweight volunteers with symptoms of metabolic syndrome (a condition similar to diabetes and PCOS).[318] Weight loss was greatest in the low-fat, complex-carbohydrate group. These data suggest that the low-fat, high-carbohydrate diet may have reduced the level of body fat, an effect that could be caused in part by a long-term increase in leptin production.

Fructose is one form of carbohydrate that is especially problematic.[319] The digestion, absorption and metabolism of fructose are different from that of glucose. Unlike glucose, fructose does not stimulate insulin secretion or enhance leptin production. Because insulin and leptin act as key signals in the regulation of food intake and body weight, dietary fructose may contribute to continued eating, increased caloric intake, and weight gain.[320]

Fructose, primarily in the form of "high-fructose corn syrup," is plentiful in the processed foods we have become accustomed to eating and drinking. Sweetened beverages tend to use high fructose corn syrup. They also pack a lot of calories, so people who consume a lot of fructose tend to also consume too many total calories.

In addition, liver metabolism of fructose favors production of triglycerides (blood fats), which are then transported to the fat cells and stored as fat. As we said earlier, elevated triglycerides may contribute to leptin resistance.

A recent study conducted at the University of Pennsylvania illustrates these points.[321] Twelve normal weight women were given test meals, one with a fructose-sweetened beverage and one with a glucose-sweetened beverage. When the fructose was consumed, the blood sugar and insulin response to the meal plummeted. But ghrelin, a hormone that stimulates hunger, did not drop as much as with the glucose beverage. And finally, the fructose meals produced a rapid and prolonged elevation of triglycerides. This is exactly the metabolic pattern you do **not** want to have. In other words, your hunger-stimulating hormone (ghrelin) is switched "on," and your hunger-suppressing hormone (leptin) is switched partially "off" because of leptin resistance.

Leptin and Exercise

A study of rats at the University of Guelph in Canada suggests that regular exercise may help to reduce leptin resistance. Rats were put on a high-fat diet and allowed to do endurance training or remain sedentary. The sedentary group developed leptin resistance. In contrast, the exercised rats were able to maintain their leptin sensitivity in spite of the high-fat diet.[322]

Another study, at the First University Faculty of Medicine in Turkey, showed that a 12-week exercise program significantly reduced leptin levels in obese women.[323]

These and other studies suggest that exercise can have a normalizing effect on leptin levels and thus reduce leptin resistance. This is good news for overweight PCOS women, who may have both abnormally high levels of leptin and leptin resistance. Regular exercise and a healthier diet will bring leptin into a more normal range. A normalized leptin level will cause leptin resistance to diminish.

Summary

There is now considerable scientific consensus that the fat cell hormone leptin and the pancreatic hormone insulin are important regulators of food intake and energy balance.

The effects of dietary fat and fructose, resulting in decreased insulin secretion and leptin production, and in reduced suppression of ghrelin, is a significant mechanism for over-consumption of calories, weight gain and obesity.

Our diet is intended to reduce both insulin resistance and leptin resistance.

A healthy diet, as outlined in this book, is a powerful tool you can use to start getting your hormones back into balance and to get them to do their job more efficiently.

Our diet helps you with hunger and energy balance in basic ways:
- Provides all of the co-factor nutrients you need to make hormones work more efficiently
- Is free of refined carbohydrates and sugars that stimulate insulin resistance and leptin resistance and that cause undesirable fluctuations in numerous hormones
- Minimizes exposure to excessive levels of fructose, which may lead to elevated triglycerides
- Minimizes undesirable dietary fats that may interfere with hormone signaling
- Contains plenty of plant fiber and healthy fats that slow down the absorption of dietary starches and sugars into the bloodstream
- Is free of chemicals and additives that may interfere with hormonal signaling
- Contains essential fatty acids that support communication between cells and hormones

16.3 Inflammation and Your Weight

In the previous chapter, we reviewed the concepts of insulin resistance and leptin resistance. We also reviewed some of the reasons why insulin and leptin resistance are likely to occur.

Systemic inflammation also plays an important role in your PCOS symptoms. This chapter reviews the link between body fat, inflammation, insulin resistance,[324] [325] leptin resistance and diet.

A growing body of evidence suggests that chronic inflammation is a trigger for insulin resistance.[326]   Insulin resistance is thought to be a primary cause of PCOS.

Contrary to what you may think, body fat is not simply an inert storehouse of unused calories encasing your body and organs.

Actually, your fat cells are metabolically very active. For example, they produce hormones (such as estrogen) and other signaling molecules that have far-reaching effects throughout your body. The signals that are sent and received by your fat cells will influence how much fat you retain and how easy or difficult it will be for you to lose weight. Some of these signals are created as the result of inflammation.

A number of studies indicate that PCOS women who are overweight tend to be in a state of chronic inflammation.[327] [328] [329] [330] Even adolescents with PCOS symptoms of high insulin and testosterone have elevated white blood counts, suggesting that the immune system is aroused and an inflammatory process may be occurring.[331] The white blood count is elevated even more when birth control pills are taken.

Chronic inflammation appears to play an under-recognized but central role in the pathology of PCOS and obesity.

The Destructive Cycle of Diet, Inflammation and Weight

The relationship of diet, inflammation and weight is summarized here:

1) A diet high in refined carbohydrates and other "fabricated" foods leads to both increased weight and increased inflammation.

2) Excess weight itself causes chronic inflammation.

3) Chronic inflammation contributes to more insulin resistance, leptin resistance and other metabolic disorders. It also decreases favorable adiponectin and increases unfavorable resistin.

4) Insulin resistance and leptin resistance stimulate accumulation of more weight, make weight loss more difficult and induce hyperandrogenism (excessive levels of male hormones) and other symptoms of PCOS.

5) The added weight induces more inflammation and thus more insulin and leptin resistance, which in turn prevents you from burning off fat stores and causes you to store even more fat.

Here is the vicious cycle of obesity and leptin resistance. Extra fat produces chronic, low-grade inflammation. Chronic inflammation produces a chronic anti-inflammatory response, led by SOCS molecules. The SOCS response stops leptin from reducing obesity. So weight goes up, which causes more inflammation. And the cycle starts all over again.

How to Break the Diet-Inflammation-Overweight Vicious Cycle

You can break this vicious cycle with three simple actions:

1) Eat a healthy diet as described in this book.
2) Get regular exercise.
3) Remove or control sources of chronic stress.

The above measures will:
- Help you lose fat weight
- Improve insulin resistance and leptin resistance
- Reduce inflammation

An Unhealthy Diet Increases Inflammation and Weight

What you eat and how much you eat affects a lot more than your weight.[332] What you eat can either stimulate inflammation or inhibit inflammation. An unhealthy diet consisting of lots of fat, refined carbohydrates and highly processed foods is not a good idea.

Refined Carbohydrates and Sugar. A diet that is high in refined carbohydrates and low in fiber can lead to excessive levels of glucose ("blood sugar") in the blood. This condition is called "hyperglycemia."

A number of studies have shown that hyperglycemia leads to inflammation. For example, in a study at the Schwartz Center for Metabolism and Nutrition at Case Western University, PCOS women consuming glucose caused immune cells to produce free radicals that caused an inflammatory response.[333] The researchers suggested that the inflammatory response induces insulin resistance and hyperandrogenism (high levels of male hormones) in PCOS women. In this study, it didn't matter whether the women were lean or overweight. In either case, the inflammatory response occurred.

Hyperglycemia (high blood sugar) also appears to increase TNF-alpha, an inflammatory biochemical that can contribute to insulin resistance, especially in lean PCOS women who have some abdominal fat.[334]

Saturated Fats and Trans Fats. A diet high in saturated fat is linked to an elevated CRP level.[335] It also induces inflammatory activity and impairs insulin signaling in the hypothalamus gland, which is your "control center" for energy balance and weight management.[336] In other words, a high-fat diet induces insulin resistance, increases inflammation and interferes with the ability of your hypothalamus gland to balance your weight.

Consumption of trans-fats has also been shown to increase inflammation.[337] [338] Trans-fats are artificially created saturated fats.

We have an extended discussion of fats and trans fats in the *Fats and Oils* section of this book.

A Healthy Diet Reduces Inflammation and Weight

A healthy diet consisting mostly of unrefined foods is the most effective way to reduce inflammation and manage weight. It also reduces insulin resistance, which reduces the tendency for hyperandrogenism (excessive male hormones), relieves various PCOS symptoms and improves fertility.

Fiber. Higher consumption of dietary fiber, as found in vegetables, fruits and legumes reduces inflammation.[339]

Omega-3 Essential Fats. Fats can directly influence production of the hormones leptin, resistin and adiponectin,[340] so the amount and type of fat you consume is important for controlling inflammation and normalizing your hormones. As discussed in the *Fats and Oils* section of this book, foods containing omega-3 fatty acids reduce inflammation.[341]

"Phyto-nutrients" in Vegetables and Fruit. Plant compounds, such as anthocyanins and bioflavonoids, generally reduce inflammation and encourage the production of anti-inflammatory adiponectin.[342] Plant pigments such as carotenoids also tend to dampen inflammation.[343] [344] The antioxidants and other "phyto-nutrients" and materials found in healthy foods play an absolutely crucial role in controlling inflammation.

The advantage of a healthy diet was borne out by a trial conducted at the Second University of Naples in Italy.[345] Half of the 120 women were put on a " Mediterranean-style" diet rich in vegetables, fruits and omega-3 fats. The other half were put on a "prudent diet" similar to the one recommended by the American Heart Association.

Not designed for weight-loss, both diets supplied over 2000 calories a day, which approximates what an average American woman consumes. Although both groups of women lost weight, the women on the Mediterranean diet lost significantly more weight and body mass than those on the "prudent diet."

Even more importantly, the Mediterranean diet group saw significant reductions in two key indicators of inflammation — CRP and IL-6. The Mediterranean diet women also had a rise in their adiponectin levels and improvement in their insulin sensitivity.

There's little question that a healthier, high-quality diet will help to reduce inflammation in women with PCOS.

The remainder of this chapter is rather technical. Continue reading if you want to deepen your understanding of the complex interplay between inflammation, hormones and body fat.

What Is Inflammation?

Inflammation is part of your body's response to injury or infection. It is a byproduct of the body's attempt to heal itself. Usually, you are aware of inflammation by its classic signs of redness, heat, swelling and pain. However, there is a very complex, hidden, powerful biochemical process that results in these classic signs of inflammation.

Inflammation is not always as obvious as pain or swelling. It can occur at a low, unnoticeable level. This is referred to as sub-clinical, chronic inflammation. In other words, the inflammatory biochemical process is occurring, but you are not aware of it. Chronic, low-grade inflammation is what we are concerned about in dealing with PCOS and weight problems.[346]

Body Fat Causes Inflammation

You can think of your fat cells as an endocrine and secretory organ, just like your ovaries, thyroid, adrenal glands, liver, hypothalamus, or any other organ or gland in your body.[347] Fat cells produce a bewildering array of biochemicals that influence what goes on in your body.[348]

One of the families of biochemicals produced by your fat cells are "cytokines," many of which are involved in the inflammatory process. They include leptin, adiponectin, tumor necrosis factor alpha (TNF-alpha) and interleukin-6 (IL-6), to name a few. Most cytokines promote inflammation while some others inhibit inflammation.

The more fat cells you have, especially around your middle, the more cytokines you will produce and the more likely it is that you are promoting inflammation.

We don't have room to review all of the possible inflammatory factors, but we'll review a few of them so that you can appreciate how complex their interrelationship is and better understand the important role they play in the outcome of PCOS.

TNF-alpha. TNF is known for producing tissue damage and pain in some autoimmune disorders. It can also interfere with the function of insulin and contributes to insulin resistance.[349]

TNF-alpha is elevated in obese women, whether or not they have PCOS. However, even lean PCOS women appear to have TNF-alpha levels higher than normal lean women.[350] PCOS women may have an unexplained tendency toward higher TNF-alpha, which is worsened by increased weight.

IL-6. IL-6 is closely related to TNF and is associated with arthritis and heart disease.

C-reactive protein (CRP), which has been associated with the development of cardiovascular disease and diabetes, is a reflection of the level of IL-6 in the body.

Fat - Immune System - Inflammation Link

Fat attracts a type of white blood cell known as a macrophage, which also produces TNF, IL-6 and other inflammatory cytokines.[351] Macrophages are scavenger cells. Their job is literally to gobble up foreign organisms and cellular debris. Macrophages seem to be drawn to body fat because fat cells tend to leak and break open, especially in people with abdominal obesity. Macrophages move into the leaky fat tissue in order to clean up debris and then they themselves begin to release TNF-alpha, IL-6 and other inflammatory factors. Macrophages appear to be a major contributor to inflammation.[352]

SOCS and Leptin Resistance

To limit the damage produced by inflammation, your body produces anti-inflammatory biochemicals that are triggered by the inflammation itself. This is a compensating mechanism that attempts to maintain a balance in the healing process.

When pro-inflammatory cytokines enter a cell to initiate or promote a biochemical processes to increase the inflammatory response, the cell simultaneously produces anti-inflammatory chemicals called "suppressors of cytokine signaling," or simply "SOCS." SOCS molecules suppress the cell's response to inflammatory cytokines. Two SOCS molecules, SOCS-1 and SOCS-3, are able to interfere with a cell's ability to respond to leptin, which increases leptin resistance.[353][354]   SOCS-3 also blocks the response to insulin, which increases insulin resistance.[355][356][357]

Some researchers believe that SOCS production is an important cause of leptin resistance and consequently contributes to the development of obesity.

SOCS may also increase fat production in the liver, helping to create a condition called "steatosis" or "fatty liver," where the liver becomes clogged with fat and does not optimally perform its many functions.[358] Your can learn more in the *Liver Health* chapter.

Adiponectin

Adiponectin is a hormone secreted by fat cells that favorably influences weight in several ways: it helps to control regulation of glucose (blood sugar), aids the metabolism of fat, improves insulin sensitivity and has an anti-inflammatory effect.[359] [360]

Unfortunately, adiponectin levels are lower in PCOS women than in other women.[361] It appears that insulin resistance, inflammation and obesity may inhibit adiponectin production.[362] [363] [364] On the other hand, leptin (in the absence of leptin resistance) increases production of adiponectin.[365]

Resistin

Fat cells and macrophages (a type of white blood cell) produce a hormone called resistin. Resistin appears to cause tissues — especially the liver — to be less sensitive to the action of insulin and thus lead to increased blood sugar levels. There is a strong association between elevated levels of resistin and obesity and diabetes.

Resistin has been shown to be a potent stimulator of inflammation, including the stimulation of TNF-alpha and IL-6.[366] [367] In experiments, increased levels of resistin also appear to induce increased SOCS-3.[368] As we said earlier, SOCS-3 contributes to leptin resistance and insulin resistance.

The amount of body fat you have may also increase resistin. While resistin in produced by fat cells, it is also produced by the macrophages that are attracted to debris leaking from fat cells. Increased macrophage activity could lead to more resistin.[369]

Although resistin levels are not elevated in all PCOS women, these women appear to be more inclined to produce resistin than those without PCOS.[370]

C-Reactive Protein (CRP)

C-reactive protein (CRP) is a protein that is a general indicator of inflammation and is associated with being overweight. CRP is a fairly common blood test that you can get from your doctor. A high level of CRP is a strong predictor of future cardiovascular disease and stroke.

In a study at the Rambam Medical Center in Israel, 36.8% of PCOS women had elevated CRP whereas only 9.6% non-PCOS women had elevated levels.[371]   Estrogen, which may be in excess in some PCOS women, is one of numerous factors that can increase CRP.[372]

Inflammation, Weight and Oxidative Stress

A condition of "oxidative stress" exists when pro-oxidant factors in the body exceed the anti-oxidant factors. The result is an accumulation of unstable, destructive molecules called "free radical" molecules, which damage components of the cell membranes, proteins or genetic material by "oxidizing" them. This process is the same chemical reaction that causes iron to rust.

Oxidative stress can result from many factors, including poor quality diet, environmental pollution, alcohol, smoking, medications, trauma, toxins, excessive exercise and inflammation, to name a few.

Oxidative stress it thought to be a primary cause of degenerative diseases and accelerated aging.

As a group, women with PCOS are more likely to experience oxidative stress than healthy women. For example, a study from the University of Harran in Turkey found an increase in oxidant status in women with PCOS. This increase was related to central obesity, age, blood pressure, serum glucose (blood sugar), insulin and triglyceride levels, and insulin resistance. In addition, their antioxidant status was found to be insufficient. The researchers said these findings suggest that oxidative stress may contribute to the increased risk of cardiovascular disease in women with PCOS.[373]

But oxidative stress does more than increase cardiovascular risk. It also promotes increased inflammation and induces insulin resistance.[374] It may also interfere with reproductive function.[375]

Oxidant stress is part of the vicious cycle of increased inflammation leading to insulin and leptin resistance and thus creating excess weight.

Women in general appear to be more likely to have oxidant stress than men, according to a research study conducted at the University of California at Berkeley.[376]

Section 17

Resources and Feedback

17.1 Resources

Here are some resources you can turn to that go beyond the scope of this book.

Get Help from Dr. Nancy Dunne

E-Mail Mini-Consultation (www.ovarian-cysts-pcos.com/db/econsult): Dr. Nancy Dunne is available to spend 15 minutes of her time to answer your specific questions or concerns about PCOS, infertility, ovarian cysts or any other health issue. She will send her response by return e-mail. Reasonable cost.

Phone Consultation (www.ovarian-cysts-pcos.com/db/pconsult): Dr. Dunne offers phone consultations for those who are too far away to visit her clinic in person. She offers extensive interviews and an in-depth review of your medical history and current concerns. When data collection is complete, Dr. Dunne will offer treatment recommendations specific to your circumstances, with a focus on natural therapies. You can choose to have an ongoing consultative relationship with Dr. Dunne for guidance and support as you follow her recommendations to optimize your health and fertility. Cost depends on the amount of time involved.

Get Other Medical Help

Find a Top PCOS Specialist in Your State (www.ovarian-cysts-pcos.com/db/specialist). It's surprisingly difficult to find a physician who understands PCOS and knows how to effectively treat it. You may be able to obtain a list of physicians in the U.S. who have a demonstrated interest in PCOS and who appear to be qualified. The list is not free but may be worth the price if you can find the right doctor for you.

American Association of Naturopathic Physicians (www.ovarian-cysts-pcos.com/db/aanp). Find a licensed naturopathic physician in your area who can help you. Licensed naturopathic physicians tend to take a natural, comprehensive, holistic approach to reproductive disorders, as contrasted to a "take this pharmaceutical pill for that problem" approach.

PCOS Support

The **Polycystic Ovarian Syndrome Association (PCOSA) (www.ovarian-cysts-pcos.com/db/ pcosa)** is a non-profit organization created by women who have PCOS. Its purpose is to serve and support you. It's an excellent resource. Become a member of PCOSA, or join one of its email lists so that you can communicate with other women who may have helpful information.

Supplements for PCOS and Infertility

Supplements Information (www.ovarian-cysts-pcos.com/db/suppinfo). Our website has some information about nutritional supplements for PCOS and infertility that is not included in this book.

Purchase of Supplements (www.ovarian-cysts-pcos.com/db/suppstore). This is where you can find out about purchasing supplements specifically for PCOS or infertility.

PCOS Information Resources

PCOS Newsletter Archives (www.ovarian-cysts-pcos.com/db/newsarchive). We publish a free newsletter about PCOS — the latest research, new developments, and other important issues and information.

Go here for a free subscription: **www.ovarian-cysts-pcos.com/db/newssubscribe**

PCOS Book List (www.ovarian-cysts-pcos.com/db/books). Popular books in print on the topic of PCOS and fertility.

PCOS Glossary (www.ovarian-cysts-pcos.com/db/glossary). If you don't know what a medical term means, please visit our online Glossary.

Health Information Resources

MedlinePlus (www.ovarian-cysts-pcos.com/db/medline). The National Institute of Health provides health news, information on any health topic, medical encyclopedia, health dictionary and more.

HealthWeb (www.ovarian-cysts-pcos.com/db/healthweb). Information links to a variety of medical topics and specialties. Includes links to academic institutions, associations, databases, consumer health resources, electronic information resources and more.

IBIDS (www.ovarian-cysts-pcos.com/db/ibids). IBIDS is the International Bibliographic Information on Dietary Supplements database, a source of medical research articles about nutritional supplements; provided by the National Institute of Health.

Additional Reading

Chapter 1.2: What Causes PCOS?

If you wish to explore more about genes and environment and how environmental pollution is affecting your health, you may find the following books helpful.

The Dependent Gene: The Fallacy of "Nature vs. Nurture by David Moore. This book reveals how all traits — even apparently straightforward characteristics like eye and hair color — are caused by complex interactions between genes and the environment at every stage of biological and psychological development, from the single fertilized egg to full-grown adulthood.

Our Stolen Future: Are We Threatening Our Fertility, Intelligence, and Survival? — A Scientific Detective Story, by Theo Colborn, Dianne Dumandski and John Myers. You MUST read this book so that you understand the severity of the chemical pollution problem and understand what a serious threat it is to your health. This book pieces together the compelling evidence from wildlife studies, laboratory experiments and human data, to lay out the emerging scientific case regarding this largely unrecognized threat. The authors trace birth defects, sexual abnormalities and reproductive failures in wildlife to their source — synthetic chemicals that mimic natural hormones, upsetting normal reproductive and developmental processes.

Living Downstream: An Ecologist Looks at Cancer and the Environment, by Sandra Steingraber. There is a growing body of evidence linking cancer to environmental pollution. Her scientific analysis ranges from the alarming worldwide patterns of cancer incidence to the sabotage wrought by cancer-promoting substances on the intricate workings of human cells. In a gripping personal narrative, she travels from hospital waiting rooms to hazardous waste sites and from farmhouse kitchens to incinerator hearings to bring to life stories of communities around the country as they confront decades of industrial and agricultural recklessness.

Chapter 5.2: The Problem with Milk

Milk And Mortality: The connection between milk drinking and coronary heart disease by David B. Gordon, 207 pages, about $185. Yes, this book is expensive!! But if you are absolutely convinced you must consume milk, maybe you should read it.

Dr. Gordon's book cites 428 scientific papers, published in peer-reviewed medical journals. His book includes 13 charts and illustrations consisting of meticulously prepared data. Charts especially worth noting are on pages 32 and 112. The first chart correlates coronary heart disease mortality rates with the consumption of milk in 23 countries. The second chart correlates milk consumption with serum cholesterol levels in 15 countries. The graphs show a convincing straight-line correlation that provides an empirical relationship between milk and heart disease.

Chapter 6.1: What's a Fat?

Fat and oils is a vast, complex topic. For additional reading on this subject, we recommend that you read *Fats that Heal, Fats the Kill*, by Udo Erasmus.

Note: You can find other relevant reading materials at our **online bookstore (www.ovarian-cysts-pcos.com/db/books).**

17.2 Feedback from You

We intend that this book be a two-way communication. What you think and feel is just as important as what we think and feel.

Please let us know about:
- Any topic that is not clear to you.
- Problems you had with the diet.
- Successes you had with the diet.
- Questions that that we didn't answer.
- Comments about the recipes - good or bad.
- A recipe you would like to share.
- How can we improve a future edition of this book?
- Anything at all!

We invite you to communicate with us by going to our feedback web page:

www.ovarian-cysts-pcos.com/db/feedback

We hope that this book will be the first step in a long-term relationship with you!

Wishing You the Best of Health,

Nancy Dunne, N.D.
Bill Slater

About the Authors

Nancy Dunne, N.D.

Hello, my name is Nancy Dunne. I'm a naturopathic physician licensed to practice primary care in the state of Montana. My specialty is the use of natural medicine to improve the health of my patients.

Over the past decade, PCOS and ovarian cysts have become especially relevant to me. My daughter's menstrual difficulties and persistent acne were diagnosed as aspects of polycystic ovary syndrome. This disturbing discovery galvanized me to do research in order to create a safe, effective treatment plan for her. The success we had with her treatment was so exciting, I began to offer similar individualized treatments to the women in my medical practice with PCOS and fertility issues. The effectiveness of this approach is clear. In addition, I have personally lost more than 50 pounds of body weight and maintained my healthy dimensions for over ten years, using the diet and exercise principles described in this book.

I've been a practicing physician since 1989. My clinic, Bitterroot Natural Medicine, is located in Missoula, Montana and offers primary care for clients of all ages. The clinic is best known for its treatment of women's health concerns, fertility issues, body reshaping, physical fitness, menopause, and polycystic ovary syndrome. Before becoming a naturopathic physician, I was a Registered Nurse, specializing in obstetrics and neonatal health.

I'm a graduate of National College of Naturopathic Medicine in Portland, Oregon. I also have a Masters degree in Applied Behavioral Science from Bastyr University in Seattle, Washington. I'm a Professional Member of the Polycystic Ovarian Syndrome Association and past President of the American Association of Naturopathic Physicians.

I want to share my experiences treating PCOS and its accompanying difficulties by using natural therapies. PCOS can be a devastating experience, with health consequences that reach deeply into a woman's life. The burden of this condition can be lightened, even erased in many cases, with your active participation, your willingness to learn and make changes. It is challenging and exhilarating to take your health in your own hands and make life the best it can be. Bill and I hope you will use this book and our website for long-term support and as an outlet for celebrating your success.

Bill Slater

In 1977, when my mother was diagnosed with cancer, I began to question my concepts of health and the causes of disease. Wanting to understand my mother's illness, I conducted extensive research in the areas of health, nutrition and disease prevention. This was the beginning of what would later become a career in health care services.

I'm the co-founder of a chiropractic clinic that became an integrative medicine center with health practitioners from different disciplines. We specialized in treating people with chronic disorders with a variety of holistic, natural therapies.

Since retiring from the clinic, I'm focusing my time on helping average people learn how to take more responsibility for their own health. My first project is polycystic ovary syndrome, because it is an under-recognized disorder that is quite serious. Unfortunately, the standard treatments are quite limited or ineffective. Dr. Dunne and I firmly believe there are some very powerful things *you* can do to effectively manage this health problem.

This diet book is the first phase of our plan to help women who have PCOS and infertility.

By the way, you may be a little shocked at the foods we are asking you to avoid. For example, we ask you to stay away from wheat and dairy products. If you find this a challenge, I understand. I have an autoimmune disorder that requires me to not eat any wheat or dairy. I can assure you that I did not die or go crazy because I could not have a cheese sandwich. It took a while, but I learned to eat different foods. Now I'm used to my new diet.

But I will admit I would love to have a pizza. Or a pastry and mocha. However, when I look at these desires rationally, I realize I would much rather keep my good health than have the momentary pleasure of a pizza. So I skip the pizza and have something else.

I have a M.B.A. from the University of California. Although I don't have a medical degree, I have studied nutrition and disease prevention for 30 years and have attended hundreds of hours of medical seminars.

References

Chapter 1.1

[1] Kiddy, DS et al, Improvement in endocrine and ovarian function during dietary treatment of obese women with polycystic ovary syndrome. Clin Endocrinol (Oxf) 1992 Jan; 36(1): 105-11

[2] Berrino, F et al, Reducing bioavailable sex hormones through a comprehensive change in diet: the diet and androgens (DIANA) randomized trial. Cancer Epidemiol Biomarkers Prev 2001 Jan; 10(1): 25-33

[3] Moran, LJ et al, Dietary composition in restoring reproductive and metabolic physiology in overweight women with polycystic ovary syndrome, J Clin Endocrin & Metab, 88(2): 812-819

[4] Stamets, K et al, A randomized trial of the effects of two types of short-term hypocaloric diets on weight loss in women with polycystic ovary syndrome, Fertil Steril, 2004, 81(3): 630-7

[5] Butzow, TL et al, The decrease in luteinizing hormone secretion in response to weight reduction is inversely related to the severity of insulin resistance in overweight women, J Clin Endocrinol Metab, 2000, 85(9): 3271-5

[6] Moran, LJ et al, Ghrelin and measures of satiety are altered in polycystic ovary syndrome but not differentially affected by diet composition, J Clin Endocrinol Metab, 2004, 89(7): 3337-44

Chapter 1.2

[7] Holte, J, Polycystic ovary syndrome and insulin resistance: thrifty genes struggling with over-feeding and sedentary life style?, J Endocrinol Invest, 1998, 21(9):589-601

[8] San Millan, S et al, Association of the polycystic ovary syndrome with genomic variants related to insulin resistance, type 2 diabetes mellitus, and obesity, J Clin Endocrinol Metab, 2004, 89(6): 2640-6

[9] Diao, FY et al, The molecular characteristics of polycystic ovary syndrome (PCOS) ovary defined by human ovary cDNA microassay, J Mol Endocrinology, 2004, 33:59-72

[10] *The Dependent Gene: The Fallacy of "Nature vs. Nurture* by David Moore

[11] Seli E et al, Optimizing ovulation induction in women with polycystic ovary syndrome. Curr Opin Obstet Gynecol 2002 Jun; 14(3): 245-54

[12] Sozen, I et al, Hyperinsulinism and Its Interaction With Hyperandrogenism in PCOS, Obstet Gynecol Survey, 2000; 55(5): 321-328

[13] Colagiuri, S et al, The 'carnivore connection' — evolutionary aspects of insulin resistance, Eur J Clin Nutr, 2002, 56: Suppl 1:S30-5

[14] Colagiuri S et al, The "carnivore connection" - evolutionary aspects of insulin reistance, Eur J Clin Nutr, 2002, 56 Suppl 1:S30-5

[15] Lovejoy, JC, Dietary fatty acids and insulin resistance, Curr Atheroscler Rep, 1999, 1(3): 215-20

[16] Tatarai T, et al, Alteration of insulin-receptor kinsase activity by high-fat feeding, Diabetes, 1988, 37(10): 1397-1404

[17] Kelly GS, Insulin resistance: lifestyle and nutritional interventions. Altern Med Rev., 2000, 5(2): 109-32

[18] Odea, K, Marked improvement in carbohydrate and lipid metabolism in diabetic Australian aborigines after temporary reversion to traditional lifestyle, Diabetes, 1984, 33(6): 596-603

[19] Smith JD et al, Relief of fibromyalgia symptoms following discontinuation of dietary excitotoxins. Ann Pharmacother 2001 Jun; 35(6): 702-6

[20] Inkster SE et al, Pituitary receptors for LH-releasing hormone (LHRH) and responsiveness to LHRH in adult female rats after neonatal monosodium L-glutamate treatment. J Endocrinol. 1985 Oct; 107(1):9-13

[21] Nemeroff, CB et al, Marked reduction in gonadal steroid hormone levels in rats treated neonatally with monosodium L-glutamate: further evidence for disruption of hypothalamic-pituitary-gonadal axis regulation. Neuroendocrinology. 1981 Nov; 33(5): 265-7.

[22] Crinnion, WJ, Environmental medicine, part 1: the human burden of environmental toxins and their common health effects, Altern Med Rev. 2000 Feb; 5(1): 52-63

[23] Lovekamp-Swan, T et al, Mechanisms of phthalate ester toxicity in the female reproductive system. Environ Health Perspect. 2003 Feb; 111(2): 139-45.

[24] Crinnion, WJ, Environmental medicine, part 1: the human burden of environmental toxins and their common health effects, Altern Med Rev. 2000 Feb; 5(1): 52-63.

[25] Crinnion, WJ, Environmental medicine, part 2 - health effects of and protection from ubiquitous airborne solvent exposure, Altern Med Rev. 2000 Apr; 5(2): 33-43.

[26] Crinnion, WJ, Environmental medicine, part 4: pesticides - biologically persistent and ubiquitous toxins, Altern Med Rev. 2000 Oct; 5(5): 432-47.

[27] Foster WG, Environmental toxicants and human fertility, Minerva Ginecol, 2003, 55(5): 451-7

[28] Ptak A et al, Comparison of the actions of 4-chlorobiphenyl and its hydroxylated metabolites on estradiol secretion by ovarian follicles in parimary cells in culture, Reprod Toxicol, 2005, 20(1): 57-64

[29] Lovekamp-Swan T et al, Mechanisms of phthalate ester toxicity in the female reproductive system, Environ Health Perspect, 2003, 111(2): 139-45

[30] Gauger KJ et al, Polychlorinated biphenyls (PCBs) exert thyroid hormone-like effects in the fetal rat brain but do not bind to thyroid hormone receptors, Environ Health Perspect, 2004, 1212(5): 516-23

[31] He J et al, Alternations of FSH-stimulated progersterone production and calcium homeostasis in primarily cultured human luteinizing-granulosa cells induced by fenvalerate, Toxicology, 2004, 203(1-3): 61-8

[32] Hoyer, Damage to ovarian development and function, Cell Tissue Res, 2005, April 23, [Epub ahead of print]

[33] Pocar P et al, The impact of endocrine disruptors on oocyte competence, Reproduction, 2003, 125(3): 313-25

[34] Troisi, GM et al, PCB-associated alteration of hepatic steroid metabolism in harbor seals (Phoca vitulina). J Toxicol Environ Health A. 2000 Dec 29; 61(8):649-55

[35] Windham GC, et al, Exposure to organochlorines compounds and effects on ovarian function, Epidemiology, 2005, 16(2): 182-90

[36] Stewart P et al, Prenatal PCB exposure, the corpus callosum, and response inhibition, Environ Health Perspect, 2003, 111(13): 1670-7

[37] Vreugdenhil HJ et al, Effects of perinatal exposure to PCBs on neuropsychological functions in the Rotterdam cohort at 9 years of age, Neuropsychology, 2004, 18(1): 185-193

[38] Soechitram SD et al, Fetal exposure to PCBs and their hydroxylated metabolites in a Dutch cohort, Environ Health Perspect, 2004, 112(11): 1208-12

[39] Janssen, OE et al, High prevalence of autoimmune thyroiditis in patients with polycystic ovary syndrome, Eur J Endocrinol, 2004, 150(3): 363-9

[40] Reimand K, et al, Autoantibody studies of female patients with reproductive failure J Reprod Immunol 2001; 51(2): 67-76

[41] Kelly CC, et al, Low grade chronic inflammation in women with polycystic ovarian syndrome J Clin Endocrinol Metab 2001; 86(6):2453-5

[42] Navarra, P et al, Increased production and release of prostaglandin-E2 by human granulose cells from polycystic ovaries, Prostaglandins, 1996, 52(3): 187-97

Chapter 2.1

[43] www.mypyramid.gov

Chapter 2.2

[44] Layman D, et al, A reduced ratio of dietary carbohydrate to protein improves body composition and blood lipid profiles during weight loss in adult women. J Nutr. 2003 Feb, 133(2): 411-17

[45] Due A et al, Effect of normal-fat diets, either medium or high in protein, on body weight in overweight subjects: a randomised 1-year trial, Int J Obes Relat Metab Disord. 2004; 28(10): 1283-90

[46] Brehm B et al, A randomized trial comparing a very low carbohydrate diet and a calorie-restricted low fat diet on body weight and cardiovascular risk factors in healthy women, J Clin Endocrinol Metab. 2003, 88(4): 1617-23

[47] Bravata, D et al, Efficacy and safety of low-carbohydrate diets: a systematic review. JAMA. 2003 Apr 9, 289(14): 1837-50

[48] Stubbs RJ: Macronutrient effects on appetite. Int J Obes, 1995, 19 (Suppl 5): S11-19

[49] Ma Y et al, Association between dietary carbohydrates and body weight, Am J Epidemiol, 2005, 161(4): 239-67

[50] Piatti, PM et al, Hypocaloric high-protein diet improves glucose oxidation and spares lean body mass: comparison to hypocaloric high-carbohydrate diet, Metabolism, 1994, 43:1481-1487

[51] Yancy, WS et al, A low-carbohydrate, ketogenic diet versus a low-fat diet to treat obesity and hyperlipidemia: a randomized, controlled trial, Ann Intern Med. 2004 May 18; 140(10): 769-77

[52] Martin, W, Annual 2002 Experimental Biology Conference of the Federation of American Societies for Experimental Biology (FASEB), New Orleans, LA April 21, 2002

[53] Wiederkehr M et al, Metabolic and endocrine effects of metabolic acidosis in humans, Swiss Med Wkly 2001, 131:127–32

[54] Stamets K et al, A randomized trial of the effects of two types of short-term hypocaloric diets on weight loss in women with polycystic ovary syndrome, Fertil Steril. 2004 Mar; 81(3): 630-7

[55] Moran, LJ et al, Dietary composition in restoring reproductive and metabolic physiology in overweight women with polycystic ovary syndrome, J Clin Endocrinology & Metabolism, 2003, 88:812-9

Chapter 2.3

[56] Bravata DM et al, Efficacy and safety of low-carbohydrate diets, JAMA, 2003, 289:1837-1850

[57] Dansinger ML et atl, Comparison of the Atkins, Ornish, Weight Watchers, and Zone Diets for weight loss and heart disease risk reduction, JAMA. 2005; 293:43-53

Chapter 2.4

[58] O'Keefe JH Jr, et al, Cardiovascular Disease Resulting From a Diet and Lifestyle at Odds With Our Paleolithic Genome: How to Become a 21st-Century Hunter-Gatherer, Mayo Clin Proc, 2004; 79:101-108

[59] Eaton, SB et al, Paleolithic vs. modern diets—selected pathophysiological implications, Eur J Nutr 2000 Apr; 39(2): 67-70

Chapter 2.5

[60] Yunsheng, M et al, Association between dietary carbohydrates and body weight, Am J Epidemiology, 2005 161(4): 359-367

Chapter 3.1

[61] Wright, CE et al, Dietary intake, physical activity, and obesity in women with polycystic ovary syndrome, Int J Obes Relat Metab Discord, 2004, 28(8): 1026-32

[62] Holte, J, Polycystic ovary syndrome and insulin resistance: thrifty genes struggling with over-feeding and sedentary life style?, J Endocrinol Invest, 1998; 21(9):589-601

[63] Friedman JM, A war on obesity, not the obese. Science. 2003 Feb 7; 299(5608): 856-8

[64] Harris, RB, Role of set-point theory in regulation of body weight. FASEB J. 1990 Dec; 4(15): 3310-8

[65] Exercise and Sport Nutrition Laboratory, Baylor University

Chapter 3.2

[66] Stubbs RJ et al, Covert manipulation of the dietary fat to carbohydrate ratio of isoenergetically dense diets: effect on food intake in feeding men ad libitum. International Journal of Obesity, July 1996, 20(7): 651-60

[67] Rolls BJ et al, Energy density but not fat content of foods affected energy intake in lean and obese women. American Journal of Clinical Nutrition, 1999 May, 69(5): 863-71

[68] Shide, DJ et al, Information about the fat content of preloads influences energy intake in healthy women. J Am Diet Assoc. 1995 Sep; 95(9): 993-8

[69] Rolls, BJ, et al, Salad and satiety: energy density and portion size of a first-course salad affect energy intake at lunch. J Am Diet Assoc. 2004 Oct; 104(10): 1570-6

[70] Rolls, BJ et al, Water incorporated into a food but not served with a food decreases energy intake in lean women. Am J Clin Nutr. 1999 Oct; 70(4): 448-55

[71] Rolls, BJ et al, What can intervention studies tell us about the relationship between fruit and vegetable consumption and weight management? Nutr Rev. 2004 Jan; 62(1):1-17

Chapter 3.5

[72] Nielsen, SJ et al, Patterns and trends in food portion sizes, 1977-1998. JAMA. 2003 Jan 22-29; 289(4):450-3

[73] Rolls BJ et al, Portion size of food affects energy intake in normal-weight and overweight men and women, Am J Clin Nutr, 2002, 76(6): 1207-13

[74] Kral, TV et al, Combined effects of energy density and portion size on energy intake in women. Am J Clin Nutr. 2004 Jun; 79(6): 962-8

[75] McCluskey, SE, et al, Binge Eating and Polycystic Ovaries, The Lancet, September 19, 1992; 340:723

Chapter 3.6

[76] Dansinger ML et al, Comparison of the Atkins, Ornish, Weight Watchers, and Zone diets for weight loss and heart disease risk reduction: a randomized trial. JAMA. 2005 Jan 5; 293(1): 43-53

[77] Kiddy, DS et al, Improvement in endocrine and ovarian function during dietary treatment of obese women with polycystic ovary syndrome, Clin Endocrinol (Oxf), 1992, 36(1): 105-111

[78] Moran, LJ et al, Dietary composition in restoring reproductive and metabolic physiology in overweight women with polycystic ovary syndrome, J Clin Endocrin & Metab, 88(2): 812-819

[79] Stamets, K et al, A randomized trial of the effects of two types of short-term hypocaloric diets on weight loss in women with polycystic ovary syndrome, Fertil Steril, 2004, 81(3): 630-7

[80] Butzow, TL et al, The decrease in luteinizing hormone secretion in response to weight reduction is inversely related to the severity of insulin resistance in overweight women, J Clin Endocrinol Metab, 2000, 85(9): 3271-5

Chapter 4.1

[81] Wolever TMS et al, The glycemic index: methodology and clinical implications. Am J Clin Nutr 1991;54: 846–54

[82] Brand-Miller, J et al, The New Glucose Revolution: The Authoritative Guide to the Glycemic Index – The Dietary Solution for Lifelong Health. New York: Marlowe & Company, 2003

[83] Teff, KL et al, Dietary fructose reduces circulating insulin and leptin, attenuates postprandial suppression of ghrelin, and increases triglycerides in women, 2004, J Clin Endocrinol Metab, 89(6): 2963-72

[84] Bray, GA et al, Consumption of high-fructose corn syrup in beverages may play a role in the epidemic of obesity, Am J Clin Nutr, 2004, 79(4):537-543

[85] Basciano H et al, Fructose, insulin resistance, and metabolic dyslipidemia.Nutr Metab (Lond). 2005 Feb 21;2(1): 5

[86] Elliot, S et al, Fructose, weight gain, and the insulin resistance syndrome, Am J Clin Nutr, 2002, 76(5): 911-922

[87] Pereira MA et al, Types of carbohydrates and risk of cardiovascular disease, J Womens Health,2003, 12(2):115-22

Chapter 4.2

[88] Schulze MB et al, Glycemic index, glycemic load, and dietary fiber intake and incidence of type 2 diabetes in younger and middle-aged women, Am J Clin Nutr, 2004, 80(2):348-56

[89] Willett W et al, Glycemic index, glycemic load, and risk of type 2 diabetes, Am J Clin Nutr, 2002, 76(1):274S-80S

[90] Liu S et al, A prospective study of dietary glycemic load, carbohydrate intake, and risk of coronary heart disease un US women, Am J Clin Nutr, 2000, 71(6):1455-61

[91] Liu S et al, Relation between a diet with a high glycemic load and plasma concentrations of high-sensitivity C-reactive protein in middle-aged women, Am J Clin Nutr, 2002, 75(3):492-8

[92] Wolever TM et al, Long-term effect of varying the source or amount of dietary carbohydrate on postprandial plasma glucose, insulin, triacylglycerol, and free fatty acid concentrations in subjects with impaired glucose tolerance, Am J Clin Nutr, 2003, 77(3):612-621

Chapter 4.3

[93] Cordain, Loren, "Cereal grains: humanity's double-edged sword," Word Rev Nutr Diet, Basel, Karger, 1999, 84:19-73 (Evolutionary Aspects of Nutrition and Health, Simopoulos AP, ed.)

[94] Liener, IE, Implications of antinutritional components in soybean foods, Crit Rev Food Sci Nutr, 1994, 34(1):31-67

[95] Kilpatrick DC, Immunological aspects of the potential role of dietary carbohydrates and lectins in human health, Eur J Nutr, 1999, 38(3):107-17

[96] Greer F et al, Effect of kidney bean (Phaseolus vulgaris) toxin on tissue weight and composition and some metabolic functions of rats, Br J Nutr, 1985, 54(1):95-103

[97] Pusztai A, Characteristics and consequences of interactions of lectins with the intestinal mucosa, Arch Latinoam Nutr, 1996, 44(4 Suppl 1):10S-15S

[98] Coppo R et al, Dietary antigens and primary immunoglobulin A nephropathy, J Am Soc Nephrol, 1992, 2(10 Suppl):S173-S180

[99] Pusztai A et al, Antinutritive effects of wehat-germ agglutinin and other N-acetylglucosamine-specific lectins, Br J Nutr, 1993, 70(1):313-321

[100] Pusztai A, Dietary lectins are metabolic signals for the gut and modulate immune and hormone functions, Eur J Clin Nutr, 1993, 47(10):691-699

[101] Adamo, Peter D, Townsend Letter For Doctors, August 1990

[102] Gray AM et al, Insulin-releasing and insulin-like activity of Agaricus campestris (mushroom), J Endocrinol, 1998, 157(2):259-66

[103] Swanston-Flatt SK et al, Glycaemic effects of traditional European plant treatments for diabetes. Studies in normal and streptozotocia diabetic mice, Diabetes Res, 1989, 10(2):69-73

[104] Auricchio R, In vitro-deranged intestinal immune response to gliadin in type 1 diabetes. Diabetes. 2004 Jul;53(7):1680-3

[105] Kucera P, Gliadin, endomysial and thyroid antibodies in patients with latent autoimmune diabetes of adults (LADA). Clin Exp Immunol. 2003 Jul;133(1):139-43

Chapter 4.4

[106] Divi RL, Chang HC, Doerge DR Anti-thyroid isoflavones from soybean: isolation, characterization, and mechanisms of action. National Center for Toxicological Research, Jefferson, AR 72079, USA.

[107] Fukutake, M et al, Quantification of genistein and genistin in soybeans and soybean products, Food Chem Toxicol. 1996 May;34(5):457-61

[108] Ishizuki, Y. et al., "The effects on the thyroid gland of soybeans administered experimentally in healthy subjects," Nippon Naibunpi Gakkai Zasshi (1991) 767:622-629

[109] Haddow, J. E. Maternal Thyroid Deficiency During Pregnancy and Subsequent Neuropsychological Development of the Child, NEJM 341: 549-555: 1999

[110] Allan, W.C. Maternal Thyroid Deficiency and Pregnancy Complications: Implications for Population Screening, J Med Screen 2000: 7: 127-130

[111] Rosenthal, M.S. The Thyroid Sourcebook, Lowell House, Los Angeles, 1996 (pp. 37-38)
Wood, L.C. Your Thyroid: A Home Reference Ballantine Books, New York, 1995 (pp. 175)

[112] Cassidy, A. et al., "Biological Effects of a Diet of Soy Protein Rich in Isoflavones on the Menstrual Cycle of Premenopausal Women," American Journal of Clinical Nutrition (1994) 60:333-340

[113] Anderson, J et al, Meta-analysis of the effects of soy protein intake on serum lipids. N Engl J Med 1995 Aug 3;333 (5): 276-82

[114] Cramer DW et al, A case-control study of galactose consumption and metabolism in relation to ovarian cancer, Cancer Epidemiol Biomarkers Prev, 2000, 9(1):95-101

[115] Carmer DW et al, Adult hypolactasia, milk consumption, and age-specific fertility, Am J Epidemiol, 1994, 139(3):282-9

[116] Tobacman JK et al, Consumption of carrageenan and other water-soluble polymers used as food additives and incidence of mammary carcinoma, Med Hypotheses, 2001, 56(5):589-98

Chapter 4.5

[117] Rock CL et al, Effects of a high-fiber, low-fat diet intervention on serum concentrations of reproductive steroid hormones in women with a history of breast cancer, J Clin Oncol. 2004 Jun 15;22(12):2379-87

[118] McKeown NM et al, Carbohydrate nutrition, insulin resistance, and the prevalence of the metabolic syndrome in the Framingham Offspring Cohort. Diabetes Care. 2004 Feb;27(2):538-46

[119] Davey BM et al, The effect of fiber-rich carbohydrates on features of Syndrome X. J Am Diet Assoc. 2003 Jan;103(1):86-96

[120] Burton-Freeman B et al, Plasma cholecystokinin is associated with subjective measures of satiety in women. Am J Clin Nutr. 2002 Sep;76(3):659-67

[121] Tsai CJ et al, Long-term intake of dietary fiber and decreased risk of cholecystectomy in women. Am J Gastroenterol. 2004 Jul;99(7):1364-70

Chapter 4.6

[122] Stefano GB, et al, Communication between animal cells and the plant foods they ingest: Phyto-zooidal dependencies and signaling, Int J Mol Med 2002 Oct;10(4):413-21

[123] Jenkins DJ et al, Type 2 diabetes and the vegetarian diet, Am J Clin Nutr. 2003 Sep;78(3 Suppl):610S-616S

[124] Pereira MA et al, Types of carbohydrates and risk of cardiovascular disease, J Womens Health (Larchmt). 2003 Mar;12(2):115-22

[125] Barnard ND et al, Diet and sex-hormone binding globulin, dysmenorrhea, and premenstrual symptoms, Obstet Gynecol, 2000 Feb;95(2):245-50

[126] Schweigert, FJ et al, Concentrations of carotenoids, retinol and a-tocopherol in plasma and follicular fluid of women undergoing IVF, 2003, Human Reproduction, 18(6):1259-1264

[127] Vega M et al, Functional luteolysis in response to hydrogen peroxide in human luteal cells, J Endocrinol. 1995 Oct;147(1):177-82

[128] Endo T et al, Hydrogen peroxide evokes antisteroidogenic and antigonadotropic actions in human granulosa luteal cells, J Clin Endocrinol Metab. 1993 Feb;76(2):337-42

[129] Weng BC et al, Beta-carotene uptake and changes in ovarian steroids and uterine proteins during the estrous cycle in the canine, J Animal Sci, 2000, 78(5):1284-90

[130] Ford, ES et al, Diabetes mellitus and serum carotenoids: findings from the third national health and nutrition examination survey, Am J Epidemiol, 1999, 149:168-176

[131] Ivorra MD, et al, Antihyperglycemic and insulin-releasing effects of ß-sitosterol 3-ß-D-Glucoside and its aglycone, ß-sitosterol, Arch Int Pharmacodyn Ther 1988;296:224-231

[132] Klippel KF et al, A multicentric, placebo-controlled, double-blind clinical trial of beta-sitosterol (phytosterol) for the treatment of benign prostatic hypertrophy, Br J Urol 1997;80:427-432

Chapter 5.1

[133] Layman DK, Protein quantity and quality at levels above the RDA improves adult weight loss. J Am Coll Nutr. 2004 Dec;23(6 Suppl):631S-636S

[134] Layman DK, Protein quantity and quality at levels above the RDA improves adult weight loss. J Am Coll Nutr. 2004 Dec;23(6 Suppl):631S-636S

[135] Anderson, GH et al, Dietary Proteins in the Regulation of Food Intake and Body Weight in Humans, 2004, J. Nutr. 134:974S-979S

[136] Halton, TL et al, The Effects of High Protein Diets on Thermogenesis, Satiety and Weight Loss: A Critical Review, J American College of Nutrition, 2004, Vol. 23, No. 5, 373-385

[137] Nuttall FQ et al, Metabolic response of people with type 2 diabetes to a high protein diet. Nutr Metab (Lond). 2004 Sep 13;1(1):6

[138] Layman DK et al, A reduced ratio of dietary carbohydrate to protein improves body composition and blood lipid profiles during weight loss in adult women. J Nutr. 2003 Feb;133(2):411-7

Chapter 5.2

[139] Segall, J, Dietary Lactose as a Possible Risk Factor for Ischaemic Heart Disease: Review of Epidemiology, International Journal of Cardiology, 1994, 46(3):197-207

[140] Alamgir, F et al, Survival Trends, Coronary Event Rates, and the MONICA Project, The Lancet, 1999, 354 (4):862-863

[141] Seely, S, Diet and Coronary Heart Disease: A Survey of Female Mortality Rates and Food Consumption Statistics of 21 Countries, Medical Hypotheses, 1981, 7(9):1133-1137

[142] McLachlan CN, Beta-casein A1, ischaemic heart disease mortality, and other illnesses, Med Hypotheses, 2001, 56(2):262-72

[143] Tailford KA et al, A casein variant in cow's milk is atherogenic, Atherosclerosis, 2003, 170(1):13-9

[144] Broxmeyer L, Thinking the unthinkable: Alzheimer's, Creutzfeldt-Jakob and Mad Cow disease: the age-related reemergence of virulent, foodborne, bovine tuberculosis or losing your mind for the sake of a shake or burger. Med Hypotheses. 2005;64(4):699-705

[145] Sandals WC et al, Prevalence of bovine parvovirus infection in Ontario dairy cattle. Can J Vet Res. 1995 Apr;59(2):81-6

[146] StCyr Coats K et al, Bovine immunodeficiency virus: incidence of infection in Mississippi dairy cattle, Vet Microbiol, 1994, 42(2-3):181-9

[147] Epstein, Samuel S. Unlabeled milk from cows treated with biosynthetic growth hormones: a case of regulatory abdication. International Journal of Health Services, Vol. 26, No. 1, 1996, pp. 173-85

[148] Bauer ER et al, Characterisation of the affinity of different anabolics and synthetic hormones to the human androgen receptor, human sex hormone binding globulin and to the bovine progestin receptor. APMIS. 2000 Dec;108(12):838-46

[149] Petti L et al, Activation of the platelet-derived growth factor receptor by the bovine papillomavirus E5 transforming protein, EMBO J (England), 1991, 10(4):845-55

[150] Larsson SC et al, Milk and lactose intakes and ovarian cancer risk in the Swedish Mammography Cohort. Am J Clin Nutr. 2004 Nov;80(5):1353-7

[151] Fairfield, KM, et al, A prospective study of dietary lactose and ovarian cancer, Int J Cancer, 2004, 110(2):271-7

[152] Ostman EM, et al, Inconsistency between glycemic and insulinemic responses to regular and fermented milk products, Am J Clin Nutr 2001 Jul;74(1):96-100

[153] Liljeberg E, et al, Milk as a supplement to mixed meals may elevate posprandial insulinaemia, Eur J Clin Nutr, 2001, 55(11):994-9

[154] Cramer D, et al, Adult hypolactasia, milk consumption, and age-specific fertility, Am J Epidemiol 1994 Feb 1;139(3):282-9

[155] Heaney, RP et al, Dietary changes favorably affect bone remodeling in older adults, J Am Dietetic Assn, 1999, 99(10):1228-33

[156] Wu, XK et al, Selective ovary resistance to insulin signaling in women with polycystic ovary syndrome, Fertil Steril, 2003, 80(4):954-65

Chapter 6.1

[157] Salmeron J et al, Dietary fat intake and risk of type 2 diabetes in women, Am J Clin Nutr, 2001, 73(6)L1019-26

[158] Oh K et al, Dietary fat intake and risk of coronary heart disease in women: 20 years of follow-up of the Nurse's Health Study, Am J Epidemiol, 2005, 161(7):672-9

[159] Mozaffarian D et al, Dietary intake of trans fatty acids and systemic inflammation in women, 2004, Am J Clin Nutr, 79(4):606-12

[160] Elias SI et al, Bakery foods are the major dietary source of trans-fatty acids among pregnant women with diets providing 30 percent energy from fat, J Am Diet Assoc, 2002, 102(1):46-51

[161] Booyens J, The presence of trans unsaturated fatty acids in ruminant meat and milk is unnatural, Med Hypotheses, 1986, 21(3):249-52

[162] Mosca, CL et al, Insulin resistance as a modifier of the relationship between dietary fat intake and weight gain. Int J Obes Relat Metab Disord. 2004 Jun;28(6):803-12

Chapter 6.2

[163] Navarra, P et al, Increased production and release of prostaglandin-E2 by human granulose cells from polycystic ovaries, Prostaglandins, 1996, 52(3):187-97

[164] Storlien, LH et al, Fatty acids, triglycerides and syndromes of insulin resistance. Prostaglandins Leukot Essent Fatty Acids. 1997 Oct;57(4-5):379-85

[165] Puri, BK et al, Eicosapentaenoic acid in treatment-resistant depression, Arch Gen Psychiatry, 2002, 59:91-92

Chapter 6.3

[166] Kasim-Karakas SE et al, Metabolic and endocrine effects of a polyunsaturated fatty acid-rich diet in polycystic ovary syndrome. J Clin Endocrinol Metab. 2004 Feb;89(2):615-20

[167] Louheranta AM et al, Association of the fatty acid profile of serum lipids with glucose and insulin metabolism during 2 fat-modified diets in subjects with impaired glucose tolerance. Am J Clin Nutr 2002 Aug;76(2):331-7

[168] Soares MJ et al, The acute effects of olive oil v. cream on postprandial thermogenesis and substrate oxidation in postmenopausal women. Br J Nutr. 2004 Feb;91(2):245-52

[169] Votruba SB et al, Prior exercise increases subsequent utilization of dietary fat. Med Sci Sports Exerc. 2002 Nov;34(11):1757-65

[170] Kratz M, et al, The impact of dietary fat composition on serum leptin concentrations in healthy nonobese men and women. J Clin Endocrinol Metab 2002 Nov;87(11):5008-14

[171] Harding, AH et al, Fat consumption and BhA1c levels: the EPIC-Norfolk study. Diabetes Care, 2001, 24(11):1911-1916

[172] Vessby B, Dietary fat, fatty acid composition in plasma and the metabolic syndrome, Curr Opin Lipidol, 2003, 14(1):15-19

[173] Storlien LH et al, Fatty acids, triglycerides and syndromes of insulin resistaqnce, Prostaglandins Leukot Essent Fatty Acids, 1997, 57(4-5):379-85

[174] Riccardi G et al, Dietary fat, insulin sensitivity and the metabolic syndrome. Clin Nutr. 2004 Aug;23(4):447-56

[175] Vessby B et al, Substituting dietary saturated for monounsaturated fat impairs insulin sensitivity in healthy men and women: the KANWU study, Diabetologia, 2001, 44(3):312-9

[176] Walker KZ et al, Body fat distribution and non-insulin-dependent diabetes: comparison of a fiber-rich, high-carbohydrate, low-fat (23%) diet and a 35% fat diet high in monounsaturated fat. Am J Clin Nutr 1996;63:254-260

Chapter 8.4

[177] Hope BK et al, An overview of the Salmonella enteritidis risk assessment for shell eggs and egg products, Risk Anal. 2002 Apr;22(2):203-18

[178] Shang H et al. "A high biotin diet improves the impaired glucose tolerance of long-term spontaneously hyperglycaemic rats with non-insulin-dependant diabetes mellitus." J Nutr Sci Vitamin.1996;42:517-526

[179] Furukawa Y, [Enhancement of glucose-induced insulin secretion and modification of glucose metabolism by biotin], Nippon Rinsho, 1999 57(10):2261-9

[180] Chung HY et al, Lutein bioavailability is higher from lutein-enriched eggs than from supplements and spinach in men. J Nutr. 2004 Aug;134(8):1887-93

[181] Schweigert, FJ et al, Concentrations of carotenoids, retinol and a-tocopherol in plasma and follicular fluid of women undergoing IVF, 2003, Human Reproduction, 18(6):1259-1264

[182] A'Damo, P, "Type O with Polycystic Ovaries," http://www.dadamo.com/ask/ask2.pl?20040506.txt

[183] Stefano GB et al, Communication between animal cells and the plant foods they ingest: Phyto-zooidal dependencies and signaling, Int J Mol Med 2002 Oct;10(4):413-21

Chapter 8.11

[184] Jaceldo-Siegl K et al, Long-term almond supplementation without advice on food replacement induces favourable nutrient modifications to the habitual diets of free-living individuals. Br J Nutr. 2004 Sep;92(3):533-40

[185] Fraser GE,Nut Consumption, Lipids, and Risk of a Coronary Event, Asia Pacific J Clin Nutr, 2000;9(Suppl.):S28-S32

[186] Jiang R et al, Nut and peanut butter consumption and risk of type 2 diabetes in women,JAMA. 2002 Nov 27;288(20):2554-60

[187] Ellsworth JL et al, Frequent nut intake and risk of death from coronary heart disease and all causes in postmenopausal women: the Iowa Women's Health Study, Nutr Metab Cardiovasc Dis 2001;11(6):372-7

[188] Wien MA et al, Almonds vs complex carbohydrates in a weight reduction program, Int J Obes Relat Metab Disord, 2003, 27(11):1365-72

Chapter 9.1
[189] http://www.aquasana.com
[190] Schliess F et al, Cell volume and insulin signaling, Int Rev Cytol, 2003, 225:187-228
[191] Schliess F et al, Insulin resistance induced by loop diuretics and hyperosmolarity in perfused rat liver, Biol Chem, 2001, 382(7):1063-9
[192] Somponpun SJ et al, Depletion of oestrogen receptor-beta expression in magnocellular arginine vasopressin neurons by hypovalaemia and dehydration, J Neuroendocrinol, 2004, 16(6):544-9
[193] Haussinger D ete al, Cell volume in the regulation of hepatic function: a mechanism for metabolic control. Biochim Biophys Acta. 1991 Dec 12;1071(4):331-50
[194] Schliess F et al, Cell hydration and insulin signaling, Cell Physiol Biochem, 2000, 10(5-6):403-8
[195] Keller U et al, Effects of changes in hydration on protein, glucose and lipid metabolism in man: impact on health, Eur J Clin Nutr, 2003, 57(Suppl 2):S69-74
[196] Shannon J et al, Relationship of food groups and water intake to colon cancer risk. Cancer Epidemiol Biomarkers Prev. 1996 Jul;5(7):495-502

Chapter 9.2
[197] Windham GC et al, Chlorination by-products in drinking water and menstrual cycle function. Environ Health Perspect. 2003 Jun;111(7):935-41
[198] Swan SH et al, A prospective study of spontaneous abortion: relation to amount and source of drinking water consumed in early pregnancy. Epidemiology. 1998 Mar;9(2):126-33

Chapter 9.3
[199] Wilcox A et al, Caffeinated beverages and decreased fertility, Lancet, 1988, 2(8626-8627):1453-6
[200] Bolumar F et al, Caffeine intake and delayed conception: a European multicenter study on infertility and subfecundity. European Study Group on Infertility Subfecundity. Am J Epidemiol. 1997 Feb 15;145(4):324-34
[201] Joesoef MR et al, Are caffeinated beverages risk factors for delayed conception? Lancet. 1990 Jan 20;335(8682):136-7
[202] Fenster, L et al, Rate of caffeine metabolism and risk of spontaneous abortion. Am J Epidemiol. 1998 Mar 1;147(5):503-10
[203] Christensen B et al, Abstention from filtered coffee reduces the concentrations of plasma homocysteine and serum cholesterol—a randomized controlled trial, Am J Clin Nutr, 2001, 74(3):302.7
[204] Verhoef P et al, Contribution of caffeine to the homocysteine-raising effect of coffee: a randomized controlled trial in humans. Am J Clin Nutr. 2002 Dec;76(6):1244-8
[205] van Dam RM et al, Coffee consumption and incidence of impaired fasting glucose, impaired glucose tolerance, and type 2 diabetes: the Hoorn Study, Diabetologia. 2004 Dec;47(12):2152-9

Chapter 9.4
[206] Chen JH et al, Green tea polyphenols prevent toxin-induced hepatotoxicity in mice by down-regulating inducible nitric oxide-derived prooxidants. Am J Clin Nutr. 2004 Sep;80(3):742-5
[207] Wu AH, Tea and circulating estrogen levels in postmenopausal Chinese women in Singapore, Carcinogenesis, 2005, Jan 20, 2005 [Epub ahead of print]
[208] Liao S, The medicinal action of androgens and green tea epigallocatechin gallate, Hong Kong Med J, 2001, 7(4):369-74
[209] Ren, F et al, Tea polyphenols down-regulate the expression of the androgen receptor in LNCaP prostate cancer cells. Oncogene. 2000 Apr 6;19(15):1924-32
[210] Liao S et al, Selective inhibition of steroid 5 alpha-reductase isozymes by tea epicatechin-3-gallate and epigallocatechin-3-gallate. Biochem Biophys Res Commun. 1995 Sep 25;214(3):833-8
[211] Tian WX et al, Weight reduction by Chinese medicinal herbs may be related to inhibition of fatty acid synthase. Life Sci. 2004 Mar 26;74(19):2389-99
[212] Kao YH et al, Modulation of endocrine systems and food intake by green tea epigallocatechin gallate, Endocrinology, 2000, 141(3):980-7

Chapter 9.5
[213] Jacqmain M et al, Calcium intake, body composition, and lipoprotein-lipid concentrations in adults. Am J Clin Nutr. 2003 Jun, 77(6):1448-52
[214] Wyshak, G, Teenaged girls, carbonated beverage consumption, and bone fractures. Arch Pediatr Adolesc Med. 2000 Jun;154(6):610-3
[215] Christian B et al, Chronic aspartame affects T-maze performance, brain cholinergic receptors and Na+,K+-ATPase in rats. Pharmacol Biochem Behav. 2004;78(1):121-7
[216] Trocho, C et al, Formaldehyde derived from dietary aspartame binds to tissue components in vivo. Life Sci. 1998;63(5):337-49
[217] Randerath, K et al, Flavor constituents in cola drinks induce hepatic DNA adducts in adult and fetal mice. Biochem Biophys Res Commun, 1993;192(1):61-8

[218] Farber TM, The toxicity of brominated sesame oil and brominated soybean oil in miniature swine. Toxicology. 1976 Mar;5(3):319-36

[219] Vorhees CV et al, Behavioral and reproductive effects of chronic developmental exposure to brominated vegetable oils in rats, Teratology, 1983, 28(3):309-18

[220] Horowitz BZ, Bromism from excessive cola consumption, J Toxicol Clin Toxicol, 1997, 35(3):315-20

Chapter 9.6

[221] Freiberg MS, et al, Alcohol consumption and the prevalence of the Metabolic Syndrome in the US.: a cross-sectional analysis of data from the Third National Health and Nutrition Examination Survey, Diabetes Care. 2004 Dec;27(12):2954-9

[222] Lazarus R et al, Alcohol intake and insulin levels. The Normative Aging Study. Am J Epidemiol. 1997 May 15;145(10):909-16

[223] Kiechl S et al, Insulin sensitivity and regular alcohol consumption: large, prospective, cross sectional population study (Bruneck study). BMJ. 1996 Oct 26;313(7064):1040-4

[224] Harding AH et al, Cross-sectional association between total level and type of alcohol consumption and glycosylated haemoglobin level: the EPIC-Norfolk Study. Eur J Clin Nutr 2002 Sep;56(9):882-90

[225] Daly ME et al, Dietary carbohydrates and insulin sensitivity: a review of the evidence and clinical implications. Am J Clin Nutr. 1997 Nov;66(5):1072-85

Chapter 10.1

[226] Gomi T et al, Strict dietary sodium reduction worsens insulin sensitivity by increasing sympathetic nervous activity in patients with primary hypertension. Am J Hypertens 1998, 11:1048-1055

[227] Fliser D et al, The effect of dietary salt on insulin sensitivity. Eur J Clin Invest 1995, 25:39-43

[228] Feldman RD, Schmidt ND. Moderate dietary salt restriction increases vascular and systemic insulin resistance. Am J Hypertens 1999;12:643-647

Chapter 11.1

[229] Smith BL, Organic foods vs. supermarket foods: element levels, J App Nutr, 1993, 45(1):35-39.

[230] Lauridsen, C et al, Organic diet enhanced the health of rats, March 29, 2005, Danish Institute of Agricultural Sciences, www.darcof.dk/research/health.html

[231] Baker, BP et al, Pesticide residues in conventional, integrated pest management (IPM)-grown and organic foods: insights from three US data sets, Food Addit Contam, 2002, 19(5):427-446

Chapter 11.2

[232] McCrory, M, Overeating in America: association between restaurant food consumption and body fatness in healthy adult men and women ages 19 to 80, Obesity Res, 1999, 7(6):564-571

Chapter 11.5

[233] Layman DK, Protein quantity and quality at levels above the RDA improves adult weight loss. J Am Coll Nutr. 2004 Dec;23(6 Suppl):631S-636S

[234] Farschchi HR et al, Beneficial metabolic effects of regular meal frequency on dietary thermogenesis, insulin sensitivity, and fasting lipid profiles in healthy obese women, Am J Clin Nutr, 2005, 81(1):16-24

[235] Forslund BH et al, Snacking frequency in relation to energy intake and food choices in obese men and women compared to a reference population, Int J Obes Relat Metab Disord, 2005, Apr 5: [Epub ahead of print]

Chapter 12.3

[236] Freeland-Graves J, Mineral adequacy of vegetarian diets, Am J Clin Nutr, 1988, 48:859-862.

[237] Barkeling, B et al, Effects of a high-proteinmeal (meat) and a high cerbohydrate meal (vegetarian) on satiety measured by automated computeriezed monitoring of subsequent food intake, motivation to eat and food preferences, Int J Obes 1990; 14:743-751

[238] Eaton, S et al, An evolutionary perspective enhances understanding of human nutritional requirements, J Nutr, 1996, 126:1732-1740.

[239] Klein, SL, The effects of hormones on sex differences in infection: from genes to behavior, Neurosci Biobehav Rev. 2000 Aug;24(6):627-38

Chapter 14.1

[240] Huber-Buchholz MM et al, Restoration of reproductive potential by lifestyle modification in obese polycystic ovary syndrome: role of insulin sensitivity and luteinizing hormone. J Clin Endocrinol Metab 1999 Apr;84(4):1470-4

[241] Giannopoulou I, et al, Exercise is required for visceral fat loss in postmenopausal women with type 2 diabetes, J Clin Endocrinol Metab, Dec 14, 2004

[242] Randeva HS et al, Exercise decreases plasma total homocysteine in overweight young women with polycystic ovary syndrome, J Clin Endocrinol Metab, 2002. 87(10):4496-501

[243] McAuley K et al, Intensive lifestyle changes are necessary to improve insulin sensitivity: A randomized controlled trial, Diabetes Care. 2002 Mar;25(3):445-52

[244] Duncan GE et al, Exercise training, without weight loss, increases insulin sensitivity and postheparin plasma lipase

activity in previously sedentary adults. Diabetes Care. 2003 Mar;26(3):557-62

[245] Ross R et al, Exercise-induced reduction in obesity and insulin resistance in women: a randomized controlled trial. Obes Res. 2004 May, 12(5):789-98

[246] Bryner RW et al, The effects of exercise intensity on body composition, weight loss and dietary composition in women, J Am Coll Nutr, 1997, 16(1):68-73

[247] Okura T et al, Effects of exercise intensity on physical fitness and risk factors for coronary heart disease, Obes Res, 2003, 11(9):1131-39

[248] Saris W et al, How much physical activity is enough to prevent unhealthy weight gain? Outcome of the IASO 1st stock conference and consensus statement, Obes Rev, 2003, 4(2):101-14

[249] Schoeller DA et al, How much physical activity is needed to minimize weight gain in previously obese women?, Am J Clin Nutr, 1997, 66(3):551-6

[250] Hu F et al, Television watching and other sedentary behaviors in relation to risk of obesity and type 2 diabetes mellitus in women, JAMA, 2003, 289(4):1785-91

[251] Mertens DJ et al, Exercise without dietary restriction as a means to long-term fat loss in the obese cardiac patient, J Sports Med Phys Fitness, 1998, 38(4):310-6

[252] Jeffery RW et al, Physical activity and weight loss: does prescribing higher physical activity goals improve outcome?, Am J Clin Nutr, 2003, 78(4):684-89

Chapter 14.2

[253] Berga, SL et al, The diagnosis and treatment of stress-induced anovulation, Minerva Ginecol, 2005, 57(1):45-54

[254] Kalantaridou SN et al, Stress and the female reproductive system, J Reprod Immunol, 2004, 62(1-2):61-8

[255] Rosmond R, Role of stress in the pathogenesis of the metabolic syndrome. Psychoneuroendocrinology. 2005 Jan;30(1):1-10

[256] Genazzani AR et al, Neuroendocrine correlates of stress-related amenorrhea, Ann N Y Acad Sci. 1991;626:125-9

[257] Seematter G, Relationship between stress, inflammation and metabolism. Curr Opin Clin Nutr Metab Care. 2004 Mar;7(2):169-73

[258] Epel ES, et al, Stress and body shape: stress-induced cortisol secretion is consistently greater among women with central fat, Psychosom Med 2000 Sep-Oct;62(5):623-32

[259] Epel, E, et al, Stress may add bite to appetite in women: a laboratory study of stress-induced cortisol and eating behavior, Psychoneuroendocrinology 2001 Jan;26(1):37-49

[260] Berga SL et al, Women with functional hypothalamic amenorrhea but not other forms of anovulation display amplified cortisol concentrations. Fertil Steril. 1997 Jun;67(6):1024-30

[261] Nepomnaschy PA et al, Stress and female reproductive function: a study of daily variations in cortisol, gonadotrophins, and gonadal steroids in the rural Mayan population, Am J Hum Biol, 2004, 16(5):523-32

[262] Dole N et al, Maternal stress and preterm birth. Am J Epidemiol. 2003 Jan 1;157(1):14-24

[263] Oths KS et al, A prospective study of psychosocial job strain and birth outcomes. Epidemiology. 2001 Nov;12(6):744-6

[264] Mulder EJ et al, Prenatal maternal stress: effects on pregnancy and the (unborn) child. Early Hum Dev. 2002 Dec;70(1-2):3-14

[265] Gallinelli A et al, Immunological changes and stress are associated with different implantation rates in patients undergoing in vitro fertilization-embryo transfer, Fert Steril, 2001, 76(1):85-91

[266] Paredes A et al, Stress promotes development of ovarian cysts in rats: the possible role of sympathetic nerve activation, Endocrine, 1998, 8(3):309-315

[267] Kitzinger, C et al, The thief of womanhood: women's experience of polycystic ovarian syndrome, Soc Sci Med 2002 Feb;54(3):349-61

[268] Cysarz D, et al, Oscillations of heart rate and respiration synchronize during poetry recitation. Am J Physiol Heart Circ Physiol. 2004 Aug;287(2):H579-87. Epub 2004 Apr 08

Chapter 14.4

[269] Clarke SD, The multi-dimensional regulation of gene expression by fatty acids: polyunsaturated fats as nutrient sensors. Curr Opin Lipidol. 2004 Feb;15(1):13-8

Chapter 15.1

[270] Willett, WC et al, Clinical practice. What vitamins should I be taking, doctor? N Engl J Med. 2001 Dec 20;345(25):1819-24

[271] Fairfield KM et al, Vitamins for chronic disease prevention in adults: scientific review. JAMA. 2002 Jun 19;287(23):3116-26

[272] Fletcher RH et al, Vitamins for chronic disease prevention in adults: clinical applications. JAMA. 2002 Jun 19;287(23):3127-9

Chapter 15.3

[273] Kelly GS, Insulin resistance: lifestyle and nutritional interventions. Altern Med Rev. 2000 Apr;5(2):109-32

[274] Thys-Jacobs S, et al, Vitamin D and calcium dysregulation in the polycystic ovarian syndrome, Steroids. 1999 Jun;64(6):430-5

[275] Boucher BJ et al, Hypovitaminosis D is associated with insulin resistance and beta cell dysfunction. Am J Clin Nutr. 2004 Dec;80(6):1666; author reply 1666-7

[276] Ames, BN et al, High-dose vitamin therapy stimulates variant enzymes with decreased coenzyme binding affinity (increased Km): relevance to genetic disease and polymorphisms, Am J Clin Nutr, 2002, 75(4):616-658

[277] Shils, ME et al, Modern Nutrition in Health and Disease, 8th ed., Lea & Febiger, Philadelphia, 1994

Chapter 16.1

[278] Cummings DE et al, A preprandial rise in plasma ghrelin levels suggests a role in meal initiation in humans, Diabetes, 2001, 50(8):1714-9

[279] Cummings, DE et al, Plasma ghrelin levels after diet-induced weight loss or gastric bypass surgery. N Engl J Med. 2002 May 23;346(21):1623-30

[280] English, PJ et al, Food fails to suppress ghrelin levels in obese humans. J Clin Endocrinol Metab. 2002 Jun;87(6):2984

[281] Monteleone P et al, Differential responses of circulating ghrelin to high-fat or high-carbhoydrate meal in healthy women, J Clin Endocrinol Metab, 2003, 88(11):5510-14

[282] Weigle, DS et al, Roles of leptin and ghrelin in the loss of body weight caused by a low fat, high carbohydrate diet, J Clin Endocrinol Metab, 2003, 88(4):1577-86

[283] Teff KL et al, Dietary fructose reduces circulating insulin and leptin, attenuates postprandial suppression of ghrelin, and increases triglycerides in women. J Clin Endocrinol Metab. 2004 Jun;89(6):2963-72

[284] Wasko, R et al, Elevated ghrelin plasma levels in patients with polycystic ovary syndrome, Horm Metab Res. 2004 Mar;36(3):170-3

[285] Schofl C, Circulating ghrelin levels in patients with polycystic ovary syndrome, J Clin Endocrinol Metab, 2002, 87(10):4607-10

[286] Moran, LJ et al, Ghrelin and measures of satiety are altered in polycystic ovary syndrome but not differentially affected by diet composition, J Clin Endocinol Metab, 2004, 89(7):3337-44

[287] Pagotto, U et al, Plasma ghrelin, obesity, and the polycystic ovary syndrome: correlation with insulin resistance and androgen levels, J Clin Endocrinol Metab, 2002, 87(12):5625-9

[288] Linden-Hirschberg AL et al, Impaired cholecystokinin secretion and disturbed appetite regulation in women with polycystic ovary syndrome, Gynecol Endocrinol. 2004 Aug;19(2):79-87

[289] Linden-Hirschberg AL et al, Impaired cholecystokinin secretion and disturbed appetite regulation in women with polycystic ovary syndrome, Gynecol Endocrinol. 2004 Aug;19(2):79-87

[290] Wu XK, Responses of somatostatin, beta-endorphin and dynorphin A to a glucose load in two groups of women with polycystic ovarian syndrome. Horm Res. 1996;46(2):59-63

[291] Martinez-Guisasola J et al, Plasma beta-endorphin levels in obese and non-obese patients with polycystic ovary disease. Gynecol Endocrinol. 2001 Feb;15(1):14-22

[292] Seifer DB et al, Current concepts of beta-endorphin physiology in female reproductive dysfunction. Fertil Steril. 1990 Nov;54(5):757-71

[293] Martinez-Guisasola, J et al, Circulating levels of immunoreactive beta-endorphin in polycystic ovary syndrome, Gynecol Endocrinol, 1999, 13(1):26-35

Chapter 16.2

[294] Havel, PJ, Peripheral signals conveying metabolic information to the brain: short-term and long-term regulation of food intake and energy homeostasis, Exp Biology and Medicine, 2001, 226:963-977.

[295] Schwartz MW et al, Reduced insulin secretion: an independent predictor of body weight gain. J Clin Endocrinol Metab, 1995, 80:1571–1576

[296] Kaiyalam KJ et al, Obesity induced by a high-fat diet is associated with reduced brain insulin transport in dogs, Diabetes, 2000, 49(9):1525-33

[297] Figlewicz DP et al, Intraventricular insulin enhances the meal-suppressive efficacy of intraventricular cholecystokinin octapeptide in the baboon. Behav Neurosci, 1995, 109:567–569

[298] Proietto, J, Mechanisms of insulin resistance caused by nutrient toxicity, Hepatol Res. 2005 Sep 30; [Epub ahead of print]

[299] Jequier E, Leptin signaling, adiposity, and energy balance, Ann N Y Acad Sci, 2002, Jun,967:379-88

[300] Kawai K et al, Leptin as a modulator of sweet taste sensitivities in mice, Proc Natl Acad Sci USA, 2000, 97(20):11044-9

[301] Benoit SC et al, Insulin and leptin as adiposity signals. Recent Prog Horm Res. 2004;59:267-85

[302] Niswender KD et al, Insulin and its evolving partnership with leptin in the hypothalamic control of energy homeostasis. Trends Endocrinol Metab. 2004 Oct;15(8):362-9

[303] Niswender KD et al, Insulin and leptin revisited: adiposity signals with overlapping physiological and intracellular signaling capabilities. Front Neuroendocrinol. 2003, 24(1):1-10

[304] McMinn JE et al, Leptin deficiency induced by fasting impairs the satiety response to cholecystokinin. Endocrinology,2000, 141:4442–4448

[305] Castracane, VD et al, When did leptin become a reproductive hormone?, Semin Reprod Med, 2002, 20(2):89-92

[306] Sir-Petermann, T et al, Are circulating leptin and luteinizing hormone synchronized in patients with polycystic ovary syndrome?, Human Reproduction, 1999, 14(6):1435-39

[307] Spritzer, PM et al, Leptin concentrations in hirsute women with polycystic ovary syndrome or idiopathic hirsutism: influence on LH and relationship with hormonal, metabolic, and anthropometric measurements. Hum Reprod 2001 Jul;16(7):1340-6

[308] Shimizu H et al. Estrogen increases in vivo leptin production in rats and human subjects. J Endocrinol 1997;154:285-292

[309] Behre HM et al, Strong association between serum levels of leptin and testosterone in men. Clin Endocrinol (Oxf) 1997;47:237-240

[310] Remsberg, K et al, Evidence for competing effects of body mass, hyperinsulinemia, insulin resistance, and androgens on leptin levels among lean, overweight and obese women with polycystic ovary syndrome, Fertil Steril, 2002, 78(3): 479

[311] Weigle DS et al, Roles of leptin and ghrelin in the loss of body weight caused by a low fat, high carbohydrate diet. J Clin Endocrinol Metab. 2003 Apr;88(4):1577-86

[312] Micic D et al, Leptin levels and insulin sensitivity in obese and non-obese patients with polycystic ovary syndrome, Gynecol Endocrinol, 1997, 11(5):315-20

[313] Laughlin GA et al, Serum leptin levels in women with polycystic ovary syndrome: the role of insulin resistance/hyperinsulinemia, J Clin Endocrinol Metab, 1997, 82(6):1692-6

[314] Mastorakos G et al, The hypothalamic-pituitary-adrenal axis in the neuroendocrine regulation of food intake and obesity: the role of corticiotropin releasing hromeone, Nutr Neurscci, 2004, 7(5-6):271-80

[315] Cha et al, Dietary fat type and energy restriction interactively influence plasma leptin concentration in rats, J Lipid Res, 1998, 39:1655-60

[316] Tulipano, G et al, Characterization of the resistance to the anorectic and endocrine effects of leptin in obesity-prone and obesity-resistant rats fed a high fat diet, J Endocrinol, 2004, 183(2): 289-98

[317] Banks, WA et al, Triglycerides induce leptin resistance at the blood-brain barrier. Diabetes. 2004 May; 53(5): 1253-60

[318] Poppitt SD et al, Long-term effects of ad libitum low-fat, high-carbohydrate diets on body weight and serum lipids in overweight subjects with metabolic syndrome. Am J Clin Nutr. 2002 Jan;75(1):11-20

[319] Bray, GA et al, Consumption of high-fructose corn syrup in beverages may play a role in the epidemic of obesity. American Journal of Clinical Nutrition, 2004, 79(4): 537-543

[320] Teff KL et al, Dietary fructose reduces circulating insulin and leptin, attenuates postprandial suppression of ghrelin, and increases triglycerides in women. J Clin Endocrinol Metab. 2004 Jun ;89(6):2963-72

[321] Teff KL et al, Dietary fructose reduces circulating insulin and leptin, attenuates postprandial suppression of ghrelin, and increases triglycerides in women. J Clin Endocrinol Metab. 2004 Jun ;89(6):2963-72

[322] Steinberg GR et al, Endurance training partially reverses dietary-induced leptin resistance in rodent skeletal muscle, Am J Physiol Endocrinol Metab, 2004, 286(1):E57-63

[323] Ozcelik O et al, Effects of different weight loss protocols on serum leptin levels in obese females, Physiol Res, 2004, Dec 9 2004 [epub ahead of print]

Chapter 16.3

[324] Festa, A et al, Chronic subclinical inflammation as part of the insulin resistance syndrome: the Insulin Resistance Atherosclerosis Study (IRAS), Circulation 2000 Jul 4;102(1):42-7

[325] Temelkova-Kurktschiev, T et al, Subclinical inflammation is strongly related to insulin resistance but not to impaired insulin secretion in a high risk population for diabetes, Metabolism 2002 Jun;51(6):743-9

[326] Grimble, RF, Inflammatory status and insulin resistance, Curr Opin Clin Nutr Metab Care, 2002 Sept; 5(5):551-9

[327] Kelly, CC et al, Low grade chronic inflammation in women with polycystic ovarian syndrome, J Clin Endocrinol Metab. 2001 Jun;86(6):2453-5

[328] Mohlig, M et al, The polycystic ovary syndrome per se is not associated with increased chronic inflammation, Eur J Endocrinol. 2004 Apr;150(4):525-32

[329] Puder, JJ et al, Central fat excess in polycystic ovary syndrome: relation to low-grade inflammation and insulin resistance, J Clin Endocrinol Metab. 2005 Nov;90(11):6014-21

[330] Orio Jr., F et al, The increase of leukocytes as a new putative marker of low-grade chronic inflammation and early cardiovascular risk in polycystic ovary syndrome, J Clin Endocrinol Metab. 2005 Jan;90(1):2-5

[331] Ibanez, L et al, High neutrophil count in girls and women with hyperinsulinaemic hyperandrogenism: normalization with metformin and flutamide overcomes the aggravation by oral contraception, Hum Reprod. 2005 Jun 23; [Epub ahead of print]

[332] Sonnenberg, L et al, Dietary patterns and the metabolic syndrome in obese and non-obese Framingham women, Obes Res. 2005 Jan;13(1):153-62.

[333] Gonzalez, F et al, Reactive oxygen species-induced oxidative stress in the development of insulin resistance and hyperandrogenism in polycystic ovary syndrome, J Clin Endocrinol Metab. 2005 Oct 25; [Epub ahead of print]

[334] Gonzalez, F et al, Hyperglycemia alters tumor necrosis factor-alpha release from mononuclear cells in women with polycystic ovary syndrome, J Clin Endocrinol Metab. 2005 Sep;90(9):5336-42

[335] King, DE et al, Relation of dietary fat and fiber to elevation of C-reactive protein, Am J Cardiol. 2003 Dec 1;92(11):1335-9

[336] De Souza, CT et al, Consumption of a fat-rich diet activates a proinflammatory response and induces insulin resistance in the hypothalamus, Endocrinology. 2005 Oct;146(10):4192-9

[337] Mozaffarian, D et al, Dietary intake of trans fatty acids and systemic inflammation in women. Am J Clin Nutr. 2004 Apr;79(4):606-12

[338] Lopez-Garcia, E et al, Consumption of trans fatty acids is related to plasma biomarkers of inflammation and endothelial dysfunction. J Nutr. 2005 Mar;135(3):562-6

[339] Ajani, UA et al, Dietary fiber and C-reactive protein: findings from national health and nutrition examination survey data. J Nutr. 2004 May;134(5):1181-5.

[340] Drevon, CA, Fatty acids and expression of adipokines, Biochim Biophys Acta. 2005 May 30;1740(2):287-92

[341] Lopez-Garcia, E et al, Consumption of (n-3) fatty acids is related to plasma biomarkers of inflammation and endothelial activation in women. J Nutr. 2004 Jul;134(7):1806-11.

[342] Tsuda, T et ai, Anthocyanin enhances adipocytokine secretion and adipocyte-specific gene expression in isolated rat adipocytes. Biochem Biophys Res Commun. 2004 Mar 26;316(1):149-57.

[343] Walston, J et al, Serum Antioxidants, Inflammation, and Total Mortality in Older Women, Am J Epidemiol. 2005 Nov 23; [Epub ahead of print]

[344] van Herpen-Broekmans, WM et al, Serum carotenoids and vitamins in relation to markers of endothelial function and inflammation. Eur J Epidemiol. 2004;19(10):915-21

[345] Esposito, K et al, Effect of a mediterranean-style diet on endothelial dysfunction and markers of vascular inflammation in the metabolic syndrome: a randomized trial. JAMA. 2004 Sep 22;292(12):1440-6

[346] Sonnenberg, GE et al, A novel pathway to the manifestations of metabolic syndrome, Obes Res. 2004 Feb;12(2):180-6

[347] Miner JL, The adipocyte as an endocrine cell. J Anim Sci. 2004 Mar;82(3):935-41

[348] Trayhurn, P et al, Signalling role of adipose tissue: adipokines and inflammation in obesity, Biochem Soc Trans. 2005 Oct;33(Pt 5):1078-81

[349] Grimble, RF, Inflammatory status and insulin resistance, Curr Opin Clin Nutr Metab Care. 2002 Sep;5(5):551-9

[350] Gonzalez, F et al, Elevated serum levels of tumor necrosis factor alpha in normal-weight women with polycystic ovary syndrome, Metabolism 1999 Apr;48(4):437-41

[351] Skurk, T et al, Production and release of macrophage migration inhibitory factor from human adipocytes, Endocrinology. 2005 Mar;146(3):1006-11

[352] Weisberg, SP et al, Obesity is associated with macrophage accumulation in adipose tissue, J Clin Invest. 2003 Dec;112(12):1796-808

[353] Bjorbaek, C et al, Identification of SOCS-3 as a potential mediator of central leptin resistance, Mol Cell. 1998 Mar;1(4):619-25

[354] Bjorbaek, C et al, The role of SOCS-3 in leptin signaling and leptin resistance. J Biol Chem. 1999 Oct 15;274(42):30059-65

[355] Farrell, GC, Signalling links in the liver: Knitting SOCS with fat and inflammation, J Hepatol. 2005 Jul;43(1):193-6

[356] Emanuelli, B et al, SOCS-3 inhibits insulin signaling and is up-regulated in response to tumor necrosis factor-alpha in the adipose tissue of obese mice, J Biol Chem. 2001 Dec 21;276(51):47944-9

[357] Senn, JJ et al, Suppressor of cytokine signaling-3 (SOCS-3), a potential mediator of interleukin-6-dependent insulin resistance in hepatocytes, J Biol Chem, 2003 Apr 18;278(16):13740-6

[358] Ueki, K et al, Central role of suppressors of cytokine signaling proteins in hepatic steatosis, insulin resistance, and the metabolic syndrome in the mouse, Proc Natl Acad Sci U S A. 2004 Jul 13;101(28):10422-7

[359] Diez, JJ et al, The role of the novel adipocyte-derived hormone adiponectin in human disease, Eur J Endocrinol. 2003 Mar;148(3):293-300

[360] Ouchi, N et al, Obesity, adiponectin and vascular inflammatory disease, Curr Opin Lipidol. 2003 Dec;14(6):561-6

[361] Carmina, E et al, Evidence for altered adipocyte function in polycystic ovary syndrome, Eur J Endocrinol. 2005 Mar;152(3):389-94.

[362] Sepilian, V et al, Adiponectin levels in women with polycystic ovary syndrome and severe insulin resistance, Soc Gynecol Investig. 2005 Feb;12(2):129-34

[363] Sieminska, L et al, Serum adiponectin in women with polycystic ovarian syndrome and its relation to clinical, metabolic and endocrine parameters, J Endocrinol Invest. 2004 Jun;27(6):528-34

[364] Bruun, JM et al, Regulation of adiponectin by adipose tissue-derived cytokines: in vivo and in vitro investigations in humans, Am J Physiol Endocrinol Metab. 2003 Sep;285(3):E527-33

[365] Delporte, ML et al, Leptin treatment markedly increased plasma adiponectin but barely decreased plasma resistin in ob/ob mice. Am J Physiol Endocrinol Metab. 2004 Sep;287(3):E446-53.

[366] Silswal, N et al, Human resistin stimulates the pro-inflammatory cytokines TNF-alpha and IL-12 in macrophages by NF-kappaB-dependent pathway, Biochem Biophys Res Commun. 2005 Sep 9;334(4):1092-101

[367] Bokarewa, M et al, Resistin, an adipokine with potent proinflammatory properties, J Immunol. 2005 May 1;174(9):5789-95

[368] Steppan, CM et al, Activation of SOCS-3 by resistin, Mol Cell Biol. 2005 Feb;25(4):1569-75

[369] Lehrke, M et al, An inflammatory cascade leading to hyperresistinemia in humans, PLoS Med. 2004 Nov;1(2):e45. Epub 2004 Nov 30

[370] Seow, KM et al, Serum and adipocyte resistin in polycystic ovary syndrome with insulin resistance, Hum Reprod. 2004 Jan;19(1):48-53

[371] Boulman, N et al, Increased C-reactive protein levels in the polycystic ovary syndrome: a marker of cardiovascular disease, J Clin Endocrinol Metab. 2004 May;89(5):2160-5.

[372] De Maat, MP et al, Determinants of C-reactive protein concentration in blood, Ital Heart J. 2001 Mar;2(3):189-95

[373] Sabuncu, T et al, Oxidative stress in polycystic ovary syndrome and its contribution to the risk of cardiovascular disease, Clin Biochem. 2001 Jul;34(5):407-13

[374] Ogihara, T et al, Oxidative stress induces insulin resistance by activating the nuclear factor-kappa B pathway and disrupting normal subcellular distribution of phosphatidylinositol 3-kinase, Diabetologia. 2004 May;47(5):794-805

[375] Iborra, A et al, Oxidative stress and autoimmune response in the infertile woman, Chem Immunol Allergy. 2005;88:150-62

[376] Block, G et al, Factors associated with oxidative stress in human populations, Am J Epidemiol. 2002 Aug 1;156(3):274-85